Micropolitics of Media Culture

Film Culture in Transition
Thomas Elsaesser: General Editor

Micropolitics of Media Culture

Reading the Rhizomes of Deleuze and Guattari

Edited by

Patricia Pisters

with assistance of Catherine M. Lord

Amsterdam University Press

The production of this book was made possible by the support of the Department of Film and Television Studies of the University of Amsterdam.

Cover illustration: Tim Gutt
Cover Design: Kok Korpershoek, Amsterdam
Lay-out: JAPES, Amsterdam

NUGI 922
ISBN 90 5356 473 x (hardcover)
ISBN 90 5356 472 1 (paperback)

Contents

Section Three
Micropolitical Becoming: Duration and Change

Introduction

Patricia Pisters

Mesdames et Monsieurs,
Bienvenue à bord de notre vol à destination

to nowhere... to you... deep inside

[...]

Beachten sie den Orbit, Mondaufgang, Sternenstaub
Beachten sie links und rechts ihre Nachbarn

We are on the way to find you...
so please forget who you are

Nous vous remercions de choisir, choisir, choisir...[1]

Philosophy and politics

When Socrates took the poisoned cup, the uneasy relationship between philosophy and politics began. Hannah Arendt traces back this emerging split
to the trial and conviction of Socrates.[2] Charged with subverting Athens'
youth, Socrates was unable to prove his innocence. He tried to convince his
accusers by engaging them in a philosophical dialogue, as a means of
searching for truth. Sadly, the problem was that it is not possible to be convincing through philosophical truth, only with opinion (*doxa*), which is part
of the political domain. Socrates' failure to win his case inspired Plato to
search for eternal truths, which according to him should govern the polis
(the philosopher as king), as opposed to the temporary truths of opinions.
After Plato, however, philosophy became famously and notoriously apoliti-
cal. The moment Aristotle was threatened with a fate similar to Socrates, he
left Athens, without feeling any responsibility for the polis. As Arendt
states, the only thing that, philosophers demanded of politics for ages, was
to have a space to protect their freedom of thought, and to be left alone.

From the French Revolution onwards, philosophy and politics regained
mutual interest. Nineteenth century philosophers historically reinterpreted

the events of 1789-1814 in politically significant ways. After the Russian Revolution in 1917, and even more so after 1945, the term 'revolution' no longer referred to the past, but came to designate a project for the future. Many philosophers engaged in this political project, but for the most part did so unsuccessfully. In the twentieth century, the gap between theory and practice seemed to grow again. Philosophers who made the step to political action very often got trapped between their ideas and their concrete effects: powerlessness or tyranny. The starting points of this book emerge from precisely these two critiques of contemporary philosophy and cultural theory. According to Richard Rorty, the academic left in general has become powerless because it does not engage in 'real' politics. In particular, the work of Gilles Deleuze and Félix Guattari has been accused by several critics of leading either to limitless individual freedom without leaving room for the social and political, or to elitist tyranny. As a film scholar and cultural theorist, I strongly felt the need to engage with these charges and critically reinvestigate the various relationships between theory and practice. Having worked with the ideas of Deleuze in the field of film studies, I felt that his work, and the work he created together with Guattari, could offer some solutions to these political impasses. However, it was necessary to inquire further into this initial intuition. The question 'what is it that we do as cultural theorists' was a central theme at an interdisciplinary symposium, 'The Politics of Gilles Deleuze', in Amsterdam.[3] A number of the articles in this book were first presented and discussed during these meetings. But, as Deleuze states, 'negotiations sometimes last so long you don't know whether they're still part of the war or the beginning of peace'.[4] This book presents a continuation of various negotiations between theory and practice, mediated by the work of Deleuze and Guattari. But before introducing the articles, let me briefly recall some of the main objections towards the relationship between politics, cultural theory and philosophy.

Most recently, Richard Rorty has been one of the important contemporary intellectuals who stirred up this unresolved issue once more. In *Achieving our Country* he deplores the fact that the intellectual left from the beginning of the twentieth century has changed from people who act into people who observe.[5] The academic left has permitted a shift from engaging in actual political life into a turn to spectatorial 'cultural politics'. This has made them powerless. There is no single academic, Rorty states, who has any policy plan to offer. While he acknowledges the merits and positive mentality changes that academics have been able to help establish in the last few decades (such as more equality for women, black people and gays), Rorty considers these changes of minor importance in respect to, for instance, continuing economic inequality. Rorty's main objection to the cultural left is the cultural pessimism since the Vietnam War. If young intellectuals see a John Wayne movie after reading Foucault or even Neal Stephenson's *Snow Crash*, Rorty argues, they get the idea that America is a terrible, violent and corrupt country.[6] In fact, Rorty deplores the fact that a common nationalistic belief in the Dream Country is no longer part of intellectual life. He praises Dewey and Whitman for their attempt to see America as the paradigmatic self-creating democracy: 'To say the United States themselves are essentially the greatest poem is to say that America will create the taste by which it will be judged. It is to envisage our nation-state as both self-creating poet and self-created poem.'[7]

According to Rorty, the mistake of the cultural left is its theorizing of difference, which opposes a sense of commonality at the level of national politics. Rorty even glorifies the 'platoon' movies ('What do our differences matter, compared with our commonality as fellow Americans?') to illustrate this point.[8] He does not seem to mind that this 'platoon-feeling' in the Vietnam war could only be created by having a 'common', national enemy, nor does he seem to acknowledge that in many platoons commonality was not as strong as it appeared to be, as shown in Oliver Stone's PLATOON.

Another major objection that Rorty has against the academic left is the level of abstraction of many academic discourses. He gives the example of Fredric Jameson's *Postmodernism, or the Cultural Logic of Late Capitalism*, which he thinks is a brilliant book. But after reading it, Rorty says, you know everything except what to do.[9] An abstract term that Rorty rejects is the Foucaultian concept of (invisible) power. When the right states that socialism has failed and that the only alternative is capitalism, the left has nothing to say, because it does not like to discuss concrete matters like money, Rorty argues.[10] Because of the emphasis on political action as such, without any acknowledgement of the many practical failures of the Left in the twentieth century, Rorty's proposal to the left to forget theory and start believing again in the American Dream is rather problematic.[11] Yet the question he asks about the relationship between cultural theory and practice remains a haunting one that invites further investigation.[12]

Contrary to Rorty, the Dutch philosopher Luuk van Middelaar does take into account the failures of political engagement of the intellectual left. In his book *Politicide* he takes a historical perspective on the relation between philosophy and politics.[13] Van Middelaar concentrates on twentieth century French philosophy, and argues that all contemporary French thinkers have made themselves guilty of 'politicide', even if they had open and strong political engagements, such as Sartre, for instance, who displayed the sort of political action that, according to Rorty, the academic left used to possess. Van Middelaar traces the *échec* of philosophy in respect to politics back to

one man, who influenced all famous French thinkers of the twentieth century, namely Alexandre Kojève. His courses on Hegel, Marx and later Nietzsche guaranteed the political impasses in generations of French thinkers.
One group of thinkers that Van Middelaar distinguishes, among whom are
neo-Kantians like Lyotard, try to reach a rational *post-political* world. They
deny the impossible end of social conflict that constitutes society and consider politics as a stage that can be overcome. Their political engagement is
moderate and has not much influence.

Another group, Existentialists and Nietzschean thinkers like Foucault
and Deleuze, have systematically denied the specific nature of political
power structures. According to Van Middelaar, they live in a *pre-political*
world. With their call for resistance, these philosophers do not acknowledge
the fact that the state, or the political power that they hate so profoundly because it interferes in social battles, has also created society and given conditions of freedom. The fact that their call for resistance can just as well lead to
tyranny they seem to take for granted. Van Middelaar analyses Deleuze as
the philosopher of 'sovereign desiring machines'. His objection to Deleuze's
'irresponsible and autonomous nomads' is twofold. On the one hand, these
'desiring machines' lead to an apology for tyranny, in that everybody, by
strictly following their own desires, is invited to become a tyrant. On the
other hand, Deleuze's philosophy would lead to political powerlessness: if
there were no connection between all these 'desiring machines', this would
lead to 'Five billion Robinson Crusoes, each King of their own islet'.[14]

Van Middelaar's overview of contemporary philosophy is brilliantly
written; he puts his finger on several sore spots. However, his concise analysis of all the thinkers he mentions does not do justice to the complexities of
their works, neither does it take into account the different meanings politics
can produce. Although their critiques are very different and even opposed,
and their solutions for intellectual political engagement as well,[15] Rorty and
Van Middelaar seem to share a conception of politics in terms of policy
plans, economic measurements and governmental organization. Their definition of politics seems to be an important indication for investigating the
possible political significance of Deleuze and Guattari's philosophy.

'Making the future different from the past': redescriptions, planes and thresholds

When they talk about politics as such, Deleuze and Guattari do not just refer
to policy plans and political organizations. They distinguish three political

lines: the molar line, the molecular line and the line of flight.[16] These different 'lines' form a complex political network (of individuals and groups, within individuals and groups). The molar line is the line of 'the binary machine', the line on which the world is divided into binary oppositions: man/ woman, adult/child, public/private, white/black. It is the line that Deleuze identifies most with representational thinking, in which identity is always formed on the basis of molar oppositions. It is also the line that organizes society in segments, strata and separate 'institutes'. It is on this level that the kind of political action Rorty and van Middelaar talk about takes place. However, Deleuze and Guattari's theory also concerns the two other lines. The molecular line works on a more invisible level: the private thoughts one can have about certain structures in society form the cracks in the system of the molar line. The line of flight is where the system really cracks, and a break is inevitable. All lines have their own internal dangers (rigid codification, microfascism and self-destruction). Always operating at the same time, these lines form complex networks of conscious and unconscious political activities.

In his book *Deleuze and the Political*, Paul Patton states that there is indeed much in *Anti-Oedipus* and *A Thousand Plateaus* that could lead to the conclusion that Deleuze and Guattari are simply anti-State and hence anti-political, as does Van Middelaar when describing desiring machines as leading to tyrannical little islands.[17] From certain passages in these books, one could conclude that Deleuze and Guattari's desiring machines are 'social suicide machines' or that Deleuze and Guattari oppose the capturing and territorializing State (bad) to the deterritorializing lines of flight (good). However, Patton argues, there are many other elements in Deleuze and Guattari's mature political philosophy which disallows a simplistic anti-political point of view: 'First, the axioms of the capitalist social machine do not simply repress a natural state of free and undirected social existence. They are also constitutive of new social forces and forms of life. Deleuze and Guattari are not romantic anarchists who believe in the realm of social being beyond the subjection to political power. It would be an error, they argue, "to take a disinterested stance toward struggle on the level of the axioms".'[18] Furthermore, to look only at the molar level of politics and the act of translating theoretical concepts directly into political actions does not do justice to both the complexity and variation of each theoretical concept nor to the indirect relationship between molar politics and micropolitics.

Of course, one can object, as does Rorty, that this indirect relationship is precisely what the cultural left has offered over the last decades, and which Rorty thinks is insufficient (politically powerless). In the article opening this book 'Redescriptive Philosophy: Deleuze and Guattari's Critical Pragmatism', Patton takes up this question by explicitly addressing Rorty and re-examining the role of philosophy. Patton argues that Rorty's pragmatism has in fact a lot in common with the work of Deleuze and Guattari. Both Rorty and Deleuze and Guattari emphasize the functional, non-representative role of texts and meaning. They also share a conception of philosophy as 'the fabrication of intellectual tools rather than the attainment of truth'. Like Rorty, Deleuze abandons the idea that philosophical descriptions of the world can or should converge on a unique or 'true' theory. Patton argues that Deleuze's method of transcendental empiricism, according to which 'what problems there are is an open question to be answered by the set of problems thrown up by history, social life or by the development of particular sciences,' is entirely consistent with Rorty's historicism.

In *What is Philosophy?* Deleuze and Guattari elaborate on the characteristics of a philosophical concept. The concept, according to Deleuze and Guattari, is never exhausted by the actual state of affairs, rather it is 'the contour of an event to come'. What is important, according to Patton, is the act of describing the events; they help to actualize particular events in a social field. Deleuze and Guattari see the invention of concepts as a means of creating new descriptions and therefore new possibilities for (political) action. They agree with Marx and Rorty that the political or even utopian job of philosophers is 'to help make the future different from the past'. Deleuze and Guattari provide a series of new concepts, such as the Body without Organs, becoming-minoritarian, (de)territorializations and many more, which can function effectively in a given social and political context.

The difference between Rorty and Deleuze is, according to Patton, the difference between complacent and critical pragmatism. For Rorty, redescriptive philosophy is a private affair that can have no bearing on public and political life. However, the invention of new concepts and new forms of description have certainly contributed to public attitudes and, as a result, eventually to changes in the law and public institutions. Patton concludes that in their common goal of freedom (instead of truth), Rorty believes freedom is to be reached within the framework of democratic society. Deleuze, on the other hand, talks about critical freedom that is our way of 'responding to what is tolerable', which is historically determined and changeable. It involves making choices that can change one's life. Redescription, made possible by the invention of new concepts, contributes to such local and specific ways in which the future will be unlike the past, be it for personal or collective 'assemblages'.[19] In *Deleuze and the Political*, Patton suggests that the 'sudden shift towards another quality of life or towards a life which is lived at another degree of intensity is one possible outcome of what they call a line of flight. It is on this kind of line that critical freedom is manifest.'[20] He adds that according to the different choices made, the individual's capacity to affect and be affected may change and give rise to what Deleuze and Guattari call 'becomings'. It is precisely because Deleuze and Guattari develop so many concepts that deal with micro-movements that determine our actions on an invisible level that their work is easily misunderstood.

While Paul Patton demonstrates the way in which philosophy is political in helping 'make the future different from the past' by creating new concepts and descriptions, Catherine M. Lord in the second article, 'The Lady Sits Between Two Long Windows, Writing', emphasizes the transformative power an encounter with art can have. More specifically, she rereads Virginia Woolf's *The Waves* with a clear question, namely the question of how theory passes into art. In Deleuze's famous conversation with Foucault, 'Intellectuals and Power', Deleuze suggests that we are in the process of experiencing a new relationship between theory and practice: 'A theorizing intellectual, for us, is no longer a subject, a representing or representative consciousness. Those who act and struggle are no longer represented, either by a group or a union that appropriates the right to stand as their conscience. Who speaks and acts? All of us are "groupuscules." Representation no longer exists; there is only action – theoretical action and practical action which serve as relays and forms of networks.'[21] In order to see how 'theoretical action' can be redefined, Lord investigates the relation between cultural theory and artistic practice, between the work of philosophers and artists, with the help of the conceptual tools offered by Deleuze and Guattari in *What is Philosophy?*.

According to Deleuze and Guattari, philosophy and art move on different planes, the plane of immanence and the plane of composition, occupied by concepts and conceptual personae and by percepts, affects and aesthetic figures. The two planes can encounter each other at several thresholds, where philosophy and art start to 'pass into each other'. In *The Waves* there is a figure, a lady writing, who seems to appear and disappear between the Deleuzian planes. Lord takes this figure, which passes from aesthetic figure to conceptual persona and back again, as her guide to disclose the secrets of such an 'experience of a new relationship between theory and practice'. From her poetical analysis it becomes clear that practice can no longer be considered an application of theory, neither can it be seen as the inspiration of theory. As Deleuze has indicated, these types of relationships are totalizing processes. The new relationship of theory and practice is far more partial, fragmentary and local.[22] Lord demonstrates that what is interdisciplinary may turn out to be the 'interdisci-planary' or even the 'transdisci-planary'. The moments in *The Waves* when self-reflection (of the characters) turns into self-reflexion (of the literary process) are the moments where one plane passes into the other. These are also the moments where becomings take place: 'the multiplicities of winds, faces, hails, rains, noises, loves, into which subjects would become.' Lord offers a new perspective on the relationship between theory and practice: 'Between philosophy and aesthetic production, the lady offers this new threshold for the future: cultural analysis as art.'

Deleuze and Guattari distinguish yet another plane that can open up to new experiences and new thoughts, that is, the plane of reference and of science. Art, philosophy and science can 'extract from chaos the shadow of "the people to come"', hence their political potential. And where philosophy, art and science become undecidable, they share this 'shadow of a people to come'.[23] In her article 'Sharing Technologies: Thought and Movement in Dancing', Maaike Bleeker is also concerned with interactions or movements between planes, using the theoretical metaphor of dance. Her question concerns thought itself. In order to investigate what is new in thinking, it is useful to look at how thought constitutes itself on the three different planes, by concepts, by percepts and affects, and by figures. On all planes, in order to think, some movement is necessary. Bleeker therefore considers three 'duets'. The first one is performed by Deleuze and Guattari; the second one is a literal duet, the choreography WHEN YOU SEE GOD TELL HIM, by dancers Itzik Galili and Jennifer Hanna; the third duet is by cognitive scientists Lakoff and Johnson, who present metaphor as a model to trace the movement of thought. By confronting these three duets, Bleeker is able to open new spaces where thought can move in different ways. The conceptual metaphor 'argument is war', for instance, both enables us to understand arguments in terms of war and prescribes how we can do so. To think of 'argument as dance' gives a new perspective on argument and all kinds of other relationships. By confronting Lakoff and Johnson's scientific figure with an aesthetic figure of a dancer (that itself passes on to the philosophical plane of immanence), Bleeker demonstrates how also the plane of reference and our knowledge starts to shift. She analyses how in the performance the dancers become friends, who set into motion the movement between them and in thinking, always moving between the three planes. In this way, Bleeker demonstrates why 'philosophy needs a non-philosophy that comprehends it, [...] just as art needs non-art and science needs non-science.'[24] Only in that way can a conception be productive.

After having seen the philosopher as writer and as dancer, Eva Jørholt presents us with a philosopher as filmmaker David Cronenberg. In her article, 'The Metaphor Made Flesh', she analyses the political and philosophical potentiality of David Cronenberg's horror movies. Jørholt makes clear what happens when philosophy, art and science meet in cinema. In looking at the visuality and sensuality of thought, Jørholt's approach is comparable to the interdisci-planary analysis of Lord and the dancing interdisciplinarity of Bleeker. Jørholt starts with a quote from David Cronenberg in which he states that by comparing imagination to disease, he hopes to illuminate some aspect of human imagination that perhaps has never been perceived before. Cronenberg's films are full of bodies that are 'out of control'. His characters are constantly seeking to invent themselves and their own lives by transgressing the boundaries of their bodily organisms. The fact that these attempts of physical and mental auto-invention usually end in disaster does not prevent the 'glimpses of utopian freedom' that Cronenberg's films offer.

Cronenberg refers to his films as 'existential drama', and the idea of 'auto-invention' would make philosophical existentialism a logic partner in dialogue with Cronenberg's films. However, Jørholt argues, the fact that Cronenberg does not consider the body as a stable centre for being in the world, but on the contrary considers it as changeable matter, means Cronenberg has more in common with Deleuze's philosophy. There is one particular Deleuzian concept that offers many points of convergence and mutual illumination: the Body without Organs. In fact, the Body without Organs is not so much a concept as a practice, something to be attained without ever reaching it. The Body without Organs can be considered as a desire producing machine, where the body (be it an individual body or any other body or 'corporation') goes beyond its traditionally defined borders of the organism. All Cronenberg's films present such bodies and spectators are invited to think new thoughts, to perceive new sensations: for instance, to become a cell in a body and to be capable of experiencing life from the cell's point of view. Jørholt pays special attention to Cronenberg's eXistenZ. This film is constructed as a computer game and asks questions about blurring the boundaries between 'real' and 'fiction'. Not only is this film 'populated' by Bodies without Organs, but also the battle that goes on between the game players and the 'realists' demonstrates why art can have a political impact. Like Salman Rushdie, Cronenberg's main character (a computer game designer) in eXistenZ is on the run because of a fatwa against her from the 'realists'. Jørholt quotes Cronenberg's commentary: 'Art is a scary thing to a lot of people because it shakes your understanding of reality, or shapes it in ways that are socially unacceptable.'

Modern utopia and the links with the epoch: capitalism and cinema

With the reference to 'the socially unacceptable', Cronenberg points to another way in which philosophy is political, which is its modern utopian vocation. Utopia and utopianism has always been a political issue. Before 1800 Utopia meant a sort of static blueprint for an ideal but far away future society. After 1800 Utopia no longer meant a perfect society, but a slow change to a better society (making the future different from the past). Since May '68, utopian ideas are mostly presented as a critical way of thinking, in which it is no longer the future that is at stake but the present. In *What is Philosophy?* Deleuze and Guattari state indeed 'that utopia is what links philosophy with its own epoch. It is with this understanding of utopia that philosophy becomes political in taking the criticism of its own time to its highest point.'[25] If we now move from the possibilities for the future (new thoughts, new sensibilities, new actions) to the present moment and look at contemporary society, we cannot avoid talking about capitalism. Obviously, almost every aspect of contemporary life is permeated by capitalism. And, as Rorty rightly suggests, the 'academic left' should not leave money matters to the right. Deleuze and Guattari, once more, agree with Rorty on this point in stating that any political philosophy should be centered on an analysis of capitalism. In *What is Philosophy?* they emphasize once more the scope of capitalism: 'A world market extends to the ends of the earth before passing into the galaxy: even the skies become horizontal.'[26]

In her article 'Micropolitics: A Political Philosophy from Marx and Beyond', Malene Busk investigates Deleuze's criticism of the epoch, and hence his analysis of capitalism. Busk first exposes the specific form of 'society of control' which capitalism today has taken. She then investigates in what ways Deleuze is an heir to Marx. The most important aspect of Marx's theory that Deleuze takes over is his idea of capitalism as an immanent system that constantly overcomes its own limits. Capitalism and philosophy, according to Deleuze, are thus both immanent systems. Both Marx and Deleuze argue that the conceptual apparatus they develop should be at the same time a presentation as well as critique of the system. Where Marx and Deleuze diverge is in their conception of Utopia. According to Deleuze, the no-where of Utopia is just as well a now-here. Therefore, Deleuze does not believe in a Revolution, but in a 'becoming-revolutionary of a people' that is available to everybody at any moment in the passing present. Deleuze's micropolitical philosophy then diverges in some significant ways from Marx's theory: Marx's contradictions become 'lines of flight'; the Party is re placed by 'war machines' and classes turn into 'minorities'. All Deleuzian terms point to the micropolitical idea that 'beliefs and desires are at the basis of every society'. However, as has been said before, all these micropolitical movements are in constant negotiations with macropolitical segmentations: 'molecular escapes and movements would be nothing if they did not return to the molar organizations to reshuffle their segments, their binary distributions of sexes, classes, and parties,' say Deleuze and Guattari.[27] A 'war machine', for instance, can be the jurisprudence that slowly has its effects on constitutional law.[28] However, Busk reminds us of Deleuze's observation that philosophy in itself is not a power. As Deleuze states in *Negotiations*: 'Philosophy isn't a Power. [...] Not being a power, philosophy cannot battle with the powers that be, but it fights a war without battles, a guerilla campaign against them. [... It] can only negotiate.'[29]

Another important aspect of the epoch, very strongly related to capitalism, is the audiovisual 'nature' of contemporary society. Images and sounds are not only increasingly dominant in contemporary life; they also have shifted from a marginal place at the periphery of economy and culture at large to the centre of the 'network society', as Manuel Castells calls contemporary culture.[30] Having seen in what way Deleuze constructs an immanent system of both philosophy and capitalism, it can now be noted that also cinema is an immanent system of images and sounds, according to Deleuze. In his two cinema books, *The Movement-Image* and *The Time-Image*, Deleuze has presented the building blocks of this audiovisual system by giving numerous formal concepts and categories with which to describe cinematographic material.[31] All the articles that deal with cinema in this book do not directly engage with the formal aspects of the cinema books.[32] Rather, they try to see how Deleuze and Guattari's political concepts can be put to work in specific films. I will come back to this point in the last section of this introduction. In my own contribution 'Glamour and Glycerine: Surplus and Residual of the Network Society', I aim to establish what the status of cinema and audiovisual culture at large is in respect to capital. Films like THE NET could be seen as examples of our contemporary capitalist society of control. However, this representative conception of cinema as a reflection of society is not sufficient to establish the importance of audiovisual culture today. Our culture has become a 'culture of real virtuality', as Castells call it. As 'real virtuality' audiovisual images have moved to the centre of society and culture. Here its relationship to capital has become so profound that capital realizes itself as cinema. Forming an immanent system with capital, cinema therefore is also the place where capital can be 'deterritorialized'. By looking at two examples of contemporary culture in which both audiovisual media and capitalism are of key importance, Bret Easton Ellis' *Glamorama* and David Fincher's

FIGHT CLUB, I try to see how Deleuze and Guattari's immanent concepts of capitalism can be used to describe this system of capital/cinema, while at the same time criticizing it. Capitalism produces and maintains itself, and at the same time it produces anti-production, what Deleuze and Guattari call 'schizophrenization'. *Glamorama* and FIGHT CLUB demonstrate how surplus ('glamour') and residual ('glycerine') are some of the ingredients that keep on circulating the schizo-flows that run through our capitalist/audiovisual society. One of the questions that is raised by Fincher's film is where 'critical freedom' and 'breaking away' turn into 'unfreedom'. This is a question that can only be dealt with at a micropolitical level, for which Deleuze gives no answers, but conceptual tools.

The next article, 'Is Bess a Bike?' also deals with capitalism and cinema. Frans-Willem Korsten looks at the mixed feelings in the reception of Lars von Trier's film BREAKING THE WAVES. He acknowledges the feminist critiques on the film that conceived the main female character, Bess, as a stereotypical example of female passivity and masochism. However, Korsten pleads for looking at the film from more perspectives. One possible other lens through which to read Bess' sacrificial behaviour is an intertextual resonance with a Dutch Medieval story that makes clear that Bess' action is not just an act of self-destruction, but also an attempt to break free. As becomes clear from the intertextual resonance, the thing that allows her to break free is faith. At another level, BREAKING THE WAVES invites an encounter with Jesus, the next 'screen' of references that Korsten elaborates. There is also the terror of capitalism and the family that put Bess' behaviour in a different light. Finally, Korsten argues that by prostituting herself Bess becomes a 'motor program of experimentation'. Bess's face, populated with intensities, becomes a Body without Organs. Bess starts to produce a schizophrenic surplus of meaning (and has nothing to do with passivity), believing that her actions will save her husband Jan. By producing a BwO, Bess' face becomes an image of combat; a combat of breaking away with the judgement of God that was capturing her. Finally, on a meta-level of the film production itself, by sentimentalizing old (melodramatic) values and bringing new ones into existence, Von Trier has resurrected Hollywood's capital and changed it at the same time, thus fitting in perfectly with the immanent system of capital/ cinema of contemporary society.

What to do with Deleuze in daily life and in cyberspace?

The next two articles deal with a very practical level of engagement with Deleuze. In 'Holy Fools: Revolutionary Elitism in Cyberspace' Richard Barbrook is very critical of the legacy of Deleuze and Guattari on the net. According to Barbrook, in cyberspace a lot of TJ's ('theory jockeys') use *A Thousand Plateaus* to provide buzzwords: 'rhizome' comes to signify any non-hierarchical network and the Body without Organs equals cyber-sex. Besides this, the libertarianism of the Sixties is eerily transformed into what Barbrook calls 'the Californian Ideology' of magazines like *Wired*. In this way 'Deleuzoguattarians' expose the weaknesses of *Anti-Oedipus* and *A Thousand Plateaus*. At least if we take Deleuze and Guattari as the romantic 'anarcho-communists' as Barbrook considers them to be. In this way Barbrook points to a few problematic aspects and effects of the heritage of Deleuze and Guattari that cannot be denied, as in for instance the impossibility of directly translating theory into practice.[33] Barbrook takes the failed experience of community radio, set up by Guattari in the early Eighties, as his representative example (that he then connects to Stalin and Pol Pot). It turned out that radio *Fréquence Libre* was not as liberal as it was intended: Guattari was more interested in lecturing his audience than in giving them direct access to the ether. Even lyrics of hip-hop songs had to be screened before airing. Barbrook reproaches Deleuze and Guattari for this avantguardistic elitism, which is precisely what has also been so problematically taken over by 'the Californian Ideology', albeit in a twisted neo-liberal version. Another reason why the community radio failed is because Guattari did not raise enough cash, because no commercial compromise could be made. Besides elitism, this 'purism' is the second disadvantage of Deleuzoguattarianism which, according to Barbrook, does not aid in understanding the non-hierarchical mixed practice and hi-tech gift-economy of the Net.

Barbrook signals a similar kind of 'politicide' in the work of Deleuze and Guattari as does Luuk van Middelaar. Both are very right in pointing out the real dangers of philosophy that enters practical life. However, both van Middelaar and Barbrook also have a rather one-dimensional view of the work of Deleuze and Guattari.[34] Although Barbrook certainly is right that elitism and purism can lead to rather disastrous effects in practice, Deleuze was very well aware of the end of the vanguardistic role of the intellectual.[35] He also has a far more complex view of capitalism, the role of the state and all the complex layers of interaction between theory and practice and between different 'political lines', and indeed, more so than is often suggested.

Furthermore, his concepts of creativity, becoming and revolution are meant for everybody. The pitfalls occur when these are taken to be an elitist 'representative' privilege, as does happen on some Net sites.

In the next article, 'How to Endure Intensity? Towards a Sustainable Nomadic Subject', Rosi Braidotti looks at another charge against Deleuze and Guattari, namely the objection of relativism and moral nihilism often made against nomadic views of subjectivity. She investigates the very concrete implications for daily life and social relations of Deleuze's philosophy. Nomadic becoming or rhizomatics is essentially an ethics of transformative forces and intensities, argues Braidotti. It is a view on subjectivity that demands the possibility of change and at the same time the 'stability' of endurance. Empowering change can occur by an imaginative investment of reason and by an aesthetic mode of 'absolute immersion of one's sensibility into the field of forces – music, color, light, speed, temperature, intensity, which one is attempting to capture'. It involves creation. And creation, Braidotti states, has different aspects. It is technological: it is about how. It is also geological: it is about where and in which territory. Ultimately, it is ethical: it is about where to set the limits and how to sustain the process of change without hurting self or other. It is especially this ethical question that Braidotti investigates more profoundly in her article.

In order to transform and change, in order to empower the actualization of virtual possibilities in the subject, memory needs imagination: some self-creation and self-invention are needed, albeit not necessarily a self-created poem of a complete Utopian Dream such as Rorty's country. Rather, one should think of micro-movements of change and creative transformation in aesthetic practice. One could recognize here the 'powers of the false' and the importance of fabulation in modern political cinema that Deleuze mentions in *The Time-Image* and that I will discuss in the next section.[36] Furthermore, contrary to some 'escape velocities'[37] that are promised in cyber-culture, Braidotti emphasizes the 'threshold of sustainability' that is necessary to find in nomadic subjectivity. According to her, the very pragmatic observation of 'I can't take it anymore' is an ethical energetic statement. With this ethical observation, the political moment of 'critical freedom' as discussed by Paul Patton is also possible.[38] Braidotti concentrates on the ethical implications. She suggests that instead of moral judgements of all kinds, the ethical (and again very pragmatic) 'what ever gets you through the day' is very important. Braidotti pleads for a less moralistic and conceptually more rigorous public debate of all problematic social issues of today. 'Whatever gets you through the day' can then be a tool to frame our thresholds of sustainability and change, both on the individual and the social level.

Becoming-minoritarian and the modern political film

Braidotti demonstrates that 'becoming' is at the heart of a Deleuzian ethics. It is also at the heart of the politics of Deleuze and Guattari. The last three articles of this book all deal more specifically with this concept. Paola Marrati analyses the problem of 'majority' and 'minority' implicated in any becoming. Sasha Vojkovic and Laleen Jayamanne both investigate how these concepts can be operative in films that deal with 'minority' positions. Paola Marrati argues in her article 'Against the Doxa: Politics of Immanence or Becoming-Minoritarian' that in one respect Deleuze has remained a Platonist, namely in his fight against opinion and common sense. Although Deleuze does not look for eternal truths or dreams of a state where the philosopher is king, he does see a breaking with the *doxa* as the ultimate philosophical and political vocation. For Deleuze this takes the shape of a struggle against the dominant image of thought that is governed by representation. According to Marrati, this critique of representation is the background to Deleuze's politics of becoming. Marrati investigates this critique of representation in the way in which it is implied in the concept of 'majority'. She then goes on to argue that the concept of 'becoming-minoritarian' creates a form of universality that is antagonistic to any representative politics. According to Deleuze a majority can never have any representative value. Not only because such a concept is not primarily defined by quantitative criteria, but also because it is a model that represents Nobody; it is an empty model. However, the emptiness of the majoritarian model is not a universal emptiness. The universal concerns everybody. And it is this kind of 'universalism' that is at work in processes of becoming where the ultimate end is a becoming-everything, a becoming-world. All processes of becoming are becoming-minoritarian and thus political: 'the shared deterritorialization and the asymmetrical movements implied by becoming must be understood in relation to the analysis of the majority as an empty model.' Contrary to Barbrook, Marrati argues that the philosopher, therefore, can represent no-one, he can only enter in a 'zone of indiscernability' with the non-philosopher and thus become-other, in the hope that something new (a thought, a sensation, a resistance to what's intolerable, 'a people') will come out of it. Becoming is always a double movement of proximity, not an invitation from an elite position to follow.

With the critique on representation, one can also ask what the consequences can be for political cinema. It is known that with his cinema books, Deleuze also develops a theory of images that goes beyond the idea of cinema as representation. The full implications of a different theory of the image are beyond the scope of this book. However, the question of representation is of course very important in considering 'political cinema' (however broadly that may be defined). In *The Time-Image* Deleuze specifically addresses the question of political cinema.[39] He distinguishes the classical political film from the modern political film. In classical political films, like BIRTH OF A NATION (Griffith, 1915) or the Russian Revolution films of Eisenstein and Pudovkin, there is always a Nation, the People, the Common Good. In modern political films, the people no longer exist, or does not yet exist: 'the people is missing'. The People has become a multiplicity of people. At best, Deleuze argues, the people is a becoming, when it is inventing itself in the suburbs and the ghettos. And all a modern political film can do is contribute to this becoming. Fragmentation and disintegration, the explosion of all unity, is therefore characteristic for the modern political film (and for contemporary political reality). There is a lot of internal violence within the different groups, which brings about a strong feeling of intolerance and impossibility.

The second difference between the classical and the modern film deals with the distinction between private and public and is related to this feeling of impossibility. In the classical political film there is still a border between private and public or political life. In the modern political film the private is immediately politically engaged. Connected to this is the fact that revolution (the change from one political belief to another, mediated by private consciousness) seems no longer possible; the modern political film is based on a feeling of the impossible and the intolerable. When Revolution is no longer possible, all that is left is a 'becoming-revolutionary'. The last characteristic of the modern political film is that it is not a place of representation (as was the classic political film, where the goals and aims of the People are represented) but a space of fabulation and 'powers of the false', an invention of the people in stories and myths that is self-creative. Cinema, seen in this perspective, can therefore be considered as comprising speech-acts.[40] They have (per)formative and hence political power, to invite becoming of all sorts, and hence to help a becoming-revolutionary, by definition minoritarian, of 'a people to come'.

However, the question of 'becoming-minoritarian' is not a straightforward process. Although virtually it is available at any moment for everybody, in certain actual historical circumstances it might not be the best political solution, as Sasha Vojkovic argues in her article 'SCHINDLER'S LIST and the Facing of History: The Return of the Promised Land'. Vojkovic analyses Spielberg's film SCHINDLER'S LIST while looking at the specific 'regimes of signs', territories and (de)territorial movements. She uses the concepts from *A Thousand Plateaus* of the four signifying systems (the signifying regime, the presignifying regime, the countersignifying semiotic and the postsignifying regime) to analyse how these regimes, as a mixed semiotic which is always the complexity of any semiotic system, function in SCHINDLER'S LIST and in respect to Jewish history. According to Vojkovic, the film problematizes the Jewish subject as exemplary of an ethnic group existing without/on an impossible territory. Since semiotics, or 'giving face' is always related to the question of territory, Vojkovic proposes a 'pragmatics of territoriality' of the film. The three 'lines of action' in the film, the line of Oscar Schindler, the line of the Jews, and the line of the Nazis, are defined by different territories. By tracing the different movements on and between these territories, Vojkovic analyses the complexities of the mixed semiotic. Becomings, in this case deterritorializations, are not always positive here. The Nazi regime is a despotic regime of the sign. It deterritorializes the 'scapegoat', the Jewish people, for whom this deterritorialization ('effacing', becoming-animal) is a negative line of flight. Reterritorialization, in the Promised Land, is therefore the only possibility of overcoming deportation and ghettoization. It is only once the arrival at the Promised Land is attained that the concept of deterritorialization needs to be reconsidered because the semiotic machines keep on moving; being a 'minority' is never a guarantee for becomings and new possibilities for the future. Vojkovic demonstrates that by offering a 'screen on which the face of history is mapped out', SCHINDLER'S LIST reminds us of how we have to review and negotiate our cultural present in order to find a zone of 'positive and absolute' deterritorialization, which is not possible at all moments. In as far as the film presents a people, the Schindler Jews represent a strong part of Jewish history, and Spielberg relies a lot on the mythical and biblical past. One could consider SCHINDLER'S LIST as a classic political film. As such it raises all the problems of representation, but functions nevertheless as a speech act that can have political impact in renegotiating the past and the present in order to create a future.

In the last article 'Forty Acres and a Mule Filmworks', Laleen Jayamanne also takes up the issue of the territory in relation to minorities and becomings. Fascinated by the aesthetic investment of the real Brooklyn location (to the point were it looks artificial) where Spike Lee's film DO THE RIGHT THING is shot, Jayamanne investigates the way in which this film is preoccupied with aesthetics. DO THE RIGHT THING has all the characteristics of a modern political film, but rather than talking about the strong polemic moments and the much discussed violence, Jayamanne looks at the preoccupation with aesthetics that is presented in this film. The many non-eventful moments in the film introduce a variety of tones, moods, temperatures and rhythms that have much more 'molecular' effects; small gestures break the sense of sensory-motor rhythms of ordinary action scenes. Jayamanne focuses on the role of Public Enemy's 'Fight the Power' by considering it as the refrain of DO THE RIGHT THING. In *A Thousand Plateaus*, Deleuze and Guattari consider the refrain as a territory marker. Considering the recurring rhythms of 'Fight the Power' as a refrain, the film gains a transformative force, both creative and destructive. As Jayamanne demonstrates, 'Fight the Power' occurs at the beginning and end of the film in a non-diegetic way, whereas in the film it is audible ten times, always blasting out of Radio Raheem's boom box, moving through the film like a moving sonic block, territorial motif or 'rhythmic character' that eventually reaches its stone wall and breaks in the final fight. However, Jayamanne suggests, the little improvised rhyme between Sal and Mookie, the day after the riot, gives in a very fragile way an opening to establish some equilibrium in the midst of terrible chaos, and hence the possibility for the creation of new sensibilities, maybe a 'new people to come' on a cross-cultural plane. With her aesthetic analysis of Lee's film, Jayamanne makes clear how a song can create a territory and how a film can be a speech act with micropolitical power.

The articles in this book interconnect at various points. In some cases I have indicated some connecting or negotiating moments in editor's notes. Of course, many other moments of dialogue are possible as well. I have chosen to emphasise the interdisciplinary character of this anthology by *not* ordering the articles by discipline. Rather, in the order of the articles, there is a theoretical and conceptual movement in thought from a more meta-theoretical level, to the level of engaging with the contemporary epoch of capital/cinema, and finally to looking at the most micro-political level of becoming. This movement in thought is reflected in the three sections that group the articles. At the same time these sections indicate the different temporal relations that the political and utopian vocation of theory can have. The articles in Section One 'Meta-Theory: The Future and the Past' deal with questions of 'how to make the future different from the past'. The fourth article in this section, Eva Jørholt's article on the cinema of David Cronenberg, makes a connection with the present, which is the temporal space of the next set of articles. In Section Two 'Engaging in the Present', utopia is defined in respect to a critical engagement with the present. In these articles the present is discussed with respect to capitalism, cinema, cyberspace and daily life. The articles in Section Three 'Micropolitical Becoming: Duration and Change', in dealing with becoming, are located in the ever escaping time of duration where everything always changes and the present is eluded.[41] This kind of time then could be seen as yet another temporal relation to 'utopia': here the complete opposite of the traditional idea of Utopia as a fixed blue print for society has been reached. No Utopia ('nowhere') can be reached forever, since the 'now here' is always mobile and transforming. In becoming, every territorialization implies possible deterritorializations and reterritorializations.

As is argued in this book, cinema and audiovisual media in general are a central concern for contemporary culture. In its immanent link with capital, audiovisual culture is the one of the most important areas from which to (re)describe, engage with and escape from contemporary culture. And as we know from Deleuze and Guattari, this can only be done in a schizophrenic way, working from within the system, producing and 'anti-producing' at the same time. Contrary to what may be expected, however, most of the articles that deal with audiovisual media do not so much tackle Deleuze's books on cinema. Although the cinema books are very important in that they offer theoretical tools to look at images from an immanent formal perspective, these formal and aesthetic concepts of the cinema books are not addressed. Instead, this anthology tries to read in a rhizomatic way the more political concepts developed by Deleuze and Guattari together in *Anti-Oedipus*, *A Thousand Plateaus* and *What is Philosophy?* to film and other contemporary issues.[42] This is because the question implicitly or explicitly addressed by all articles in this anthology is that of whether and in which respects Deleuze and Guattari offer any useful concepts to bridge the gap between theory and practice.

From the several critiques on philosophy's direct and mostly failed engagements, it is clear that we cannot ask the philosopher nor the artist nor the scientist to write a policy plan, as is suggested by Rorty. All too often this has led to 'politicide' and elitist tyranny, as is demonstrated by Van Middelaar and Barbrook. Philosophers should invent new concepts in order to redescribe the world and create new possibilities for the future. Theory should be seen as a 'practice of theory' in which it is very important that art, science and philosophy mutually illuminate their specific effects. The analysis of the current epoch, by emphasizing both the immanence of capitalism and the centrality of audiovisual media that function as speech acts, is another area where theory can become political. With the many concepts that Deleuze and Guattari have invented, it has become clear that 'politics' in contemporary society really takes place at the microlevel of beliefs and desires. It is this invisible level that is most important in a culture that at the same time increasingly depends on the visible, to the point where 'capital becomes cinema'. It is also for this reason that the micro- and macropolitics keep on influencing each other continuously, always moving and changing, demanding that everybody always be alert. All theory and philosophy can do is to give tools to sharpen our perceptions and sensibilities for grasping the complexities of the various political lines that constitute the individual and the social. With this modest mission it might be possible to see where philosophy and politics can meet again, without the risk of passing round 'a poisoned chalice'.

Section One

Meta-theory:
The Future and the Past

1 Redescriptive Philosophy

Deleuze and Guattari's Critical Pragmatism

Paul Patton

Rorty and Deleuze: a 'rendez-vous manqué'

In a recent essay on Derrida[1], Rorty advocates a 'syncretic, ecumenical perspective' which would minimise differences between his own pragmatism and the 'postmodernism' of French philosophers such as Foucault and Derrida. I propose to support this proposal by adding Deleuze and Guattari to the list of those who have much in common with Rorty's pragmatism. This may seem an implausible extension of his ecumenical perspective since Rorty has written very little on either Deleuze or Guattari and almost nothing that is favourable. A review of Deleuze's *Nietzsche and Philosophy* alongside Richard Schacht's *Nietzsche*, written quite early in his engagement with French 'postmodern' philosophers, painted a rather unflattering picture of Parisian silliness which cultivated and imitated 'the more fatuous side of Nietzsche'.[2] Deleuze's crime was to have taken Nietzsche's metaphysical system-building tendency seriously and elaborated the theory of will to power in a manner which ultimately 'dissolves everything into a mush of reactive forces in order to bring out their underlying nastiness'.[3] Apart from this brief encounter, references to Deleuze in Rorty's subsequent essays are scarce and mostly consist of adding his name to lists of French 'postmodernist' philosophers such as Foucault and Lyotard.[4]

This lack of engagement is regrettable since of all the French 'postmodernists' it is Deleuze and Guattari who come closest to many of Rorty's views. For example, we find in their work a conception of text and interpretation remarkably similar to Rorty's. Their claim that there is no philosophically significant difference between what a text is made of and what it means parallels his rejection of the distinction between using and interpreting texts and more generally the distinction between signifying bits of the world such as signs and texts and other objects such as trees and quarks. Just as Rorty claims that reading texts is a matter of placing them in relation with 'other texts, people, obsessions, bits of information or what have you',[5] so in their Introduction to *A Thousand Plateaus*, Deleuze and Guattari defend the idea of a book which should be regarded as an assemblage with the world rather than an image or representation of it: 'We will never ask what a book means, as signified or signifier, we will not look for anything to understand in it. We will ask what it functions with, in connection with what other things it does or does not transmit intensities... A book itself is a little machine'.[6] The pragmatism of their conception of philosophy is especially evident in the earlier version of this Introduction published separately as 'Rhizome', where they invoke Foucault's conception of a book as a tool-box and Proust's conception of a book as a pair of spectacles in support of their stated aim of producing 'a functional, pragmatic book'.[7]

Over and above this convergence on the issue of texts and meaning, there are a number of more far reaching similarities between their conceptions of philosophy. Deleuze and Guattari share a pragmatist conception of philosophy as the fabrication of intellectual tools rather than the attainment of truth, and a progressivist conception of the social function of philosophy. Rorty's concern with issues of material social justice is matched by their reluctance to abandon Marx's critique of the inequalities generated by capitalism. While there are also significant differences between Rorty's pragmatism and Deleuze and Guattari's critical pragmatism, the absence of any sustained engagement between them amounts to something of a *rendez-vous manqué* in contemporary social and political philosophy. In order to show this, however, we require an effort of translation between different philosophical idioms of the kind Rorty imagines when he calls for a book about Derrida that would meet analytic philosophers halfway. Reconciling idioms in this manner would contribute to breaking down barriers to international communication which are, in Rorty's view, the result of nothing more than 'the very different courses of reading that different countries demand of their philosophy students'.[8]

Take Rorty's use of the term 'ironist' to refer to those who are aware of the contingency of their own 'final vocabularies' and also aware that such vocabularies can neither be justified nor refuted by argument but only replaced by other vocabularies. Deleuze is an ironist in this sense: his solo writings display a highly developed and self-conscious ability to move from one philosophical vocabulary to another, while his collaborative work with Guattari abhors argument in favour of the invention of new vocabularies. In Rorty's account too, an ironist is a nominalist and historicist who believes that nothing has an intrinsic nature or real essence and that all our descriptions of events and states of affairs are couched in the terms of particular vocabularies which are subject to change: 'Ironists agree with Davidson about our inability to step outside our language in order to compare it with some thing else, and with Heidegger about the contingency and historicity of that language'.[9] He contrasts ironists with metaphysicians who believe that there are real essences and an intrinsic nature of things which it is the task of philosophy to discover. Deleuze also abandons the idea that philosophical descriptions of the world can or should converge on one unique true theory. On this issue, he agrees with Rorty's anti-metaphysical stance.

Anti-representationalism

Like Rorty, Deleuze rejects the idea of thought as the representation of an external reality in favour of the idea that truth is a human construct. One of the aims of *Difference and Repetition* is the elaboration of a non-representational conception of thought.[10] In that book and in *Nietzsche and Philosophy* Deleuze argues that philosophical reflection on the nature of thought has been dominated by a single 'dogmatic' image which identifies thinking with knowing and which supposes that knowledge is ultimately a form of *recognition*. One of the central presuppositions of the dogmatic image is the idea that thought has a natural affinity with the true, that thought 'seeks truth or that it loves and wills truth "by right"'.[11] Deleuze has two objections to this image of thought: first, that it is a timid and conformist model based upon the most banal acts of everyday thinking. He does not deny that recognition occurs, but he wants to retain the name of thinking for the different activity which takes place when the mind is provoked by an encounter with the unknown or the unfamiliar. Apprenticeship or learning provides him with an alternative image of thought as something to which we are driven by necessity or by the perception of a problem.

Second, he objects that the dogmatic image tells us nothing about the real conditions which give rise to thought. Thus, in *Nietzsche and Philosophy*, he takes the will to power as the basis for a 'genetic and differential' genealogical analysis of thought, with the result that the 'element' of thought is no longer truth and falsity but 'the noble and the base, the high and the low, depending on the nature of the forces that take hold of thought itself'.[12] This approach breaks the connection between thought and truth assumed by the dogmatic image. It points to a genetic analysis of thought in so far as it is concerned with the forces which determine thought to take a particular form and to pursue particular objects. Having argued that for Nietzsche the sense and value of things is determined by the qualities of the will to power expressed within them, Deleuze concludes that we 'always have the truths we deserve as a function of the sense of what we conceive, of the value of what we believe'.[13] His point is not to deny the possibility of truth, but rather to suggest that truth is no more than an 'abstract universal' the precise character of which remains 'entirely undetermined'.[14]

It is perhaps an effect of the 'different courses of reading that different countries demand of their philosophy students' that Deleuze argues in transcendentalist terms against the representational image which dominates philosophy from Plato to Descartes and Kant. Rather than abandon transcendentalism in the manner of Quine, Sellars or the later Wittgenstein, he proposes an alternative account of the transcendental conditions of thought. In *Difference and Repetition* he outlines a theory of 'transcendental' problems as the ground of thinking and the source of all truths, suggesting that 'problems are the differential elements in thought, the genetic elements in the true'.[15] Problems here are understood in a sense related to Kantian Transcendental Ideas as the specific objects of pure thought. Deleuze's conception of transcendental problems as the genetic elements of thought implies a twofold genesis: a logical genesis of truths in the form of solutions to particular problems and a transcendental genesis of the act of thinking in the discovery or constitution of Ideas or Problems. Both geneses are implicated in the activity which Deleuze takes as his model for thought: 'The exploration of Ideas and the elevation of each faculty to its transcendent exercise amounts to the same thing. These are two aspects of an essential apprenticeship or process of learning'.[16] In these terms, the task of philosophy is to specify the elements and structure of the Ideas or Problems which govern thought in a particular field.

Does this reliance upon the language of transcendental philosophy mean that Deleuze is a metaphysician in Rorty's sense of the term? On the contrary, there is no reason to believe that, for Deleuze, the transcendental problems which find expression and determination in the concepts and vocabularies of philosophers exist out there in the world independently of those forms of expression. He does not believe that the goal of philosophy is a final vocabulary of problems in terms of which we will be able to represent the world as it really is. Instead, he defends the idea of a transcendental *empiricism* according to which what problems there are is an open question to be answered by the exploration of the field of thought in a given society at a given time. Just as there are Ideas or Problems which correspond to the physical and biological realities studied by natural science, so there are Ideas of psychic structures, languages and societies which are the objects of social sciences. For Deleuze, the limits of thought are set neither by the ahistorical nature of human reason nor by the nature of reality as such, but by the set of problems thrown up by history, social life or the development of particular sciences. In this sense, his conception of philosophy is entirely consistent with Rorty's historicism.

Philosophical constructivism

Rorty suggests that since ironists do not believe in the existence of a final vocabulary which it is the aim of philosophy to discover, their descriptions of their own activity will be 'dominated by metaphors of making rather than finding, of diversification and novelty rather than convergence to the antecedently present'.[17] In his final collaboration with Guattari, *What is Philosophy?*, Deleuze proposes a definition of philosophy as the creation of concepts, where concepts are defined, following Nietzsche, as that which philosophers must 'make and create'.[18] Deleuze and Guattari's conception of philosophy resembles Deleuze's transcendental empiricism in many respects, even though it is presented in a quite different philosophical vocabulary. They propose a stipulative definition of philosophy in which the creation of concepts serves to distinguish philosophy from other forms of intellectual activity such as science and art: 'The concept belongs to philosophy and only to philosophy'.[19] In their view, science aims at the representation of states of affairs by means of mathematical or propositional functions, while art does not aim at representation but at the capture and expression in a given medium of the objective content of particular sensations. Philosophy falls somewhere in between: it is like science in that it fulfils a cognitive rather than an affective function, but it is like art, especially modern art, in that it does not seek to refer or to represent independently existing objects or states of affairs.[20] An echo of the Kantian distinctions between knowledge, thought and sensation may be heard in the differences which are spelt out in *What is Philosophy?* between science, philosophy and art; or between scientific functions, philosophical concepts and artistic 'blocks of sensation' on the one hand and their respective objects on the other.

Scientific functions and propositions are referential in the sense that they *refer to* bodies or states of affairs which are supposed to exist independently of the functions concerned. The independence of the variables on a given scientific plane of reference establishes an external relation between a function and its object, such as a particle with a given position, energy, mass and spin. This referential relation is explicit in the case of propositional functions and formalised sentences of ordinary language where the objects which constitute the extension of a given concept are also the referents of singular terms. By contrast, the objects of philosophical concepts are pure events and their relation to events is not referential but expressive. Concepts express events in the sense that Descartes' Cogito expresses the event of thought or the Social Contract expresses the event of the establishment of civil society. It is this feature of the relation between concepts and their objects that they have in mind when they claim that concepts are 'self-referential' or that the concept 'has *no reference*: it is self-referential, [in the sense that] it posits itself and its object at the same time as it is created'.[21]

In addition to this internal relation between the concept and the event that it expresses, Deleuze and Guattari maintain that concepts stand in external relations to other concepts and to the problems to which they constitute a response: 'A concept lacks meaning to the extent that it is not connected to other concepts and is not linked to a problem that it resolves or helps to resolve.'[22] Concepts therefore possess a history, which includes the variations which they undergo in their migration from one problem to another. Thus, the concept of the social contract is transformed in the shift from Hobbes's problem of the constitution and legitimation of coercive political authority to Rawls's problem of the principles of a just society. Throughout the tradition of contractarian approaches to political philosophy, the concept of the contract is transformed as a result of being rethought in relation to new problems, while retaining elements of its former incarnations. In any concept, Deleuze and Guattari suggest, 'there are usually bits or components that come from other concepts, which correspond to other problems and presuppose other planes'.[23] Although this conception of philosophy does not relate the creation of concepts to transcendental Ideas or Problems in the manner that Deleuze did in *Difference and Repetition*, the extent to which it is a successor to Deleuze's earlier account is indicated by his remark in *Difference and Repetition* that 'problems are of the order of events'.[24]

Clearly, the cognitive function of philosophy as Deleuze and Guattari define it is bound up with their concept of the pure events which philosophical concepts are supposed to express. In *The Logic of Sense*, Deleuze argued that the Stoics were the first to create a philosophical concept of the event, discovering this along with sense or the 'what is expressed' of the proposition. For the Stoics, the 'sayable' or sense which is expressed in a proposition is an incorporeal entity which subsists independently of its linguistic expression and apart from the mixtures of bodies to which it is attributed. Similarly, Deleuze conceives of sense as 'an incorporeal, complex and irreducible entity, at the surface of things, a pure event which inheres or subsists in the proposition'.[25] The concept of pure events which he and Guattari put forward in *What is Philosophy?* also relies on this Stoic distinction between corporeal states of affairs and incorporeal events that 'rise like a vapour from the states of affairs themselves'.[26] In these terms, pure events are incorporeal entities which subsist over and above the particular forms in which they are expressed in statements and actualised in bodies and states of affairs. The concept of the social contract may be considered to express the pure event of incorporation of a legal and political system. As such, the contract is irreducible to its incarnation in particular forms of political or civil society.[27] Historical events such as the social contract, war or revolution are therefore incorporeal abstractions which may be actualised in different societies at different times but which are not exhausted by such particular determinations. It is as though actual historical events were doubled by a series of ideal or virtual events: 'What History grasps of the event is its effectuation in states of affairs or in lived experience, but the event in its becoming, in its specific consistency, in its self-positing concept, escapes History'.[28]

Deleuze and Guattari contrast the effectuation of a given pure event in particular circumstances with the 'counter-effectuation' which occurs when a new concept is extracted from things. They acknowledge that, in a material sense, events are indistinguishable from the bodies and states of affairs in which they are effectuated. However, the events which are expressed in philosophical concepts are not material but pure events which exceed their actualisation in particular material processes and states of affairs. In this sense, pure events represent a 'reserve'[29] of being and the guarantee of an open future. To counter-effectuate everyday events is therefore to consider them as processes whose outcome is not yet determined. It is to relate them back to the pure event of which they appear only as one determination or specification, or to consider them in the light of the transcendental problem to which they constitute only one particular solution. Kant makes a similar point in *The Contest of the Faculties* when he distinguishes between the concept of a revolution in favour of universal rights of man as this was expressed in the 'enthusiasm' of Europeans for those ideals and the manner in which that concept and those ideals were actualised in the bloody events of 1789. In this sense, Deleuze and Guattari suggest, 'the concept is the contour, the configuration, the constellation of an event to come'.[30]

Events and descriptions

It follows from the account of incorporeals as the 'expressed' of statements that the individuation of events as events of a particular kind is dependent upon language. There is a parallel here with Elizabeth Anscombe's view that intentional actions are always actions under a description. Anscombe argues that because actions involve intentions and because having an intention presupposes some description of what it is one intends to do, it follows that the same spatio-temporal occurrence may correspond to a series of actions: moving a lever up and down, pumping water, poisoning a well and so on.[31] Human actions can be identified as actions of a particular kind only by taking descriptions into account. This thesis about the dependence of actions upon descriptions implies that the nature of actions is not exhausted by any particular description or set of descriptions. More generally, it implies that the same spatio-temporal occurrence or series of states of affairs may incarnate an open-ended series of actions. Ian Hacking explores some surprising consequences of this thesis. One is the phenomenon to which Nietzsche and Foucault drew attention, namely that new forms of description of human behaviour make possible new kinds of action. Only after the discursive characterisation of behaviour in terms of juvenile delinquency or multiple personality was established did it become possible for individuals to conceive of themselves and therefore to act as delinquents or to switch personalities: 'Inventing or molding a new kind, a new classification, of people or of behaviour may create new ways to be a person, new choices to make, for good or evil. There are new descriptions, hence new actions under a description.'[32]

The second surprising conclusion which Hacking draws from this account of the nature of actions is that there is no simple fact of the matter which enables us to say whether a given redescription of a past action is correct or incorrect: 'If a description did not exist, or was not available, at an earlier time, then at that time one could not act intentionally under that description.'[33] In order to reach this conclusion, Hacking relies upon Anscombe's doctrine that all intentional actions are actions under a description. Deleuze's Stoic conception of pure events involves no reference to intentions, but it does imply that the specification of everyday events as events of a certain kind is a function of the manner in which they are described. As a result, generalising Anscombe's thesis about the relation between actions and descriptions points in the same direction as Deleuze's Stoic thesis about the relationship between pure events and the forms of their linguistic expression. In Anscombe's view, since the same spatio-temporal occurrence may constitute more than one action and therefore be described in a variety of ways, it follows that the nature of actions is essentially indeterminate. For Deleuze, there is a similar indeterminacy associated with the event proper or pure event, since this is not reducible to the manner in which it is incarnated in particular states of affairs. Conversely, there is no limit to the variety of events which may be incarnated in a given spatio-temporal occurrence or series of states of affairs. In other words, whether we consider everyday incarnate or impure events as spatio-temporal occur-rences under a description or as the actualisation in bodies and states of af-fairs of a given pure event, their character as events of a particular kind is determined by the manner in which they are described.

Since the manner in which a given occurrence is described or 'repre-sented' within a given social context determines it as a particular kind of event, there is good reason for political actors to contest accepted descrip-tions. In their discussion of language use in *A Thousand Plateaus*, Deleuze and Guattari describe the change in status of a body, or the change in its rela-tions to other bodies, which occurs when it is subject to a new description as an 'incorporeal transformation'. The explicit performative statements which provided Austin with the point of departure for his theory of speech acts provide the clearest cases of such events. A judge's sentence transforms an accused person into a convicted felon. What took place before (the mur-der, the trial) and what takes place after (the punishment) are corporeal events. These involve changes of state which affect bodies, their passions and their interrelations, but 'the transformation of the accused into a convict is a pure instantaneous act or incorporeal attribute'.[34] Deleuze and Guattari argue that the pragmatic function of language consists in the attribution or effectuation of the incorporeal transformations current in a society at any given time: reaching adulthood, becoming unemployed, improving effi-ciency, restoring accountability and so on. Understood in these terms, lan-guage use is not primarily the communication of information but a matter of acting in or upon the world: event attributions do not simply describe or re-port pre-existing events, they help to actualise particular events in the social field. That is why politics frequently takes the form of struggle over the ap-propriate description of events.

Deleuze's Stoic conception of events not only points to the role of lan-guage and other forms of representation in the actualisation of everyday events, it also points to a critical role for philosophy in relation to the com-mon sense understanding of events. Their conception of philosophy implies a constructivist and critical engagement with what Rorty calls the final vo-cabularies that characterise a particular society at a particular time. For Rorty irony is opposed to common sense where the latter is understood as the attitude of those who take for granted 'the final vocabulary to which they and those around them are habituated'.[35] Similarly, for Deleuze and Guattari the attitude of common sense is the very antithesis of philosophy as they understand it. Common sense is the domain of opinions which are by definition wedded to the final vocabulary of a given milieu. In their view, philosophy is untimely and 'worthy of the event' when it does not simply respond to events in the terms of common sense but rather creates *new* con-

cepts which enable us to counter-actualise present events and historical processes.[36] Foucault provides another example of a philosopher who
consciously seeks to break with common sense without always attempting
to spell out a politics that might contain 'the just and definitive solution'.[37]
He describes his work as attempting to 'problematize' aspects of present social reality, by which he means proposing new concepts and new descriptions of social phenomena, such as criminal punishment or sexuality, in
order to disturb habitual ways of thinking and talking. In an interview dealing with his method of historical philosophy, he proposed the term
'eventalisation' to describe this procedure. Foremost among the several
meanings he attached to this term was the 'breach of self-evidence' that occurs, for example, when what was taken to be part of an unbroken history
turns out to be singular and contingent.[38]

Deleuze and Guattari also see the invention of concepts as a means of
breaking with self-evidence by providing new means of description of the
forces which shape our present and therefore new possibilities for action.
They agree with Marx and Rorty that the job of philosophers is 'to help
make the future different from the past'.[39] For this reason they endow it with
an explicitly political vocation and define philosophy as the creation of 'untimely' concepts in Nietzsche's sense of this term: 'acting counter to [our]
time, and therefore acting on our time and let us hope, for the benefit of a
time to come'.[40] From *Nietzsche and Philosophy* onwards, Deleuze always
aligned his conception of philosophy with that of Nietzsche on two points:
opposition to those whose ultimate aim is the recognition of what exists,
and preference for an untimely thought which seeks to invent new possibilities for life. In *What is Philosophy?*, he and Guattari suggest that 'it is with
utopia that philosophy becomes political and takes the criticism of its own
time to its highest point'.[41] Philosophy as they define it is utopian in the
sense that Rorty suggests that utopian politics has been the rule rather than
the exception among intellectuals ever since the French revolution fired the
romantic imagination of Europe, namely in setting aside questions about
the will of God or the nature of man in favour of the dream 'of creating a
hitherto unknown form of society'.[42] Deleuze and Guattari argue that philosophy should be 'utopian' in a similar sense, namely contributing to the
emergence of new forms of individual and collective identity, or as they put
it, summoning forth 'a new earth and a people that does not yet exist'.[43]

According to Rorty, philosophy helps to make the future different from
the past by providing new means of description for social and political
events and states of affairs. Redescription rather than argument is the only
appropriate method of criticism of an existing vocabulary, and as a result
ironists are those who 'specialise in redescribing ranges of objects or events

in partially neologistic jargon, in the hope of inciting people to adopt and extend that jargon'.[44] For Deleuze too, the creation of concepts is inseparable from the elaboration of new vocabularies. He points to Foucault's concept of 'disciplinary society' as one of the more successful conceptual inventions in recent years.[45] Clearly, this concept is inseparable from the vocabulary of power, strategy, forces and bodies which Foucault developed in *Discipline and Punish* and related texts. Its effectivity can be measured in part by the way in which it changed what could be said or written about prisons, but also by the degree to which elements of this vocabulary have been taken up throughout political philosophy and the social sciences. The prodigious exercise of concept creation which Deleuze undertook with Guattari provides a series of vocabularies in terms of which we can describe significant features of the contemporary landscape. These include the terminology used to describe different kinds of social, linguistic and affective assemblages (strata, content and expression, territories, lines of flight or deterritorialization); the terms employed in the elaboration of a micropolitics of desire founded on the dynamics of unconscious affect and the different ways in which this interacts with individual and collective subjectivities (body without organs, intensities, molar and molecular segmentarities); an account of capital as a non-territorially based *axiomatic* of flows of materials, labour and information (as opposed to a territorial system of overcoding); a concept of the State as an apparatus of capture which, in the forms of its present actualisation, is increasingly subordinated to the requirements of the capitalist axiomatic; a concept of abstract machines of metamorphosis (nomadic war machines) which are the agents of social and political transformation; and finally a vocabulary in which to describe processes of becoming-minor or becoming-revolutionary and which enable Deleuze and Guattari to outline a politics of difference or differentiation defined in opposition to all attempts to capture or reconfigure the position of majority.[46]

Rorty abandons talk of truth and falsity in philosophy in favour of the degree to which a new vocabulary is interesting, where 'interesting' philosophy is usually 'a contest between an entrenched vocabulary which has become a nuisance and a half-formed new vocabulary which vaguely promises great things'.[47] Deleuze and Guattari's account of the utopian vocation of philosophy is similarly linked to a pragmatic response to the question of the value of philosophical concepts. In *Difference and Repetition*, Deleuze had already described the act of thought as a 'throw of the dice', by which he meant that thinking is a form of experimentation, the success or failure of which lies outside the control of the thinker. In *What is Philosophy?* he and Guattari suggest that philosophy is a form of experimentation in the creation of new concepts: 'to think is to experiment ...'.[48] Obviously, the creation

of concepts can neither bring about nor controvert what its concepts express, whether this is political society under a rule of law, justice or equality
between the sexes. Rather, philosophical activity contributes to making the
future different from the past by affording new forms of description,
thought and action. As a result, the adequacy or inadequacy with which
philosophy performs this task is not assessable in terms of truth and falsity
but in terms of categories such as interesting or important. Philosophy can
offer guidelines for well-formed as opposed to flimsy concepts, but it cannot
offer criteria for judging the importance of concepts or events. The only criteria by which concepts may be assessed are those of 'the new, remarkable
and interesting that replace the appearance of truth and are more demanding than it is'.[49] In these terms, philosophy's utopian vocation of calling for 'a
new earth and new people' is achieved when it produces interesting concepts which can function effectively in a given social and political context.

Critical versus complacent pragmatism

We have drawn attention to the pragmatism of Deleuze and Guattari's concept of philosophy and redescribed their account of the nature and task of
philosophy in terms of Rorty's account of philosophy as providing new vocabularies and new means of description. What lesson should we draw
from this comparison? Should we conclude that, contrary to appearances
and contrary to Rorty's view of those such as Foucault who share their conception of philosophy, Deleuze and Guattari are in fact liberal ironists? In
fact, there are still differences which, at the risk of being unfair to Rorty, we
can describe as those between a complacent and a critical pragmatism. One
difference between them concerns their views of the manner in which
redescriptive philosophy can play a political role. Rorty sees the kind of
redescription which the work of philosophers such as Foucault, Deleuze or
Derrida makes possible as essentially a private affair. He thinks that there is
a tension between this kind of philosophical commitment to the cause of
freedom and the commitment to not inflicting pain on others which is part
of a liberal public political culture. Since redescription can humiliate and
cause pain in others, a liberal public political culture should not impose
such redescriptions on others. Rather, it should allow people to be taken on
their own terms.[50] But that is not sufficient to show that redescriptive philosophy should be regarded as private. The exercise of standard liberal free-
doms such as freedom of speech may also humiliate and cause pain in

others. This does not imply that these are private affairs: on the contrary, it is a reason why the forms of their exercise are subject to public control.

Rorty also thinks that redescriptive philosophy can have no bearing on the political culture of liberal democracies because this is a pragmatic culture concerned principally with issues of public policy, issues on which this kind of philosophy has little to say. Hence the view expressed in *Achieving Our Country* that 'the Left should put a moratorium on theory. It should try to kick its philosophy habit'.[51] But many of Rorty's own examples of the kinds of progress achieved by what he calls the cultural left might be taken as evidence for precisely the opposite view. The kinds of conceptual, historical and social analysis which made it possible to write about the oppression of women, blacks and gays were not carried out independently of the invention or transformation of philosophical concepts. This kind of intellectual activity made it possible to invent new concepts and develop new forms of description which have contributed to changes in public attitudes and, as a result, eventually to changes in the law and public institutions. For Deleuze and Guattari, politics is played out precisely in this kind of indirect interaction between forms of becoming-minoritarian or revolutionary and majoritarian political culture. For this reason, they agree with Foucault that the pursuit of freedom implies a constant effort to detach ourselves from past ways of thinking and acting.

By contrast, even though he shares the view that the ultimate goal of philosophy is freedom rather than truth, Rorty seems inclined to believe at least in so far as social philosophy is concerned that this goal has been reached with the conceptual framework of the liberal democratic society. At one point, he suggests that 'Western social and political thought may have had the last *conceptual* revolution it needs'.[52] Rorty misrepresents Foucault and by implication other redescriptive philosophers in attributing to him 'the conviction that we are too far gone for reform to work – that a convulsion is needed'.[53] His suggestion that Foucault yearns for a kind of autonomy that could never be embodied in social institutions is only partially correct. Foucault shares with Deleuze a conception of freedom as something which is realised in the ongoing process of pushing back the limits of what it is possible to do or to be. This is what he means by 'the undefined work of freedom'.[54] Deleuze expresses a similar view when, with deliberate reference to Kant's distinction between the Revolution and the enthusiasm which its ideals aroused throughout Europe, he distinguishes between the way in which revolutions turn out historically and the 'becoming-revolutionary' which is a permanent possibility open to all. Like Foucault, he views this kind of individual and collective self-transformation as our only way of 'responding to what is intolerable', where the limits of what is intolerable are themselves historically determined and subject to change.[55] In this manner, the redescription made possible by the invention of new concepts contributes to such local and specific ways in which the future will be unlike the past.

2 The Lady Sits Between Two Long Windows, Writing

Deleuze/Guattari and the Practice of Cultural Analysis

Catherine M. Lord

The lady sits between two long windows, writing. The gardeners sweep the lawn with giant brooms. We are the first to come here. We the discovers of an unknown land.[1]

Art thinks no less than philosophy, but it thinks through affects and percepts.[2]

Our lady of planes: cultural analysis at the threshold

How and where does cultural analysis pass into art? This question once more opens up the threshold between the theoretical and the artistic, the philosophical and the literary. The boundary between the two may require not exploration, but formation. In *What is Philosophy?* Deleuze and Guattari prove themselves to be experienced at both the analysis and the making of planes – that of 'immanence' and that of 'composition' – both guides for adventures at the threshold.[3] According to Deleuze and Guattari, the first plane belongs to the work of philosophers, the second to artists. The first enables the development of concepts, the second makes the 'aesthetic,' or what is the 'work of sensation.'[4] Both planes are always already there, permanently extending into the future. The plane of immanence is a site of chaos which becomes structured through concepts, for 'the plane is all that holds them together.'[5] The plane of composition composes flux into blocks of sensation. When percepts and aesthetic figures are constructed from the artist's material, this latter plane is in action. Just as concepts produce structures from the plane of immanence, artworks crystallise through the plane of composition.[6]

Yet as the second epigraph to my essay implies, between the two planes, some inscrutable connection is at work. Otherwise, art would not 'think'.

Deleuze and Guattari admit that the two 'entities' of 'art' and 'philosophy' can 'pass into each other'.[7] It is therefore viable to consider the 'affect' of a 'concept' or the 'concept' of an 'affect'.[8] Yet having admitted as much, Deleuze and Guattari tend towards making the two planes separate. Referring to abstract and conceptual art, the authors insist that in the attempt to bring together philosophy and art, neither succeed in substituting 'the concept for the sensation'.[9] That terrain where art and philosophy can pass into each other is enigmatic precisely because concepts and aesthetic figures are not simply interchangeable. To explore the enigma, I will bring together the planes of immanence and composition with Virginia Woolf's majestic and poetic *The Waves* (1931), where resides a figure which appears and disappears between the Deleuzian and Guattarian planes. 'She' will be able to shed much light on how concepts reform themselves through aesthetic composition. As a possible conceptual and aesthetic figure, she might illuminate the secrets of how cultural analysis can pass into the literary art of Virginia Woolf.

Taking a reading lamp into the undisclosed site requires a reminder about the interdisciplinary function of cultural analysis. For Mieke Bal, this endeavour involves both specific objects of inquiry and 'precise methodological starting points'.[10] As a 'practice,' cultural analysis is not 'methodologically eclectic, nor indifferent'. For example, philosophy might engage literature. The methodological problems produced in the encounter never simplify the terms of any one discipline. The procedures of a certain practice need not be ditched; instead, their critical strategies can be revised and enhanced. Bal underlines the self-reflexive functions of cultural analysis. Joining her, Jonathan Culler argues that what gives cultural analysis 'definition' is a 'particular sort of theoretical engagement: its reflection on the way in which its own disciplinary and methodological standpoints shape the objects that it analyses'.[11] Thus, self-reflexion is a key concept for interdisciplinary study. In initiating an encounter between a Deleuzian philosophy and Woolf's novel as a means of discovering/making new edges between the planes, I will be examining the interdisciplinary procedures which enable self-reflexion, while moving beyond it. What is demanded is nothing less than an analysis of analysis.[12]

The lady who sits writing in Woolf's *The Waves* might offer herself as a character belonging to the world of analysis, of thought under scrutiny yet protected in a garden, who 'sits between two long windows, writing'. The lady might be read as the image of the thinker at work or, equally well, the novelist, dramatist, poet or painter at her task. No precise description of her task is offered. Furthermore, 'she' can both embody a character and trope while refusing to conform comfortably to either of these labels. The two glass, transparent panes could be read as planes, one for immanence, one for composition. Glass has the potential to reflect. The lady will inspire the novel's writer-character Bernard to reflect upon himself and his insatiable drive to make the phrases of a book. Around both him and the lady, the novel's textual waves make six characters: Bernard, Susan, Jinny, Rhoda, Neville, Louis. They narrate their lives from childhood to death. While the subjectivities of the six soliloquists undulate, break into colors and lights and particles, the 'writing lady' is swallowed up in the becomings of the six; yet she surfaces to remain stubbornly writing and intransigent in her task. The two, transparent planes behind which she writes may figure more than the two glass thresholds, but with them she proffers a *mise en abyme* of great import.

This French, narratological term designates an embedded fabula revealing important layers in the primary narrative;[13] the interaction between such textual layers has analytical consequences. Bernard is a phrase maker; the lady is a writer. He is the novel's more important narrator; he produces the text's final, exuberant soliloquy. In an original version of *The Waves*, the chief narrator was a woman.[14] Between Bernard and the lady writing, therefore, is a correspondence. As a child, he first discovered her behind the wall of a private house.[15] As a recurring motif, she haunts him until the end of the book. He reflects on his 'friends' lives and, those 'fabulous presences, men with brooms, *women writing* ... clouds and phantoms of dust too, of dust that changed'.[16] Bernard the phrase maker confronts the irrepressibly productive lady as she is caught up in the flux and ceaseless transformations of existence, with its intimations of death in particles of dust. She remains immanent, even in Bernard's last days, yet she is also caught up in the flow. In formulating an earlier version of the plane of composition, Deleuze describes it as the 'intersection of all concrete forms'. As such, it enables a transaction and mixing and regrouping of different particles – dust, phantoms and presences.[17] The lady may be a focus of self-reflection (for Bernard) and of self-reflexion (for the process of literary production).

Yet the lady may also be an entity on the plane from which the stuff of concepts are made. Deleuze and Guattari propose the intervention of a 'conceptual persona'.[18] Not identical with the philosopher who produces the concepts, the conceptual persona manifests in the philosophical text as a third person, a *dramatis personae* in the fray of the conceptual field. She or he, and curiously these folk are gendered, the conceptual persona allows the agency of philosophical thought to make shifts while being allowed the privilege to act as an 'idiot', most particularly when the need to unthink thought should arise. For such a procedure hacks into the ice of the philosophical which has frozen into institutional practice. What is more, this unthinkingly thoughtful idiot not only defines a territory of concepts but simultaneously deterritorializes it.[19] One prominent example lies in the opening pages of *The Waves*, provisionally circumventing Bernard as he enters an undiscovered territory, at once enclosed, pristine and untouchable, yet waiting to be transversed for the first time. As I shall argue, the territory of the garden is one whose domain is maintained only to be collapsed then dissolved, reconstituted then washed into the unexpected along a trajectory of joy and suffering. This ebbs and flows, repeatedly. Whether the writing lady is its conceptual persona or aesthetic caretaker is one question to be tackled. Notwithstanding, she is a force to reckon with, residing at the edges into which the plane of immanence and composition interact.[20]

Here is the crux of the matter. The provisional and sometimes deceptive categories 'philosophy' and 'art' may find themselves deterritorialized and redrawn. In other words, what is interdisciplinary may turn out to be the 'inter-disci-planary' or even 'trans-disci-planary.' Yet by bringing Deleuze/ Guattari into a heuristic encounter with Woolf's novel, the writing lady may remain untouched by the philosophy raiding her figurative garden. In other words, there may be edges where she can remain immanently untouchable, even at the intersection between planes. Woolf's writing lady might operate as a moving force who questions and re-draws the very theories which traverse her. What may occur is a double process: between the Deleuze/ Guattari planes of Woolfian fiction a harmonious but dissonant interaction in which cultural analysis as a dominantly self-reflexive enterprise can be both questioned and expanded. As this occurs, certain practices of cultural analysis might themselves pass into undiscovered lands.

Between self-reflexion and becoming

The lady writing allows Bernard to figure himself through identification, or a specific mode of self-reflection. That is, as she writes so does he. In a fine examination of self-reflection as a questioning activity, Mieke Bal underlines the differences between 'self-reflection' and 'self-reflexion'.[21] Broadly speaking, argues Bal, self-reflection involves identifications between reader, characters and figures in the work, the artist, be this the painter or writer. However, there is a complicating factor in the apparently easy system of re-duplications which might arise between the different parties. Between them, details may arise which interfere with the projective processes.[22] In *The Waves*, Bernard is a man, the lady a woman; put simply, what is avoided is an easy and narcissistic fit between one character and the other, between focalizing subject and object. As Bal points out, a work's processes of self-reflection may produce a sense of fragmentation and dissimilarity between work, reader and writer. As a result, what can be enhanced is the task of 'self-reflexion,' that point when the artistic or critical work turns upon itself for the purposes of scrutiny. Thus, self-reflexion can liberate the self's capacity to recognise its differences from the Other, be this the text or the reader. To clarify this, it is important to emphasize that differences arise between theoretical and artistic objects. The two may recognise similarities in each other, but also surrender to their differences. Thus one can delve into its undiscovered facets through the other, doing so through an asymmetrical self-reflection which gives way to self-reflexion.[23] When this occurs between the lady and Bernard, when self-reflection gives way to this self-reflexion, so too does the plane of immanence begin to yield to that of composition through what is termed a 'becoming'.

⌈According to Deleuze and Guattari, subjects 'become' along specified sites, co-ordinates and vectors through which the concept of self-hood must fracture then re-form.⌋Rather than a 'person,' Deleuze and Guattari specify the 'thing, or substance', that which makes itself into the multiplicities of winds, faces, hails, rains, noises, loves, into which subjects would become.[24] Bernard asks 'how describe the world seen without a self?' answering in a jostling of colours, phantoms and phrases which, as he remarks, cannot be adequately represented by his textual compositions.[25] Nor, is the implication, can he or his friends be reduced to solid masses or points of specular identification fixed through the texture of a medium with all its protocols of signification. Everything is in flux. Persons pass into multiplicities.

So too can concepts. 'Specular identification' is a concept which has its ancestry in psychoanalysis. Deleuze and Guattari point out that 'concepts' can be defined as such because of their internal consistency, and the fact that they bear a signature.[26] Descartes' *cogito* is a prime example.[27] In her script, the lady can be defined as Bernard's specular identification, or that glimpse of self Lacan found in the mirror phase.[28] Made resonant with the Lacanian concept, Bernard idealises himself as female writer. Yet if we follow Lacan, the next move would be to interpret the lady as the one with whom Bernard will never coincide, except through the illusions of specularity. The mirror phase requires that narcissism be in place, that the human subject sell out to the *meconnaisance* that beyond the glass lies the self. For this chimera to hold, the subject must be caught by the gaze of the Other.

However, this does not occur between Bernard and the lady. In the garden or through his subsequent evocations of her image, the lady never meets his gaze. A lady rather than a gentleman writing ensures that Bernard's submersion in specular identification would have to cross the gender divide. Moreover, his frequent reference to the writing lady as opposed to the gentleman of that profession establishes a formal distance between the lady and Bernard. Self-reflection does not allow Bernard the narcissistic gratification of absorbing his counterpart. For him, the lady will remain incorrigible. In his final soliloquy, he almost laments that nothing will 'interfere with the fixity of that woman writing'.[29] She brings little consolation. Mieke Bal suggests that acts of self-portraiture which omit 'self-exultation', be this when a 'detail demonstrates a danger', do not produce self-reflectivity but rather self-reflexivity.[30]

To think self-reflexively means to question the very processes through which meanings are made. When Bernard confronts the lady through this mode of self-examination, that which he has idealised becomes the focus of challenge and disillusionment. The very act of phrase making, that which enables discourse to take place, is what Bernard questions to the core. Having spent a life dedicated to teasing out the right phrases, he admits that he would rather 'have done' without them. In fact, he claims to

> need a little language such as lovers use, words of one syllable such as children speak when they come into the room and find their mother sewing and pick up some scrap of bright wool, a feather, or a shred of chintz. I need a howl; a cry.[31]

Even though the passage evokes mothers, the lady does not act as a maternal figure. Indeed, throughout *The Waves*, no references are made to the parents of any narrator. The forces and affects of a 'howl; a cry' could suggest another connotation of to 'reflex', namely, to 'turn back'. Running from the garden, Bernard does not look back. Perhaps the escape might have roused the lady's attention. Then he might have met her gaze. Then goodness knows what cries and howls would come. The emotive forces which do emerge arrive in the wake of memories reflexively re-formed in the present. The past is understood as part of the present plane. The past as pure affect is thus prevented from shattering the text's waves and phrasal webs. Thus, the conceptual understanding of identity and the past as a psychoanalytic concept, passes into the forms of sensation and temporal percept before returning in a transformed state. In other words, the Lacanian concept of identity can be re-formed into a self-reflexive model at the poetic threshold of the lady's garden and atomic shiftings of the novel's aesthetic structure. The interaction between the Lacanian concept and the novel's poetic force takes interdisciplanarity one step further. For though, admittedly, the novel's aesthetic action unfixes the Lacanian concept, this in turn interacts with the plane of affects until this liquefies at the edges; its newly forming fluids mix with *The Waves* and the lady of the novel emerges as new, though provisionally crystallite from her medium. The shape and constitution of both planes

– the conceptual and the affective – transform each other not just through touching, but through mutual penetration, not just through the approach (interdisciplinarity) but through the planes pushing into each other, that is, through the intensity of inter-disciplanarity.

Self-reflexion, therefore, can act as a threshold between the plane of immanence and composition, enabling the mixing of forces I have just outlined above. But such mixings encounter necessary impediments, or lines of resistance between the planes. The lady writes behind two long windows through which Bernard will focalise but never cross. Neville remarks on another type of barrier, namely that between life and language. Life on Shaftesbury Avenue is 'poetry if we do not write it'.[32] Yet to 'prove' his point, Neville deploys rhythm and narrative launched between motifs from Shakespeare. In other words, Neville approaches his demonstration with poetic drama, making his case through the very procedure which unmakes it. Neville can persuade us that 'beyond' poetry is life, which is more 'poetic' when lived. Yet he admits that there this beyond will not be negotiated without poeisis.

Neville's conundrum, much like that of Bernard, finds its figure in the *mise en abyme* of the lady writing from the inner 'beyond' of her windows. She cannot be reached. She cannot be touched. She never looks out. She never stops writing. Haunted, Bernard persists in the practice of poetics as life and language. These two forces he confronts as irreducible yet irreconcilable. Despite his heroic optimism, the lady's windows cut a threshold between language functioning conceptually, on the one side, and affectively on the other.[33] As the novel dissects its own textuality, the lady as figure inscribes this particular cutting edge. She resides on the transparent blade where theory and art, epistemology and sensation bleed into each other.

The practice of self-reflexion enables *The Waves* to question the efficacy of language as that practice which redeems the subject from the inexorable quest to 'sum up', as Bernard puts it, and 'the meaning of life'.[34] Furthermore, the lady writing is difficult to pin down as a Lacanian concept. Instead, as a figure of meaning 'she' acts reflexively towards psychoanalysis, urging it to subvert the overly specific model of the mirror phase. For such specificity, refusing to yield to other models, suggests a form of theory narcissistically engaged with itself. Even though this particular caveat of psychoanalytic thought has a long history of being set into different angles of reflection through literary texts, the entrance of Deleuze and Guattari's concepts upon the psychoanalytic scene helps to re-form this territory. [35]

What Deleuze and Guattari challenge in psychoanalysis is precisely this hankering for specular identifications and mother and father imagos in general.[36] In the chapter 'Becoming Intense, Becoming Animal...', Deleuze and

Guattari make the case against Freud's 'A Child Is Being Beaten', arguing that the whodunnit of the beater and whether or not it is the 'father-figure' is irrelevant.[37] For Deleuze and Guattari, the celebrated case-history 'Wolf-Man' makes a petty, domestic Oedipal drama out of one man's drive to live fully, to engage in a 'becoming-animal', not to end up as a solitary beast but a multiplicity of charged, hairy creatures.[38] The implications of this approach are radical. Singular and personal pronouns can be unmasked as illusions. They deny what they conceal, namely the 'collective assemblages' which make human life rich and impossible to sum up through static formulations and received ideas. Individuality is a misnomer for a 'body' which is 'defined only by a longitude and a latitude' consisting of nothing but 'affects and local movements'.[39] These desires as mobilities do not signify the plane, but instead they form it. In *Anti-Oedipus: Capitalism and Schizophrenia*, Deleuze/Guattari emphasise that the 'order of desire' is

> the order of *production*; all production is at once, desiring production; all production is at once, desiring-production and social production. We therefore reproach psychoanalysis for having stifled this production, for having shunted it into *representation*.[40]

Psychoanalysis urges that we examine representational modes of desire. In contrast, Deleuze/Guattari specify desire as lines of movement through the plane of immanence. Such a domain is limitless. As the second epigraph to my article suggests, the plane allows the borderlines between qualities, elements, animals, sorcerers, women and men to function not as subjects but as movements, flows, phrases and atoms which break, fracture, and just keep on moving.[41]

It is through such leaking and mixing that the Deleuzian plane of immanence intervenes to test the lady behind panes which inspire self-reflexion. As a result, both the lady and the *mise en scene* boil in a melting pot of velocities and particles. Her self-reflexive role becomes corpuscular as she dissolves into the novel's *prima materia*. For Deleuze and Guattari, a becoming is not a simple case of taking the form of a wolf, vampire, woman, man, sorceress or crab. When becomings take place, the issue is not one of resemblance. No one is 'like' another entity. When Robert de Niro in TAXI DRIVER (Martin Scorsese, 1976) moves like a 'crab,' he vibrates with 'corpuscles' which resonate with atoms oscillating in a crab-like way.[42] Rather than imitating the thing, from it is absorbed a 'something' comprising crab fragments and forces. What is more, the territories of crab and wolf pass through each other. Hence, the plane is the site of ever changing domains and their thresholds.

It is no coincidence, then, that Deleuze and Guattari admire Woolf's poetic novel. They applaud the manner in which its territories transverse one another. Deleuze and Guattari flow with the novel's waves as 'vibrations, shifting borderlines inscribed on the plane of immanence as so many abstractions'.[43] The six narrators are more than 'characters'. Webs of thought and affect, dissolving and reforming each other, they fulfil the call that Woolf made in her diaries: 'Saturate every atom ... eliminate all deadness, weight, superfluity.'[44] The ideological markings of class and gender plunge into the 'particles emitted from the aggregate'.[45] Bernard's closing soliloquy does not absorb the 'faces' of the other five narrators. Quite differently, it gathers together starkly different qualities of glass, water, air, cold and heat, so that the domains from whence these elements come deterritorialize:

> The crystal, the globe of life as one calls it, far from being hard and cold to the touch, has walls of thinnest air. If I press them all will burst. Whatever sentence I extract whole and entire from this cauldron is only a string of six little fish that let themselves be caught while a million others leap and sizzle, making the cauldron bubble like boiling silver ... Faces recur, faces and faces – they press their beauty to the walls of my bubble –
>
> ...How impossible to order them rightly; to detach one separately, or give the effect of the whole – again like music.[46]

The syntax of the 'sentence' makes six fish which are the becoming-narrators of the novel. Six fish become millions, then recur as faces pushing at the contours of the globe. A multiple osmosis takes place between glass, air, silver and the liquid of the cauldron. The evidence that the lady is 'in' the cooking pot can be found in the reference to the crystal, the glass and their properties of being 'hard and cold to the touch.' Breaking through the plane of this passage are the lady's windows. The 'walls' of the bubble evoke the enclosure at Elvedon. Over it Bernard once climbed, making his first discovery of the unstoppable scribbler. The immanent lady on the plane mixes at the level of molecular intimacy with Bernard, his life, his friends, and the impossible task of ordering reality in its wave forms, its vibrations, its musicality.

The lady writing hinges on the edge of contradictory, critical approaches. Engaged with the psychoanalytic paradigm, she can be figured as a specular identification. Passing in and out of the Deleuze/Guattari plane of composition, pulsating with sensation, she supports a self-reflexive practice which then has consequences for her role as a conceptual persona, and one who can dramatise her psychoanalytic role in such a way that she can figure a concept of identification which is non-narcissistic and capable of flux. Pieces of her windows, walls and her *mise en scène* are deterritorialized. Miraculously, she becomes a series of entities, if not a multiplicity of 'becoming' ladies, thrust in a fray with six, narrating fish. Yet importantly, even after such atomic collisions with the philosophical methods of Deleuze and Guattari, she and her matrix reconsolidate. This happens in recurring motifs at the novel's critical junctures. Bernard's final soliloquy and swan song finds her rehoused in her garden, her task intact.[47]

Two remarks are necessary. Firstly, standing the test of durability, the lady is a trope of immanence. Even when processed through the plane, she returns to a form signifying that immanence. The fact that she can encompass two irreconcilable practices – the self-reflexive and the self-reflective – suggests that the two modes of reading can touch and intersect in such a way that compositional and conceptual practices exchange their particles. But this can only occur at the specific site of the lady writing. This 'site' loses its specularity through the plane of composition, only to regain it through an alternative paradigm. Secondly, two contrasting practices – the self-reflective and the self-reflexive – though hinged one upon another, capable of operating together, can do so only when the two operate by taking turns. As the lady loses her territorial domain but regains it, the compositional and the conceptual work together through alternation. In other words, when one is 'off', the other is 'on'. The off/on movement correlates with the alternating, undulating, fall and rise of the waves. Cultural analysis at the threshold of the two practices is not, in this respect, interdisci-planary. Self-reflexivity does not constitute its own plane. However, between the asymmetical vectors of self-reflective/self-reflexive practice, a threshold of cultural analysis has been found: it forms the moving line which waves are made of.

Our lady of immanence, our lady of composition

As I have already emphasised, *What is Philosophy?* clarifies that the plane of immanence is what belongs to philosophy proper. The becomings which fill it are not affects, but concepts. The plane of composition is the domain of aesthetic figures and the arts. The immanent plane which modulates neither affects nor percepts but concepts is designated as 'fragmentary wholes'. In other words, the plane which partakes of the infinite cannot itself be a concept.[48] Concepts are like 'multiple waves, rising and falling, but the plane of immanence is the single wave that rolls them up and unrolls them'.[49] Thus, in that Bernard crosses through and is traversed by the other narrators, the lady's text could act as a planar, single wave, rolling up the peaks and lows of the other characters.

Of course, the first objection to this line of analysis is that I have conflated the plane of immanence with that of composition. Despite this, the plane of immanence would allow the lady to be the single wave gathering up the percepts and affects of the novel's narrators. The most tricky problem is as-certaining whether the lady is better theorised as a conceptual persona or whether she is better cast an aesthetic figure belonging exclusively to the plane of composition.

According to Deleuze and Guattari, concepts are defined by their capac-ity to resonate with each other. They need not be mutually complementary.[50] Importantly, though, the concept comes into being when it posits a 'possible world' and a 'face', or when it inscribes the Other which inhabits or marks out that world. Finally, what is required is a language or speech.[51] Deleuze and Guattari test out their designation on case histories. I will do the same with Mieke Bal's concept of self-reflexivity, as theorised in her essay on cul-tural analysis,[52] engaging this theory with Woolf's writing lady. My aim will be to examine the type of role taken by the lady writing on the plane of im-manence.

The world in which Bal culls her concept is that of the museum. The type of self-reflexivity she articulates is formed through museal analysis, and ac-cording to Deleuze and Guattari's criteria for attributing concepts, the museal concept can be said to be signed by her. The 'face' is the 'second per-son', that viewing/reading Other who walks around the museum, con-structing the visual and verbal and the visual *as* verbal. Here is the third criterion of what comprises the Deleuzian/Guattarian concept of concept. Bal suggests that museal discourse is *apo-deictic*.[53] The Greek verb has a dou-ble meaning. It connotes the activities of explaining, exposing and affirm-ing, on the one hand, but opining on the other. This is where the second person comes into play. The first person who has set up an exhibition might appear invisible. The second person has been interpellated in the museum's speech act and is thus drawn into opining about the third person, or artistic object.[54] The invisibility of the first person is illusory and can be exposed by an awareness of the second and third person. Furthermore, the third person is not an inactive sign. As Bal suggests, it 'becomes an actor, or singer'.[55] Deleuze and Guattari insist that 'every concept shapes and reshapes the event in its own way'.[56] Bal's museal concept certainly reshapes conven-tional practices of the event, be this analysing a particular exhibition, where the event involves walk-around reading, or the event of exposition. Bal's concept of self-reflexivity does well on the plane of immanence.

Yet before turning back to the writing lady, an important question now arises. How would Bal's concept fare on the plane of composition? Just as concepts become on the plane of immanence, so too do percepts and affects on the plane of composition. Deleuze and Guattari deploy both planes to distinguish philosophy from art:

> Sensory becoming is the action by which something or someone is ceaselessly becom-
> ing-other (while continuing to be what they are), sunflower or Ahab, whereas con-
> ceptual becoming is in the action by which the common event eludes itself.
> Conceptual becoming is heterogeneity grasped in an absolute form.[57]

On the plane of immanence, concepts become, and there the event 'eludes' itself. The visitor to the museum might find her usual habits of assessing a painterly event elusive if armed with the self-reflexive concept. If Van Gogh's 'Sunflowers' were framed by paintings of eyes, the reading-viewer might be eluded by the framed event, considering herself the object being viewed by the sunflowers. If she experiences the event of the sunflowers on the plane of composition, then she would become into the percept of the colours and forms. These, though, do not form perceptions. Deleuze and Guattari emphasise the thought aspects of the plane of composition. Yet somehow, the becoming on this plane would require the viewer to become the sunflowers while still being herself.

Deleuze and Guattari claim that specific types of becoming occur sepa-
rately. In other words, the viewer would have to become the sunflowers without allowing conceptual events to interfere. But if blocks of affect oper-
ate through thought, how can these thoughts not intersect with the plane of immanence? In other words, Deleuze and Guattari cannot account for the event of the two planes leaking into each other. Having said this, the philos-
ophers are aware of a muddle which may solve part of the problem. There may be 'sensations of concepts' and 'concepts of sensations.'[58] The potential contained in this insight is not brought home until the final page of chapter seven. The three planes of science, art and philosophy are considered together. While insisting on their distinction, Deleuze and Guattari admit the following: 'A rich tissue of correspondences can be established between the planes.'[59] The use of the epistemic 'can be' is revealing. The choice of whether the connections are to be made is left to the second person. Thus, the tissue-making between planes becomes a matter less of an interdisciplinary, but more of an interdisciplanary choice.

It is now that the lady writing and her *mise en scène* can be approached in the wake of museal discourse. Following Bernard over the wall at Elvedon reveals the following:

> The lady sits between two long windows writing. The gardeners sweep the lawn
> with giant brooms. We are the first to come here. We are the discoverers of an un-
> known land.

Bernard the narrator and 'first person' claims himself as a second person, closely associated with a 'we' who is more than himself and his companion Susan. There is a deictic pointing to 'we' the readers. No one has visited this museum. The lady is the third person. Or perhaps she is not. Maybe she is the first person writing the image-text, the children being the third person, the signs that act, and we, the second persons. Yet if the *apo-deictic* countours are shunted around yet again, perhaps the lady is not writing, but underlining what she is reading, that is, Bernard's text or the reader/viewer's interpretation. Then the lady would pass into second personhood. The reader/ viewer would then be the third person, and Bernard the first. The geometries can turn endlessly. They can leave the reader eluded. Furthermore, the garden forms a possible world, the lady the 'face', and the focalized narrative the language. Indeed, what is provided is a concept, signed by Woolf. Thus, the lady, her writing/reading and her *mise en scène* have their place as concept on the plane of immanence.

The lady also has a place on the plane of composition, interweaving with the streams of affects which Bernard focalises. When he declares that 'it is a mistake, this extreme precision, this orderly and military progress', he refers to the habits of daily life.[60] But the lady too has her habits. The gardeners who sweep are systematic, practical and military. Years later, the garden and its inhabitants undergo a becoming. It is one which releases affects from under the force of precision. Once this has been exposed, there is

> always deep below it, even when we arrive punctually at the appointed time with our white waistcoats and polite formalities, a rushing stream of broken dreams, nursery rhymes, street cries, half-finished sentences and sights – elm trees, willow trees, gardeners sweeping, women writing – that rise and sink even as we hand a lady down to dinner.[61]

The writing lady as a concept has given way to the plane of composition. The passage comprises the sorcerers' drawings: the affects of memory, verbal vestiges, the percepts of 'half-finished sentences and sights', trees, gardeners, and women writing. Our lady of concepts has become into thoughtful blocks of sensation.

As the plane of immanence (concepts), passes into the plane of composition (percepts and affects), the lady writes in the domain of fixity and flux, renewed every time it is discovered. The lady writing and the concept within which she is embedded pass into composition, and back again. Each time the shift occurs, her domain needs to discovered for the first time. Even her fixities are constantly moving. In my reading she has been our lady of the threshold, forming and dissolving the mobile tissues. She has passed between both conceptual persona and aesthetic figure. These two roles, exchanging their substances with one another, can join together two planes which, for the most part, are irreconcilable. As a threshold, she is a site which does not eradicate the self-reflexive but allows it the conduits to pass into other events. The lady marks out the potential for one plane, say that of concepts, to set off a series of becomings which, once they begin to accrue and manifest, form another plane, that of affects; and the net result is not just a pressing, but an interlacing between the planes. Deleuze and Guattari do imply this conceptual and aesthetic possibility of profound interconnection, but they do not endeavour to develop it as yet another concept. Thus, the lady writing her possible world is the figure at not just the cutting, but the interpenetrating edge between art and philosophy. She offers to cultural analysis the opportunity to bring together not only self-reflexive approaches, which are interdisciplinary, but what I have coined as the concept of inter-planary approaches, that is, the intimate and mutually transformational interaction between artistic and theoretical practice, one which can push the horizons of critical practices to an even further threshold. Between philosophy and aesthetic production, theory and art, the lady offers this new edge at a yet untried domain for the future: cultural analysis as art.[62]

3   Sharing Technologies

Thought and Movement in Dancing

Maaike Bleeker

Movement in thought: three 'duets'

In *What is Philosophy?* Gilles Deleuze and Félix Guattari differentiate between philosophy, art and science, seeing each as a means of confronting chaos. They define philosophy, art and science as three modes of thinking that proceed in different ways: art thinks through affects and percepts; science thinks through knowledge; philosophy thinks through concepts. The three modes of thinking take place on different 'planes', and they utilize different 'elements'. The three planes along with their elements are irreducible, while the brain is the junction (not the unity) of these three planes:

> plane of immanence of philosophy, plane of composition of art, plane of reference or coordination of science; form of concept, force of sensation, function of knowledge; concepts and conceptual personae, sensations and aesthetic figures, figures and partial observers.[1]

The differences between the three planes are a recurring motive throughout their book. Deleuze and Guattari observe, however, that there are also cases in which art, science and philosophy cannot be understood as distinct in relation to the chaos the brain plunges into. After having stressed the differences between the planes throughout their book, they conclude that what seems to be more important now are the problems of *inference* between the planes that meet in the brain:

> In this submersion it seems that there is extracted from chaos the shadow of the 'people to come' in the form that art, but also philosophy and science, summon forth: mass-people, world-people, brain-people, chaos-people – nonthinking thought that lodges in the three, like Klee's nonconceptual concept or Kandinsky's internal silence. It is there that concepts, sensations, and functions become undecidable, at the same time as philosophy, art and science become indiscernible, as if they shared the same shadow that extends itself across their different nature and constantly accompanies them.[2]

In this article, I will explore this area where concepts, sensations and functions become undecidable, and I will do so through three 'duets'. Firstly, these comprise the 'duet' performed by the philosophers Deleuze and Guattari themselves, the duet that finds its expression in four books, the last of which is *What is Philosophy?* The second duet is a literal duet between dancers Itzik Galili and Jennifer Hanna in WHEN YOU SEE GOD TELL HIM (1995), a choreography by Itzik Galili.[3] The third is by George Lakoff and Mark Johnson, two cognitive scientists who claim metaphor to be a fundamental principle of human understanding that operates in all forms of our symbolic activity and, therefore, is indispensable for the practice of science and all other forms of knowledge.[4] Each of these duets deals with thinking and movement, be it in radically different ways. Deleuze and Guattari present a model of thinking as movement mediated through conceptual personae (on the plane of immanence of philosophy), aesthetic figures (on the plane of composition of art) and partial observers (on the plane of reference of science). In WHEN YOU SEE GOD TELL HIM, it is the bodies of dancers moving through a composition in time and space that mediate in thought processes. Lakoff and Johnson, starting from the point of view of the scientific observer, present metaphor as a model to trace the movement of thought.

'Thought is movement' itself could be called such a metaphor underlying the way we conceptualize thinking. In their books, Lakoff and Johnson reveal the metaphorical structure underlying different modes of thinking, and they explain its functioning in terms of inference. Furthermore, they conceive of thinking as proceeding through inferences of conceptual metaphors with bodily sensations and present a theoretical model of thinking as proceeding through the body.

It is not my intention to erase the differences between these three duets and paste them together into one coherent model or story. Instead, I will use the inferences between them as a starting point to explore the relation between thinking and movement. I propose the duet as a model of the movement of thought as the product of shared technologies in which the three planes as defined by Deleuze and Guattari function as partners in interaction rather than as separate entities or distinct categories.

Friends of wisdom

'Philosophy, art and science are not the mental objects of an objectified brain but the three aspects under which the brain becomes subject, Thought brain. They are the three planes, the rafts on which the brain plunges into chaos', write Deleuze and Guattari in *What is Philosophy?*.[5] They describe the brain as a 'state of survey without distance' and subjectivity as its effect.[6] At the same time that the brain becomes subject, the concept becomes object as created, as event or creation itself. Within this movement subjectivity appears as an 'eject'. On each plane these 'ejects' appear in a different way: on the plane of immanence of philosophy as the subject of creation of concepts ('I conceive'), on the plane of composition of art as the subject of feeling ('I feel'), on the plane of reference or coordination of science as the subject of knowledge ('I know'). Deleuze and Guattari conceive of these 'ejects' in terms of speech act theory. In everyday life speech acts refer back to psychosocial types who actually attest to a third person: 'I decree mobilization as President of the Republic', 'I speak to you as father', and so on. In the same way the philosophical shifter is a speech act in the third person where it is always the conceptual persona who says 'I'. This leads them to a reformulation of speech acts, pointing attention to the way speech acts produce positions and the way these positions mediate in the movement of thoughts: 'In philosophical enunciations, we do not do something by saying it but produce movement by thinking it through the intermediary of a conceptual persona.'[7]

Conceptual personae are complicated entities that lead a hazy existence somewhere in between the concept and the pre-conceptual plane.[8] They are part of the implicit presuppositions forming images of thought. Sometimes they appear with a proper name, like Socrates, who is the principal conceptual persona of Platonism. Yet the conceptual persona is not to be confused with a character. Conceptual personae and characters only nominally coincide and do not have the same role. The character of a dialogue sets out concepts. Conceptual personae, on the other hand, carry out the movements that describe the author's plane of immanence, and they play a part in the very creation of the author's concepts. They can have all kinds of features. In *What is Philosophy?* Deleuze and Guattari distinguish between pathic features (the idiot, the maniac), relational features (the friend), dynamic features (the diver, the dancer), juridical features (the claimant, the judge, the plaintiff) and existential features (the bourgeois). These features of conceptual personae do have relationships with the epoch or historical milieu in which they appear that only psychosocial types enable us to asses. Through these features, conceptual personae and psychosocial types refer to each other and combine, yet without ever merging. Unlike a psycho-social type, the 'I conceive' of philosophy is not an empirical circumstance but instead has to be understood as a presence that is intrinsic to thought, a condition of possibility of thought itself, a living category, a transcendentally lived reality. Conceptual personae appear as the agents of philosophical enunciation. Deleuze and Guattari speak of 'intercessors, crystals or *seeds of thought'*.[9]

Deleuze and Guattari propose to understand the 'I' of philosophy in terms of friendship. They refer to the Greek origin of philo-sophy, the friends of wisdom, those who seek wisdom but do not formally possess it. Friendship appears as a precondition of thought; it is part of a relational model of thinking as taking place between friends. Friendship, as Deleuze explains, is not based on having the same ideas. Rather, it is the condition of having something to say to one another as a result of which thought starts to move. Friendship carries something of a mystery within itself, and this mystery Deleuze understands in terms of being possessed by a certain 'charme'. This 'charme' is the spark that lightens up between the friends, turning them into friends.[10] In *What is Philosophy?* Deleuze and Guattari present friendship as the most outstanding feature of the conceptual personae. Yet, here, they define the relationship between the friends of wisdom in slightly different terms. The friends as they appear as mediators of movement in philosophical thought are claimant and rivals striving for the same object. Friendship here designates a form of competent intimacy that involves love as well. Love, not for one another, but for the goal both friends are striving towards. Friendship, therefore, involves competitive distrust of the rival as much as an amorous striving towards the object of desire. Striving and rivalry are part and parcel of philosophy as a continuous state of becoming, of thought as movement. It is, according to Deleuze and Guattari, in this sense that philosophy has to be understood as something Greek that coincides with the contribution of cities: the formation of societies of friends or equals, but also the promotion of relationships of rivalry between and within them, the contest between claimants in every sphere, in love, the games, tribunals, judiciaries, politics, and even in thought. Friendship designates 'the rivalry of free men and a generalized athleticism'.[11]

What is Philosophy? is the fourth and last book Deleuze and Guattari wrote together. It is 'the last achievement of a form of experimental "authorship" that has few precedents in philosophy', as translators Hugh Tomlinson and Graham Burchell put it.[12] They quote Deleuze's own account of this extraordinary collaboration, saying: 'We don't work, together, we work between the two. ... We don't work, we negotiate. We were never in the same rhythm, we were always out of step.'[13] Deleuze describes his philosophical 'duet' with Guattari in terms of movement, in terms of dance, but only in order to disqualify them as dance partners. Instead of moving along in the same rhythm naturally, every step had to be won through negotiation. His intellectual partnership with Guattari thus seems to conform to their model of philosophical thinking as the product of competent intimacy between claimant and rival, a friendship that has to be won time and again over competitive distrust.

In the books that are the expression of this 'duet', however, it is hard to distinguish between the two competitors. The differences in rhythm have dissolved into a collective movement presented under the double name that has become their trade mark. Their books thus express a collectivity that is absent from their conception of conceptual personae and their role in thought as movement. At this point, I think, the model of the duet as performed on stage presents a useful alternative to Deleuze and Guattari's generalized athleticism. Both the duet and athleticism point attention to the inferences between mental and physical movements, between movement as performed in thinking and movement as performed by bodies in space. In either case, this movement is acted out in different ways, staged on different 'planes'. Unlike the movement of dancing bodies on stage, the movement of conceptual personae does not refer to spatiotemporal coordinates that define the successive positions of a moving object and the fixed reference points in relation to which these positions vary. Nevertheless, I will argue, comparing the movements performed in philosophical thought with the duet as performed in the theatre may be helpful to further explore the character of the movement performed in thinking either of them. What kind of movement are we talking about? And who is moved by it in what way?

Argument as dance

Imagine a culture where an argument is viewed as a dance, the participants are seen as performers, and the goal is to perform in a balanced and aesthetically pleasing way. In such a culture, people would view arguments differently, experience them differently, carry them out differently, and talk about them differently.[14]

With this invitation in the first chapter of *Metaphors We Live By*, Lakoff and Johnson demonstrate the extent to which our conception of argument and argumentation is structured by the conceptual metaphor 'argument is war'. According to them, all of our most basic abstract concepts are defined by clusters of often inconsistent metaphors, most of which operate unconsciously and automatically in our understanding. What we think of a 'literal' language is actually based on underlying conceptual metaphors that define its conceptual structure and the inferences we draw from that structure. Thinking proceeds in and through these metaphorical structures that are reflected in our everyday language by a wide variety of expressions. These expressions not only structure the way we talk about – for example –

argument: many of the things we actually do in arguing are structured by them. We do not just talk about arguments in terms of war, the metaphor is in our very concept of argument. It is a metaphor we live by.

Lakoff and Johnson do not feel comfortable with the idea of argument as dance. They think it would change the concept of arguing to such an extent that they would find it hard to talk of arguing at all:

> In such a culture, people would view arguments differently, carry them out differently, and talk about them differently. But we would probably not view them as arguing at all: they would simply be doing something different. It would seem strange even to call what they are doing 'arguing'. Perhaps the most neutral way of describing this difference between their culture and ours would be to say that we have a discourse form structured in terms of battle and they have one structured in terms of dance.[15]

As Lakoff and Johnson point out, in a culture where argument is viewed as dance, people would not dance arguments but rather the discourse through which they would proceed while arguing would be organized along different metaphorical structures. Discourse implies a set of semiotic and epistemological habits that enable and prescribe ways of communicating and thinking. It entails epistemological attitudes and also includes unexamined assumptions about meaning and about the world. Discourse, therefore, both enables and prescribes ways of thinking. In our discourse structured in terms of battle, the conceptual metaphor 'argument is war' both enables us to understand argument in terms of war *and* prescribes us to do so.

For Lakoff and Johnson discourse understood in terms of dance can only exist as a hypothesis. Probably, this is informed not only by their concept of argument but also by their concept of dance: dance as a performance with the goal to move in a balanced and aesthetically pleasing way. As such, dance appears as the 'other' of argument, just as art and the aesthetic function as the repressed other of the cognitive in their later undertaking *Philosophy in the Flesh: The Embodied Mind and Its Challenge to Western Thought*. In this book they call into question central themes of the Western philosophical tradition from the point of view of cognitive science. They take the cognitive in the richest possible sense to describe any mental operations and structures that are involved in language, meaning, perception, conceptual systems and reason. Since according to them our conceptual systems and our reason arise from our bodies, they also use the term cognitive for our sensory-motor system that contributes to our abilities to conceptualize and reason. They present metaphor as a structural model for the inferences that take place between sensory-motor operations and subjective experiences.

Surprisingly, however, in their rereading of the philosophical tradition from the classical Greeks through Kantian morality to modern analytical philosophy, they leave out aesthetics, the terrain of making meaning through the body from way back, altogether.

Deleuze and Guattari do conceive of art as a mode of thinking. A mode of thinking, however, that moves in a fundamentally different way than science or philosophy. In art, thinking proceeds through sensations, and these sensations are formed by contracting that which composes it. This contraction is not an action but a pure passion, 'a contemplation that preserves the before in the after'.[16] Art, therefore, takes place on a plane that is altogether different from mechanisms, dynamisms and finalities. Art takes place on the plane of composition, and this plane is populated not with conceptual personae but with aesthetic figures. The difference between conceptual personae and aesthetic figures is that the former are the power of concepts and the latter are the power of affects and percepts. In art, it is not the conceptual persona that says 'I conceive' but the aesthetic figure that says 'I feel'. Through the speech acts 'I feel' and 'I conceive', philosophy is defined in terms of thinking as conceiving while art is defined in terms of thinking as feeling. Or, to put it in Lakoff and Johnson's terms, in Deleuze and Guattari's account art is lived by the conceptual metaphor 'thinking is feeling' and philosophy is lived by the conceptual metaphor 'thinking is conceiving'.

Notwithstanding the fact that art and philosophy constitute fundamentally different modes of thinking taking place on different planes and utilizing different elements, it is according to Deleuze and Guattari possible to think on one plane through the elements of the other. They understand these moments that cross-overs take place not in terms of new types of objects but in terms of new modes of thinking:

> The plane of composition of art and the plane of immanence of philosophy can slip into each other to the degree that parts of one may be occupied by entities of the other. In fact, in each case the plane and that which occupies it are like two relatively distinct and heterogeneous parts. A thinker may therefore decisively modify what thinking means, draw up a new image of thought, and institute a new plane of immanence. But, instead of creating new concepts that occupy it, populate it with other instances, with other poetic, novelistic, or even pictorial or musical entities.[17]

I take WHEN YOU SEE GOD TELL HIM to be an example of such a moment where aesthetic figures, the dancers, are carried onto the plane of immanence; where the plane of composition of art and the plane of immanence of philosophy start to slip into one another, and thought begins to move in new ways. In a parallel movement also the plane of reference and our knowledge about thinking itself start to shift.

Dancing on the plane of immanence

WHEN YOU SEE GOD TELL HIM is set to an extraordinary musical score. This score consists of part of a lecture given by I.F. Stone at the Ford Hall Forum and is set to music by Scott Johnson. Stone's text invokes us to stop turning argument into war, to stop settling arguments with war and to find a different way of dealing with arguments other than having recourse to war.[18] The dancers propose this through their bodily movements in the dance, while the text proposes to do so through a reconceptualization of human relationships and interactions in terms of family: 'We have to begin to think of ourselves as a family' in order to overcome 'those reversions to barbarity and tribalism, who are still hung up in ancient, anachronistic hatreds like we see in Ulster, like we see in Israel, Palestine. That we can see in many parts of the world'. Stone argues for a change in the way we live and deal with one another, and argues that what is needed is that we begin to understand ourselves as part of one family. Once we start conceiving of ourselves as part of one family -once we begin to understand the relationships between different peoples in terms of family relationships – we will start living these relationships in a different way as well. This possibility of the active and intentional use of metaphor to change the way we perceive the world remains implicit in Lakoff and Johnson's theory. Lakoff and Johnson's interest is in the unintended consequences of metaphorical structures underlying our everyday experiences. Nevertheless, their theoretical framework also allows for a conscious use of metaphor as a 'searchlight' to lighten up aspects of conceptual fields that had remained invisible before, or even as a means of transforming behavior. We can take a metaphor to reorganize a familiar conceptual field in ways that were unimaginable before the use of this metaphor. Following Lakoff and Johnson's claims, this would not only change the way we talk about this conceptual field, but change the very nature of what is performed in thinking it. This is what happens in WHEN YOU SEE GOD TELL HIM.

When the light goes up we see a man and a woman living in separate worlds, each in a small beam of light on either side of the stage. He is examining a flower, she is running around in circles. After a little while, she breaks away from 'her' beam of light and runs toward him, turns her back towards him and bends over in what I take to be a sexual invitation. He does not accept the invitation and turns away. She repeats the gesture three times until he literally jumps over her, picks her up on his shoulders and puts her in a different place. He starts doing some frantic dance on his own with his face turned away from her towards the backside of the stage. Nevertheless, her gesture did catch his eye, or so it seems, for after a little while he turns around and imitates her pose in what appears to be an attempt at conciliation. It is the start of an interaction in which they get acquainted with one another.

According to Deleuze, it is the perception of a certain 'charme' that marks the moment of the appearance of friendship. The perception of this 'charme' is the spark that sets into motion the movement of thought between the two friends of wisdom.[19] The opening sequence of WHEN YOU SEE GOD TELL HIM shows such a moment that marks the beginning of movement of thought. Thought that in this case literally proceeds through movement. The appearance of friendship here is shown in terms of 'becoming family'; this is a process in which the dancers become familiar with each other, and thereby inspired by the invitation to intimacy implied by the text. The first line of Stone's text reads: 'You know, I have so little here to say this evening, but there's so many things that have been said over and over again, that need to be said again and again.' In the performance it is the perception of this certain 'charme' that turns the situation of 'having so little to say here this evening' into a situation of collaborative movement where things 'need to be said again and again'.

The interaction between the two partners in movement on stage does not always proceed harmoniously. When Stone's voice observes that 'it is too small a planet – it grows smaller and smaller all the time', the dancers are physically in each other's way, one blocking the movement of the other. There are moments when they fall back in what the text calls 'ancient, conditioned reflexes and psychoses of mankind and his homocidal tendencies'. Nevertheless, as they become more familiar with one another they seem to 'begin to enjoy the differences in the human family like we enjoy the differences in a garden of flowers. There is very little time to muster this broader vision,' Stone says, but 'Either we live together, or we die together' and the dancers drop 'dead' on the floor. Stone ends his text with the question: 'Is it necessary – is it necessary?' During these final words, the dancers walk away together towards a single beam of light, facing a common goal. She picks the petals from the flower he had been holding at the beginning of the piece, as if to indicate that what the future will be remains the question but nevertheless they will face it together.

The choreography thus presents a reading of Stone's text in terms of a relationship between a man and a woman, translating the big words of the text into embodied situations we live by. Yet to understand the performance solely as a visualization of the argument made in the text would mean to ignore the many moments in which the dance presents a critique of, or an elaboration on, the text. The performance does much more than translating the argument made in the text into dance movement. It offers a reconceptualization of the argument made in the text – as well as a reconceptualization of what it means to argue – in terms of dance, and through this reconceptualization the performance breaks open the argument as made in the text, undermines it, and expands on it. In doing so, the performance can be read as an example of what Deleuze and Guattari describe as art's ambiguous relationship with chaos. Art, science and philosophy cast planes over the chaos, but at the same time they want us to tear open the firmament and plunge into chaos: 'It is as if *the struggle against chaos* does not take place without an affinity with the enemy, because another struggle develops and takes on more importance – the struggle *against opinion*, which claims to protect us from chaos itself.'[20] Deleuze and Guattari refer to D.H. Lawrence's *Chaos in Poetry* in which he explains what produces poetry:

> People are constantly putting up an umbrella that shelters them and on the underside of which they draw a firmament and write their conventions and opinions. But poets, artists, make a slit in the umbrella, they tear open the firmament itself, to let in a bit of free and windy chaos and to frame in a sudden light a vision that appears through the rent.[21]

Art can do so through creating structures that at the same time break up existing ones. This way, art can illuminate the chaos for a moment and render it sensory. Understood this way, art can perform what Stone's text argues for, namely to break through the opinions and presuppositions we hide ourselves behind and open up to a new vision. What the performance also demonstrates is that these new visions imply new points of view as well, as a result of which thought starts to move in new ways.

Tearing open the firmament

In Johnson's musical score, Stone's text is literally cut up and the pieces framed in new ways. His first sentence – 'You know, I have so little here to say this evening, but there's so many things that have been said over and over again that need to be said again and again' – is cut into pieces, some of which are repeated and transformed into a rhythmic structure. This is further elaborated on in the performance, in which the movement of the dancers presents a visual equivalent to this process of cutting up. When the text says 'There are so many things that have been said', the man and the woman face the audience together. During 'that need to be said' they raise their arms. During 'that have been said' they move backwards, and during 'That need to be said' they raise their arms again while moving forward. The movement pattern enhances the rhythmical structure of the text and the musical score, while at the same time the meaning of the text and the movements performed start to interfere with one another. Through these inferences of the argument performed through the text with the movements performed on stage, attention gets directed in new ways as a result of which Stone's first sentence turns into an ambiguous statement. The composition of the performance opens up the possibility of different readings of the same text at the same time offering different points of view from which this text could be read. Central to this ambiguity is the question of agency: who is the agent mediating in the movement of thought performed in and through the duet?

Stone's first sentence 'You know, I have so little here to say this evening, but there's so many things that have been said over and over again that need to be said again and again.' now can be read as a self-reflexive remark about the theatre situation. Its position at the beginning of the performance turns his statement into a commentary on performing the same performance night after night. At the same time it remains an integral part of Stone's ongoing argument as made in the text. A third layer is added when the text begins to interfere with the individual performance of the dancers. Right after the man has jumped over the woman, the text begins with 'You know'. After a minute or so, this 'you know' is repeated, then followed by 'I have so little to say here this evening'. At that moment the man walks away from the woman towards the back of the stage as if 'having so little to say this evening' is the reason why he walks away from her. While the text says 'but there are so many things that have been said', he starts doing his frantic dance, moving from left to right and back again, again and again, following the rhythm of the textmontage: 'that have been said, so many so many things, that have been said, that need to be said, over and over again, over and over again, over and over again, over and over again'. Thoughts that might be playing through his head and find a physical expression in his movement, showing him hovering between the fact that these things 'have been said' already so many times, yet that they 'need to be said again and again'. His movement comes to a stop as he bends over in imitation of the woman's pose, marking the beginning of yet another old story starting all over again, the old story of love.

With their performance, the dancers present partnership as an alternative to the rivalry, violence and tribalism the text speaks of. The piece shows development of this partnership represented through the interaction of the dancers on stage. Like it is the case with the friends of wisdom, this relationship does involve love. Love, in this case, not only for the object both friends are striving towards, but for one another as well. The development of the interaction between the partners in movement does include moments of rivalry; moments they interact as claimant and rival striving for the same goal, driven by desire for the same object. However, what the duet also demonstrates is that in order for these personae of claimant and rival to appear partnership is required, partnership that is needed to execute the movements that produces the two figures on stage as claimant and rival. As dancers they are the condition of possibility of movement itself, like the conceptual personae are the condition of possibility of philosophical thought. They are a presence intrinsic to movement. Yet it is only within these movements that they appear as claimant and rival, positions that appear as points of view implied by the sequence of movements.

It is within this collaborative effort and as a result of shared technologies that claimant and rival appear as points of view. Furthermore, in the duet the two figures on stage appear as claimant and rival at the very same moment that they also appear as partners in the execution of the movement. It depends on how one wants to look at it. The performance demonstrates that points of view as constituted in and by the movements performed at the same time imply a point of view from where they can be perceived as such. In Deleuze and Guattari's account, these two points of view threaten to get conflated as a result of which the 'I conceive' of philosophy can appear as the immaculate conception of and by a lonely thought athlete surfing the plane of immanence. Here, the duet presents an alternative model in which both aspects of friendship – sharing and rivalry – are shown in relation to one another and as different moments mediating in the movement of thought between the two partners and between both partners and the audience.

At one point in the performance, there is a minute-long sequence in which the only text is a continuous repetition of 'again and again'. During this minute the dancers execute an intricate series of highly energetic movements in which they constantly change place yet remain very close to one another. They move around each other figured in entanglement, engaged in an ongoing series of collisions, which release force of action and reaction. This repetitive movement in the rhythm of 'again and again' not only presents a visual equivalent to the words 'again and again'. More than that, it brings to mind the reason why 'these things' that have been said 'over and over again' still have to be said again and again: the many actions and reactions that collide time and again 'that we can see in many parts of the world'. This way, the contraction on the plane of composition not only shows the before in the after, but also, the other way round, the performance foreshadows what in the linear argument of the text still has to come.

Furthermore, the impact of the collisions and the force of action and reaction on these bodies makes one *feel* how tiresome this situation is more than the words of the text. The performance mediates in a movement of thought in which thinking as conceiving and thinking as feeling begin to interfere. In the theatrical duet these inferences take place through the involvement of a third party, namely the audience. It is the point of view of the observer that marks the 'place' where thinking as feeling and thinking as conceiving start to interfere as concepts, sensations and functions become undecidable. The argument as represented in dance movement is made sensible again as the words begin to interfere with the energy as evoked by the execution of the movements. When finally the man lays his head to rest on the woman's shoulder, with a movement of longing, stretching towards her, this feels like relief. This gesture not only puts an end to a representation of human conflicts as we can see them in many parts of the world. It also resolves the emotional impact caused by the collision of these two bodies here and now on stage involved in a conflict that addresses the viewer on an emotional and sensational level, and these emotions and sensations get mixed up with the conception of the story represented. Here Lakoff and Johnson's theory of primary metaphor offers a model to understand the 'I' as it emerges from the confrontation with the composed chaos that is the performance.

The feeling of meaning

'If the mental objects of philosophy, art and science (that is to say, vital ideas) have a place, it will be in the deepest of the synaptic fissures, in the hiatuses, intervals, and meantimes of a non-objectifiable brain, in a place where to go in search for them will be to create,' write Deleuze and Guattari.[22] According to them it is the brain that thinks and not man – the latter being only a 'cerebral crystallization'.[23] Lakoff and Johnson search for this moment where subjectivity appears as a cerebral crystallization. They look for it within the deepest synaptic fissures, and they come up with a model in which subjectivity is the effect of complex processes of inferences taking place between reasoning, conceptual thinking, perception and motor control.

According to Lakoff and Johnson, the basic level of reasoning is categorization. Every living being categorizes. Even the amoeba categorizes the things it encounters into food and non-food, what it moves toward or moves away from. The amoeba cannot choose whether to categorize; it just does. The same is true at every level of the animal world. Animals categorize food, predators, possible mates, members of their own species, and so on. How animals categorize depends upon their sensing apparatus and their ability to move themselves and to manipulate objects. Categorization is therefore a consequence of embodiment. We categorize as we do because we have the brains and bodies we have and because we interact in the world in the way we do. Think of the properties of the human body that contribute to the peculiarities of our conceptual system. We have eyes and ears, arms and legs, that work in certain, very definite ways and not in others. We have a visual system with topographic maps and orientation-sensitive cells that provides structure for our ability to conceptualize spatial relations. Our abilities to move in the ways we do and to track the motion of other things give motion a major role in our conceptual system. The fact that we have muscles and use them to apply force in certain ways leads to the structure of our system of causal concepts. It is not just that our bodies and brains determine that we categorize; they also determine what kinds of categories we will have and what their structure will be.

What we call concepts are therefore in fact neural structures that allow us to characterize our categories mentally and reason about them. This makes them embodied in the trivial sense that any mental construct is realized neurally. But there is a deeper and more important sense in which our concepts are embodied. What makes concepts concepts is their inferential capacity, their capacity to be bound together in ways that yield inferences, and these inferences are, according to Lakoff and Johnson, best understood in terms of metaphor. In *Metaphors We Live By*, they proposed metaphor as a model to describe the co-activation of two conceptual fields. In *Philosophy in the Flesh* they turn to metaphor again, but this time as a model to describe the co-activation of sensory-motor operations and subjective experiences. The conflation of these two is the simultaneous activation of their respective neural networks. In this model, the shared technology of the neural network provides a bodily basis for the inferences between thinking as feeling and thinking as conceiving.

Like Deleuze and Guattari, Lakoff and Johnson conceive of subjectivity as the effect of the brain, emerging as an effect of the survey of chaos. Like Deleuze and Guattari, they conceive of a sense of self as the product of the movement performed in thinking, as a by-product of reasoning. With their theory of primary metaphor, however, they present an alternative account of the movement performed in thinking, an account that undercuts the con-ception–perception distinction. They oppose the view that conceptual structure, although it must have a neural realization in the brain which hap-pens to reside in a body, is not crucially shaped or given any significant in-ferential content by the body. While perception has always been accepted as bodily in nature, just as movement is, conception – the formation and use of concepts – has traditionally been seen as purely mental and wholly separate from and independent of our abilities to perceive and to move. According to Lakoff and Johnson, however, much conceptual inference is sensory-motor inference. This is a radical claim from the perspective of faculty psychology, a philosophy that posits a radical separation between the rational abilities and the sensory-motor system. However, Lakoff and Johnson argue, it is not at all radical from the point of view of the brain, which is the joint locus of reason, perception and movement.

Deleuze and Guattari too point out that it is the same brain that says 'I conceive' and 'I feel'. It is the same brain, yet subjectivity emerges in a differ-ent way on different planes. In their account, the 'I' functions as a shifter be-tween the planes, between different instances of subjectivity appearing in different ways on different planes. These differences they understand in terms of different movements performed in thinking as proceeding through concepts (on the plane of philosophy), affects (on the plane of art) or knowl-edge (on the plane of science). Lakoff and Johnson come up with a model to understand the relationships between these instances as well as between the planes in terms of metaphorical structures connecting these instances in a non-unitary way. Furthermore, with their notion of primary metaphor, they present an account for the ways in which bodies are involved in the process of constitution and reconstitution of points of view both of the 'I conceive' of philosophy and the 'I feel' of art, making both of them sensory again. Their model suggests that the distinction between the planes itself might be part of the firmament we draw on the underside of the umbrella that shelters us, i.e. a historically and culturally determined formation that is the product of the discourse through which we proceed while thinking and as a result of which the particular 'I's of philosophy, art and science emerge. Finally, their model suggests that these 'I's could begin to emerge differently once we start conceiving of the movement performed in thinking through different conceptual metaphors. At this point, a fragment of WHEN YOU SEE GOD TELL HIM can serve as a searchlight highlighting aspects of the 'I conceive' that re-main in the dark in Deleuze and Guattari's concept of the conceptual per-sona as mediator in the movement of thought.

Sharing technologies

In a philosophical enunciation, movement is produced through thinking, and this happens through the intermediary of a conceptual persona. In a philosophical enunciation, it is the conceptual persona who says 'I conceive' and thus constitutes a point of view according to which planes of immanence are distinguished from one another or brought together. These points of view, the seeds of thought as Deleuze and Guattari call them, then have to be reconstituted by a reader. In the duet, it is the two dance partners who produce an ongoing flow of movement – a constant state of becoming – in which movements of one partner are generated by movements of the other. The partners need one another, depend on one another, for it is their interaction that produces the movement just as they are produced as partners in and by it. This ongoing flow of movement constitutes points of view as well, points of view that can be reconstituted by an audience as a result of which the audience can move along with what is presented. However, how a particular audience will reconstitute these points of view and move along with what is presented will not only depend on the points of view as constituted by the performance, but also on conventions, knowledge and experience that they share with it, or not. The duet as performed in the theatre thus points attention to the seed of thought and the 'I conceive' of the conceptual persona as two different, yet intimately related moments. In the duet, their relationship is visualized in a way that renders the 'I conceive' of philosophy sensory again in a way that stirs the imagination.

When Stone speaks of how the world gets smaller in terms of travel time, and how we are becoming one family through sharing each other's technology, culture, poetry and philosophy, the dancers begin performing a collective movement that at first looks like a representation of a vehicle, a wheelbarrow perhaps. They act out progress and reduction of travel time through the portrayal of a shared technology in bodily movement. Yet when the voice of Stone says 'we share each other's technology', this visually becomes represented in an entirely different way. At this moment, the woman repeats the sexual invitation the performance started with, and this time the man responds without hesitation. Sharing technologies is not shown through the embodiment of technology, but by means of a reference to a much more bodily or physical technique. They show thinking to be an embodied activity that, like Deleuze and Guattari's athleticism, may include moments of rivalry. In the end, however, it is the collaborative effort that makes this productive, both in terms of pleasure and of offspring. Furthermore, they demonstrate that the constitution of the 'I conceive' represented by the conceptual personae – Deleuze and Guattari's seed of thought – is not sufficient for conception to take place. The duet thus argues for a more radical notion of thinking in terms of partnership, in which the two friends are involved as desiring bodies sharing technologies of various kinds. It is this body that allows for the metaphorical jump between different planes, and as a result thought can begin to move in new ways. It is this body that is the site of the desire as involved in the conception of both philosophical ideas and children.[24]

4   The Metaphor Made Flesh

A Philosophy of the Body Disguised as Biological Horror Film

Eva Jørholt

To make a metaphor in which you compare imagination to disease is to illuminate some aspect of human imagination that perhaps has not been seen or perceived that way before. I think that imagination and creativity are completely natural and also, under certain circumstances, quite dangerous. The fact that they're dangerous doesn't mean that they are not necessary and should not be repressed.[1]

Generic 'wrapping' of philosophy

The Canadian filmmaker David Cronenberg is usually classified as a director of horror films. His *aficionados* have nicknamed him for example 'The Baron of Blood' or 'The King of Schlock Horror'. Others – including Cronenberg himself – have referred to his films as biological horror and even as venereal horror. The horror genre is usually considered inferior to art cinema, but to Cronenberg there is no difference; both aim at disturbing any false sense of security and at questioning our most basic notions of stability:

> I think of horror films as art, as films of confrontation. Films that make you confront aspects of your own life that are different [sic] to face. Just because you're making a horror film doesn't mean you can't make an artful film. Tell me the difference between someone's favourite horror film and someone else's favourite art film. There really isn't any. Emotions, imagery, intellect, your own sense of self.[2]

And with reference to his own work, Cronenberg specifies that the phrase 'biological horror'- often attached to his work – really refers to the fact that his films are very body-conscious. They are very conscious of physical existence as a living organism, rather than other horror films or science fiction films which are very technologically oriented or concerned with the supernatural, and in that sense are very disembodied.[3] But if Cronenberg's films

do belong to the horror genre at all – he prefers to think of them as constitut-
ing their own genre or subgenre – they certainly are horror films with a difference. What is important, however, is not so much the generic
classification of his work as the fact that from his very first commercially
distributed feature film, SHIVERS (1975), to his latest, EXISTENZ (1999), he
has continuously been discussing highly philosophical issues which have
been fleshed out in extremely visceral imagery. It would, therefore, be quite
appropriate to conceive of his films as philosophical essays disguised as
horror films. According to the director himself, the horror genre has in fact
functioned as a kind of protective shelter for him, a generical wrapping
which has allowed him to make the kind of philosophical films he wanted to
make.

Cronenberg's films focus on the human body which, according to the
filmmaker himself, is 'the first fact of human existence':

> For me, everything comes out of that: philosophy, religion. Everything comes out of
> the body. And the fact of human mortality, it's natural that my films would focus on
> that. Even from my first writings as a young kid, death and dealing with it was very
> strongly present. So it seemed natural to deal with the body and what happens to the
> body and then for me to invent some fantasmagoria, to create metaphors for the body
> and the things that happen to the body, and have part of the body brought outside of
> the body so we could look at it and so on. And that brings me into the genre of body
> horror.[4]

The physicality – and mortality – of our bodily existence as human beings
who sense, think, and act in this world is at the centre of Cronenberg's philosophical film-making. In a certain sense, he might, consequently, be labeled
an existentialist filmmaker – a notion which seems to be supported by the
very title of his latest film, EXISTENZ. Cronenberg often refers to his films as
existentialist dramas, just as he sees the concept of 'auto-invention' as a key
to his work. The philosophy of existentialism may, therefore, seem an obvious path when approaching Cronenberg's work. There are, however, significant differences between the existentialism(s) of, say, Sartre, Camus, and
Merleau-Ponty on the one hand and that of Cronenberg on the other.

Whereas existentialist philosophy regards the human body as a stable
basis for our being in the world, Cronenberg tends to see the body as something ephemeral, as material flesh which may be sculpted in numerous
ways. In Cronenberg's work – as in many recent horror films – the flesh is
flesh in a very literal and materialist sense. His films are full of cancerous
flesh, mutant flesh, bloody flesh, psychic flesh, erotic flesh, etc. That is, pure
matter engaged in constant transformations. At the same time, however, the
flesh in Cronenberg's films is also a metaphor for thought, an embodied

philosophy. Cronenberg admits to being obsessed with finding a way of expressing metaphors cinematographically. In contradistinction to the writer who expresses himself and his ideas through the abstraction of the written word, the filmmaker, according to Cronenberg, is under the obligation to make the word flesh:

> I have an obsessiveness with metaphor. Metaphor is really the bedrock of all prose, of all literature. How do you do metaphor in film? For me, I realize that it's through the creation of monstrous imagery. If you talk about pure ideas... Pure ideas are invisible. You don't have anything to photograph. This is of course something you can do in literature, and you cannot do it on screen in the same way. I have to make the word be flesh and then photograph the flesh because I can't photograph the word. [...] I'm looking for the metaphor, and that leads me to a certain monstrousness. [5]

Consequently, the omnipresence of the flesh in Cronenberg's work should also be seen as an attempt to bring philosophy back to the body, to the flesh from where it originated. The flesh functions as pure matter and as pure thought! A kind of physicality of thought which is aptly expressed through the sensuous medium of cinema:

> The cinema feels very tactile to me. It's not just visual. It's sensual in many many ways. I have even wondered about the sensuality of thought. How physical is thought? On the surface, it seems to be very disembodied. But I don't think it is disembodied. You can't have thought without a body, which is why I always return to the idea of the body being the primary fact of human existence. When I think of imagery and metaphor and thought, it seems a very sensual thing to me. It needs to be embodied physically somehow. [6]

With these views on the flesh and the physicality of thought, Cronenberg seems much closer to the philosophy of Gilles Deleuze and Félix Guattari than to ('classical') existentialism. Deleuze's and Guattari's so-called Bodies without Organs (BwO's), as expressed in *A Thousand Plateaus*, appear to constitute a particularly illuminating and thought-provoking conceptual framework for entering the seemingly bizarre world of David Cronenberg. In the following pages, I shall develop this line of thought further. And I will end with an attempt at an experimental reading of eXistenZ along the lines of the Deleuzian/Guattarian BwO. A reading which does not pretend to present a correct image or even an interpretation of what the film is actually about, but a reading which will attempt to illuminate the film through two seemingly related philosophies of the body in order to, perhaps, produce new thoughts. In this sense, my experimental fusion of Deleuze and Cronenberg fully adopts Deleuze's paraphrase of Godard's famous dictum: 'Pas une idée juste, juste une idée'.

Bodies without Organs – the field of immanence of desire

> No organ is constant as regards either function or position,... sex organs sprout any-
> where,... rectums open, defecate and close,... the entire organism changes color and
> consistency in split-second adjustments.[7]

Human beings could swap sexual organs, or do without sexual organs per
se, for procreation. We are free to develop different kinds of organs that
would give pleasure, and that have nothing to do with sex. The distinction
between male and female would diminish, and perhaps we would become
less polarized and more integrated creatures. I'm not talking about trans-
sexual operations. I'm talking about the possibility that human beings
would be able to physically mutate at will, even if it took five years to complete that mutation. Sheer force of will would allow you to change your
physical self.[8]

> Why not walk on your head, sing with your sinuses, see through your skin, breathe
> with your belly: the simple Thing, the Entity, the full Body, the stationary Voyage, An-
> orexia, cutaneous Vision, Yoga, Krishna, Love, Experimentation.[9]

William Burroughs is in many ways a connecting link between David
Cronenberg and Gilles Deleuze. Both are highly inspired by his writings,
and by *Naked Lunch* in particular. Against all odds, unfilmable as it may
seem, Cronenberg made this bizarre novel into a (very Cronenbergian) film
in 1991, and Deleuze and Guattari use it as a cornerstone in their presentation of the BwO. In fact, the Burroughsian phantasmagoria of *Naked Lunch*
seems to incarnate the very essence of the BwO. Deleuze never mentions
Cronenberg in his two volumes on cinema. Given his predilection for rather
elitist art cinema, it is possible that he was not familiar with Cronenberg's
films; but it is equally possible that he simply did not like them. I do not
know, and neither do I know whether Cronenberg is familiar with the philosophy of Deleuze.

In his film books, Deleuze does not speak of BwOs either. And as I shall
try to argue below, it is exactly through the concept of the BwO that the philosophy of Gilles Deleuze may be said to converge most strongly with that
of David Cronenberg. In his second volume on cinema, *The Time-Image*,
Deleuze does, however, present a couple of ideas on the human body which
may be of interest even with regard to the films of Cronenberg. He opens
chapter 8 with the words '"Give me a body then": this is the formula of
philosophical reversal' – and proceeds to elucidate the relationship between
'Cinema, body and brain, thought', as this chapter is entitled.[10] To Deleuze,
as well as to Cronenberg, the flesh is thought, just as the mind is flesh, for

contrary to the Cartesian mind-body split, Deleuzian materialism sees the brain simply as part of the body. And the body forces us to think the unthinkable, he claims, stressing that 'it is through the body (and no longer through the intermediary of the body) that cinema forms its alliance with the spirit, with thought.'[11] This statement is fully in line with Cronenberg's view of cinema as a materialization of thought. According to Deleuze – and Cronenberg would hardly disagree – the flesh is our only possible object of belief. After the death of God, it no longer makes sense to believe in another world:

> What is certain is that believing is no longer believing in another world, or in a transformed world. It is only, it is simply believing in the body. It is giving discourse to the body, and, for this purpose, reaching the body before discourses, before words, before things are named [...] Our belief can have no object but 'the flesh' [...] We must believe in the body, but as in the germ of life, the seed which splits open the paving-stones, which has been preserved and lives on in the holy shroud or the mummy's bandages, and which bears witness to life, in this world as it is.[12]

Throughout his books on cinema, Deleuze carefully distinguishes his own philosophy from that of the phenomenologists, for whereas phenomenology privileges man over matter, Deleuzian materialism simply places man in matter. Following Bergson, Deleuze conceives matter as being made up of innumerable 'images' which keep 'bumping' into one another in a dynamic flow of action and reaction. In this context, the only particularity about man, the only thing that distinguishes him from the rest of matter, is the delay, the slight hesitation between action and reaction which Deleuze refers to as a 'centre of indetermination'. Although he does stress the fleshy materiality of the body, I would claim that the body to which Deleuze is referring in the first part of the above quoted passage does not differ essentially from the phenomenological body. Both are distinctly human bodies, and both are the foundation or the source of thought. This is also (one of) the way(s) in which the human body is depicted in Cronenberg's existentialist dramas.

But there is more. For when Deleuze speaks of the body as 'the seed which splits open the paving-stones' etc., we sense that maybe this body is not quite human after all. Rather, this 'revolutionary' body reaches out of Deleuze's film books and into *A Thousand Plateaus* and the Deleuzian/ Guattarian concept of the BwO. How are we to understand this Body without Organs? Is it made of flesh, blood and bone, or is it merely a metaphor? In a peculiar sense it seems to be lodged in an 'interzone' between the two: both physical body and metaphor and yet not quite either of them. Just as

Cronenberg's bodies are at the same time metaphorical and highly material, and actually neither.

Deleuze and Guattari only inform us that the BwO is not a concept but a practice. The BwO is something that you must seek to attain without the prospect of ever reaching it: 'You never reach the Body without Organs, you can't reach it, you are forever attaining it, it is a limit', they say.[13] As I shall try to make clear a little later, the same may be argued for the existential bodily experimentations performed in Cronenberg's films. So, on the one hand, the BwO is profoundly physical, albeit in a highly spiritual way, because of the intimate bonds between mind and body. And on the other hand, it is (probably) to be seen as a metaphor for (almost) any kind of deterritorializing practice – whether this practice be directly linked to the body or not. Deleuze and Guattari mention several examples of (near) BwOs: the hypochondriac body, the paranoid body, the schizo body, the drugged body, and the masochist body. They pay special attention to the masochist who reaches out for the BwO by suffering physical pain and to the drug addict whose driving force is an overwhelming physical cold. But also, e.g., Taoist Yin-Yang lovemaking (in which the man does not ejaculate) qualifies as a BwO.

What is of importance here, however, is neither the pain nor the cold or the lack of ejaculation, for these are only means of reaching a higher goal. What matters are the free-flowing intensities produced by these various conditions, for the BwO is nothing but pure intensity, desire in and for itself, a desire which will lose its intensity if fulfilled. According to Deleuze and Guattari, the 'BwO is the *field of immanence* of desire, the *plane of consistency* specific to desire (with desire defined as a process of production without reference to any exterior agency, whether it be a lack that hollows it out or a pleasure that fills it)'.[14]

To reach for the Body without Organs does not mean to empty your carcass of its organs. If you have your liver, your kidneys, your spleen, etcetera removed, the most probable result is that you will die. But there is nothing suicidal about the BwO, and it 'is not at all the opposite of the organs. The organs are not its enemies. The enemy is the organism. The BwO is opposed not to the organs but to that organization of the organs called the organism.'[15]

'The enemy is the organism' – to readers familiar with Deleuze's work, this rings familiar and recalls the 'rhizome'. Like the rhizome, the BwO would thus appear to be a figurative term, a metaphor for a dynamic, non-hierarchical network. When Deleuze and Guattari claim that 'the organs distribute themselves on the BwO, but they distribute themselves independently of the form of the organism; forms become contingent, organs are no longer anything more than intensities that are produced, flows, thresholds, and gradients',[16] the organism under attack is not so much the physical human body as it is a way of organizing things to function within an organism in a wider, more general sense – society at large, the army, a business corporation, the educational system, a university thesis edited according to 'the rules', etc.

In both the physical and the metaphorical sense, the BwO is best defined as pure, still unformed, energetic matter characterized by an unbridled flow of intensities. In this sense, Deleuze and Guattari compare the BwO to an egg, a sort of highly productive zero degree intensity:

> The BwO causes intensities to pass; it produces and distributes them in a *spatium* that is itself intensive, lacking extension. It is not space, nor is it in space; it is matter that occupies space to a given degree – to the degree corresponding to the intensities produced. It is nonstratified, unformed, intense matter, the matrix of intensity, intensity = 0; but there is nothing negative about that zero, there are no negative or opposite intensities. Matter equals energy. Production of the real as an intensive magnitude starting at zero.[17]

Just as the egg eventually develops into, e.g., a bird or a human being, the BwO stratifies or coagulates to become an organism. The BwO constantly 'swings between two poles, the surfaces of stratification into which it is recoiled, on which it submits to the judgment, and the plane of consistency in which it unfurls and opens to experimentation'.[18] If stratification is the ever present flip side to the BwO's dynamic, free-flowing desire, its three worst menaces are the organism, signification, and subjectification.

Deleuze and Guattari are well aware of the dangers of experimenting with the BwO, and they emphasize that if you free the BwO 'with too violent an action, if you blow apart the strata without taking precautions, then instead of drawing the plane you will be killed, plunged into a black hole, or even dragged toward catastrophe'.[19] When reaching out for the uninhibited desire of the BwO, you should never OD, not by drugs or physical punishment from your 'master', nor by a total dissolution of signification or self. Death is not the ultimate BwO, as death will inevitably put a final stop to the flow of intensities:

> Dismantling the organism has never meant killing yourself, but rather opening the body to connections that presuppose an entire assemblage, circuits, conjunctions, levels and thresholds, passages and distributions of intensity, and territories and deterritorializations measured with the craft of a surveyor.[20]

But there are other dangers as well, for if the BwO is always desire, not all BwO's are desirable. Proliferating cancer and unbridled inflation, for instance, also qualify as BwOs. Deleuze and Guattari state that each instant, each second, a cell becomes cancerous, mad, proliferates and loses its con-figuration, takes over everything; the organism must resubmit it to its rule or restratify it, not only for its own survival, but also to make possible an es-cape from the organism, the fabrication of the 'other' BwO on the plane of consistency.[21]

These cancerous BwOs, however, are 'totalitarian and fascist BwO's, ter-rifying caricatures of the plane of consistency'. It would seem that with this talk of fascist BwO's, we have moved away from the physical level and re-turned to metaphor; but Deleuze and Guattari carefully emphasize that the fascist BwO 'is a problem not of ideology but of pure matter, a phenomenon of physical, biological, psychic, social, or cosmic matter'.[22] According to Deleuze and Guattari, the tumour, whether social or physical, is a BwO which can just as well be seen as a stratification that has run wild. Hence, it should not be confused with the true and positive BwO.

Disintegrating organisms and productive diseases of many kinds are prominent in David Cronenberg's work in which the flesh is seen both as a promise of freedom and as a threat to the organism, in the metaphorical as well as in the physical sense. Cronenberg's characters are constantly seeking to invent themselves and their own lives through a transgression of the boundaries of their bodily organisms. These attempts at physical and/or mental auto-invention usually end in disaster, however, either because the characters' physical organisms are destroyed, resulting in death, or because the experiments are taken over by more or less fascist corporations. But still, Cronenberg's films do offer glimpses of a utopian freedom, towards which his characters are constantly reaching out, without ever attaining it.

The independence of the flesh – philosophical body sculptures

I don't think that the flesh is necessarily treacherous, evil, bad. It is cantankerous, and it is independent. The idea of independence is the key. It really is like colonialism. The colonies suddenly decide that they can and should exist with their own personality and should detach from the control of the mother country. At first the colony is per-ceived as being treacherous. It's a betrayal. Ultimately, it can be seen as the separation of a partner that could be very valuable as an equal rather than as something you dominate. I think that the flesh in my films is like that.[23]

In Cronenberg's films, heads explode and turn their insides out (SCANNERS, 1980); women give birth to abnormal children through huge external cancer tumours (THE BROOD, 1979); anuses talk (NAKED LUNCH, 1991); people develop new sexual organs all over their bodies (RABID, 1976; VIDEODROME, 1982; and CRASH, 1996); human flesh fuses with insects and/or machines (THE FLY, 1986; and VIDEODROME); the mind is made flesh (SCANNERS, THE BROOD, VIDEODROME), etc. And in almost all his films, the flesh is highly erotic and shivering with uninhibited sexual desire.

Although accused by Robin Wood, among others, of being a reactionary director[24] – because of the way women and their sexuality are presented in his early films – Cronenberg is, in fact, far more radical or even transgressive than Wood can even begin to imagine. The point is, though, that Cronenberg is not progressive in the traditional, ideological sense. But when it comes to the way we usually think of, e.g., morals, gender, and sex, his films are highly deterritorializing in a very Deleuzian sense.

Cronenberg is convinced that 'we have never been natural creatures in a natural setting. We create our own reality, not only in the field of technology. Humans have never accepted the world as it is, they always try and change it'.[25] Biomedical gender has become 'irrelevant', for in Cronenberg's opinion, the body is not necessarily given once and for all but should rather be seen as pure matter open to any kind of transformations. Translated into Deleuzian terms, Cronenberg's philosophy would read something like this: although the body may have stratified into a certain kind of organism with a certain gender, etcetera, this stratifiction should never be conceived of as absolute for in some way or other, the body can always be resculpted or reinvented.

In Cronenberg's films, the human body is sometimes transformed as the result of experiments conducted by more or less mad scientists and sometimes because the characters themselves want to change their physical appearances or because they are hungry for new kinds of stimulation, new forms of erotic desire. Within its low budget horror format, even Cronenberg's first feature film, SHIVERS, explored this theme in a highly visceral manner. Here, the inhabitants of a modern apartment complex are taken over by strange parasites which have been created by a scientist who saw them as 'a combination of an aphrodisiac and a venereal disease that will hopefully turn the world into one beautiful, mindless orgy'.

Once the parasites have found a human body to host them, they do exactly what the professor wanted them to do, i.e. they relieve their hosts of all rational constraints and turn them into mindless, instinct-driven animals hungry for love. In Deleuzian terms, you might say that the characters as well as the apartment complex undergo a radical transformation from stratified organisms to (different levels of) uncontrolled Bodies without Organs. The inhabitants are brought to a state of pure matter tingling with highly erotic shivers, and in a Deleuzian sense, SHIVERS may therefore be seen as a most radical film about the revolutionary power of sheer sexual intensity.

In VIDEODROME, Cronenberg went even further as he launched the so-called 'New Flesh'. At first sight, the 'new flesh' would appear to be the result of a fusion of a man and a machine. In the film, the organic flesh of the protagonist's hand meshes with the metal of a gun to become a 'handgun' in the most literal sense imaginable, and at the same time he becomes a sort of human VCR as he develops an abdominal slit into which you may insert video cassettes which shape his perception of reality and make him act accordingly. On this level, the new flesh expresses that the human body as we know it may be transformed through an act of will:

> The most accessible version of the 'New Flesh' in VIDEODROME would be that you can actually change what it means to be a human being in a physical way. We have certainly changed in a psychological way since the beginning of mankind. In fact, we have changed in a physical way as well. We are physically different from our forefathers, partly because of what we take into our bodies, and partly because of things like glasses and surgery. But there is a further step that could happen, which would be that you could grow another arm, that you could actually physically change the way you look – mutate.[26]

According to the protagonist himself, he is 'the video word made flesh', and I would argue that in fact the new flesh should be understood rather as a complete fusion of mind and body rather than as a fusion of man and machine. The physical alterations were just the first phase. The protagonist must kill himself, leave his body as organism in order to 'enter the next phase and become the new flesh'.

On a perhaps less accessible level, another version of the new flesh would therefore be that it is a Deleuzian BwO. It is pure desire, desire which is never fulfilled and keeps craving still stronger stimulation, whether sexual, tactile, or emotional. The new flesh is a Body without Organs in the truest sense of the term. Not an organism, not organs, not even a body, only energy floating through space, producing 'the real as an intensive magnitude starting at zero'. The new flesh is the egg before it stratifies into an organism, a subject, a signification. It is the true field of immanence of desire.

At the same time, however, Cronenberg follows the phenomenologists in seeing the human body as the basis for our perception of reality. But convinced as he is of the intimate bond between mind and matter, this leads him to the rather radical conclusion that reality is as evanescent and subject to change as are our bodies:

> One of our touchstones for reality is our bodies. And yet they too are by definition ephemeral. So to whatever degree we center our reality – and our understanding of

reality – in our bodies, we are surrendering that sense of reality to our bodies' ephemerality. [...] By affecting the body – whether it's with TV, drugs (invented or otherwise) – you alter your reality. Maybe that's an advance. I don't know if I'm evolving at all in terms of the struggle.[27]

Throughout his work, Cronenberg has firmly rejected the Cartesian mind/body split. Not only are visions and other mental phenomena made flesh on the plot level of several of his films (e.g. THE BROOD, SCANNERS, and VIDEODROME), but thematically his films are also constantly oscillating between the body as physical matter and as metaphor. It is, of course, quite normal to see society at large from an individual's point of view. But if you conceive of society as a large organism and return this metaphor to the body from which it was taken, while at the same time maintaining the individual's point of view, strange things happen; by this reversal of the metaphor, one is suddenly invited to adopt an individual cell's point of view:

> I often wonder what it's like to be a cell in a body. Just one cell in the skin or in a brain or an eye. What is the experience of that cell? It has an independent existence, and yet it seems to be part of something that doesn't depend on it, and that has an existence quite separate from it. When you think of colonies of ants or bees, they aren't physically joined the way an organism made up of cells is, but it's the same thing. They have an independent existence, an independent history. But they are part of a whole that is composed of them. That's what fascinates me about institutions. An institution is really like an organism, a multi-celled animal in which the people are the cells. The very word 'corporation' means body. [28]

Within the organism – whether this organism be the human body, an institution, or society at large – each cell has its own place and function. This well-ordered state of affairs may, of course, be highly satisfactory – not least when the organisms in question are our own physical bodies. Although we are used to regarding independence as a positive concept, it is the last thing we would want for our liver, our heart, our spleen, our kidneys, or the cells of our bodily tissue in general.

If, however, as a thought experiment, we take another round-trip from our own physical bodies to the organism as a metaphor and back, the result is as disturbing as it is illuminating. For not only does the usually very positive concept of independence become highly relative, but the same goes for the equally very negative concept of disease. When related to, e.g., society as an organism, disease may be welcomed as an equally dynamic and subversive process in which the individual 'cells' or 'organs' achieve independence. But just as Deleuze and Guattari stress that the BwO is a limit which can (or should) never be reached, Cronenberg warns us that the complete independence of the organs may be equal to chaos and destruction:

People are fascinated by little sections of the CIA, which might be said to develop independent of the body of the CIA. It's like a tumor or a liver or a spleen that decides it
will have its own independent existence. It still needs to share the common blood that
flows through all the organs, but the spleen wants to go off and do a few things. It'll
come back. It has to. But it wants to have its own adventures. That's fascinating to me.
I don't think of it as a threat. It's only a real threat if all your organs decide to go off in
different directions. At a certain point the chaos equals destruction. But at the same
time the potential for adventure and creative difference is exciting.[29]

Disease is a recurrent feature of Cronenberg's films – on a physical as well as
on a metaphorical level. In this context, the unsolved enigmas of cancer and
Aids become interesting in so far as they represent some of the last avatars
of uncontrollable flesh which have not (yet) been completely mapped out
by medical science. In Deleuzian/Guattarian terms, they are bad BwOs but
BwOs nevertheless, and as such they constitute a challenge not only to science but to rational thinking in general. For like Deleuze/Guattari and Burroughs, Cronenberg would like to 'exterminate rational thought', to quote
the protagonist of his NAKED LUNCH, or to cut down the trees which most of
us have planted in our heads, according to Deleuze and Guattari.

Cronenberg sees rational thought as related to fascism, whereas uninhibited imagination is as subversive to totalitarian regimes/organisms as is
physical disease to the human body. But he goes even further, for if a human
being is actually nothing but pure matter, flesh, then we have no privilege
over cancer cells or a virus, for the only difference becomes the way in which
matter is organized. But, as we have seen, matter can be reshaped and reor-
ganized. So why not compare ourselves to cells in a cancerous tissue? Why
not try to see the world from the point of view of a virus?

Cancer and viruses may be understood as highly energetic BwOs, as uncontrolled intensity embedded in the flesh itself. A virus makes its way
through the organism which hosts it, it functions as pure desire. From the
organism's point of view, a virus is of course not very desirable, but if you
try to look at the viral activity from the point of view of the virus – as
Cronenberg does – the perspective changes radically. In fact, the characters
of his films may in many ways be seen as uncontrollable cancer cells or as viral agents threatening to overthrow the established order by their unbridled
sexual desire. Dystopia or Utopia? It is only a question of perspective:

To understand physical process on earth requires a revision of the theory that we're
all God's creatures – all that Victorian sentiment. It should certainly be extended to
encompass disease, virus and bacteria. Why not? A virus is only doing its job. It's trying to live its life. The fact that it's destroying you by doing so is not its fault. It's about
trying to understand interrelationships among organisms, even those we perceive as

disease. To understand it from the disease's point of view, it's just a matter of life. It has nothing to do with disease. I think most diseases would be very shocked to be considered diseases at all. It's a very negative connotation. For them, it's very positive when they take over your body and destroy you. It's a triumph. It's all part of trying to reverse the normal understanding of what goes on physically, psychologically and biologically to us. [...] Naturally, we're interested in human diseases. But how does the disease perceive us? That illuminates what we are.[30]

We are used to thinking of disease in highly negative terms and do not, when we are ill, experience it as energy. On the contrary. If we do make any connection at all between disease and sexual energy, we will presumably see the two as precluding one another, and I suppose that when Cronenberg is suffering from influenza, even he does not conceive of the flu as 'the love of two alien kinds of creatures for each other', as one of the characters puts it in SHIVERS. But as a truly deterritorializing thought experiment, it is indeed highly interesting to look upon disease as energetic matter and as pure intensity.

Although Deleuze and Guattari tend to view disease in somewhat more negative terms, it would seem that Cronenberg's concept of both imagination and disease is in fact equivalent to the Deleuzian/Guattarian figure of the rhizome which they themselves compare to weeds, to virus and to cancer. Like the rhizome – and the BwO – imagination and disease destratify established order through their uncontrollable activity, tracing truly deterritorializing 'lines of flight' in an ever ongoing dynamic process which can be stopped only if the disease is cured and the organic order of the organism restored, or if the 'molecular' imagination ossifies into 'molar' subjects and/or fixed significations.

Does this mean that we should start to think of disease as something healthy? Well, not necessarily, for it all depends on whether you look at it from a metaphorical or a physical point of view. But in Cronenberg's films, the metaphor is made flesh in such a way that we are never quite sure which is which. In fact, it may be precisely this constant oscillation between a metaphorical and a physical understanding of the body which makes his films as unsettling as they are illuminating.

The name of the game is eXistenZ: What's mind? No matter. What's matter? Never mind.

People are programmed to accept so little but the possibilities are so great. eXistenZ is not just a game, it's an entirely new game system.[31]

In Chris Rodley's interview book *Cronenberg on Cronenberg*, the director states that 'part of my cinematic voyage has been to try and discover the connection between the physical and the spiritual: what we are physically; what is the essence of physical life and existence. It's still a conundrum that drives me mad: the old Bertrand Russell riddle. What's mind? No matter. What's matter? Never mind.'[32] In eXistenZ this philosophical riddle has been materialized in a Chinese box-structured story about people engaging in a kind of virtual reality game which ends up by completely blurring the frontiers between their own imagination, the design of the game, and what is usually known as reality. In a very literal sense, the film is a playful staging of mind as matter and matter as mind. And, at the same time, it is once more the metaphor made flesh, eXistenZ being a highly sensual metaphor for the director's ideas about the human condition with its potentials as well as its restraints.

eXistenZ is the name of a new interactive game invented by the renowned game designer Allegra Geller (Jennifer Jason Leigh) for Antenna Research, a large corporation with a lot of money behind it. eXistenZ may recall some already existing computer games but as the film plays in an undefined future where bio-technology has replaced technological hardware and software as we know them today, there are significant differences. In order to play the game, the players must 'connect' but not through modems nor through hi-tech gloves or glasses. An umbilical cord made of flesh-like organic material is plugged into their so-called 'bioport', a hole in each player's back through which the game is connected directly to his or her spinal cord. At a test launch of this new game, Allegra Geller is shot down by a fanatic. She does not die from her wounds, however, but escapes with a young guy, Ted Pikul (Jude Law), who has never before been plugged into these kinds of games. But she invites him to have a bio-port installed, and together they enter the world of eXistenZ where they allow repressed sides of themselves to come out. At the same time, they are pursued both by other corporations hungry to take over Allegra's new game from Antenna Research, and by realist fanatics who are strongly opposed to the spreading of imaginary worlds like that of eXistenZ.

In the film's complex structure, Allegra and Pikul enter still further into new games. Inside the world of eXistenZ, they venture on another game, in relation to which eXistenZ becomes a kind of reality level. And at the end of the film, it is disclosed that what we have taken to be a reality world outside the game eXistenZ is in fact just the imaginary world of another game, transCendenZ, which transcends or encompasses all the other games. When the transCendenZ players quit the game, however, the film leaves us in doubt as to whether the players have in fact returned to the reality of the film or just to another game level. The boundaries between reality and the imaginary game worlds are completely blurred. Within the framework of the film, it has become impossible to tell truth from lie, actuality from virtuality, reality from imagination. In a very Deleuzian sense, the virtual and the actual have become indistinguishable. And we are invited to ask ourselves whether this kaleidoscopic questioning of reality stops at the end of the film. Can we be sure that we who are watching the film are not also just players in some game which we take for reality?

The idea for EXISTENZ, for which Cronenberg wrote the screenplay himself, originated in 1995 when he was interviewing Salman Rushdie for the Canadian magazine *Shift*. Among many other things, the filmmaker and the writer discussed whether computer games could be a new art form. Whereas Cronenberg expressed great enthusiasm for games like MYST, Rushdie was considerably more reserved, arguing that a computer game could not qualify as true art, just as a game designer could not qualify as an artist. Rushdie's argument was that a game will always to a large extent follow a preordained path that does not leave as much space for the player's completion as does, for instance, a novel *vis-à-vis* its readers.

Some interesting remnants of this conversation have survived in the finished film. When Allegra Geller is pursued by realist fundamentalists who actually issue a *fatwa* against her, the link to Rushdie is, of course, quite obvious. But, at the same time, the Allegra Geller character is probably also modelled after Cronenberg himself. As a director of horror films, he – like the game designer – has never been considered a true artist, and the film sets out to prove that computer games may qualify as art for much the same reasons as Cronenberg considers horror films to be a true art form. To Cronenberg, the game players are existentialists who are being pursued by realists for their deforming of reality:

> I'm talking about the existentialists, i.e. the game players, versus the realists. The deforming of reality is a criticism that has been levelled against all art, even religious icons, which has to do with Man being made in God's image, so you can't make images of either. Art is a scary thing to a lot of people because it shakes your understanding of reality, or shapes it in ways that are socially unacceptable. As a card-carrying existentialist I think all reality is virtual. It's all invented. It's collaborative, so you need friends to help you create a reality. But it's not about what's real and what isn't.[33]

In this existentialist sense, the game players are closely related to all the auto-inventing characters of Cronenberg's other movies. In EXISTENZ the characters just engage in a game in which they live out their innermost fantasies and even their subconscious, at least to a certain extent. The game world which the players enter resembles the real world, just as the players bring their actual physical appearances and senses into this fantasy world. It is the imagination made flesh, so to speak. Only when you are inside the game's virtual lookalike reality, can you make things happen which you would not ordinarily allow yourself to do or take part in. In this sense, the games may be seen as yet another instance of that search for ever more titillating stimulation which Cronenberg has investigated in earlier films like SHIVERS, VIDEODROME, and CRASH.

In VIDEODROME, the character Nicki Brand (played by Deborah Harry) expresses it this way: 'We live in overstimulated times. We crave stimulation for its own sake. We gorge ourselves on it. We always want more, whether it's sexual, tactile, or emotional.' And when the characters of CRASH get sexually aroused by car crashes, it is explained by the fact that their nervous systems are so deadened that they have to experience this kind of extreme situation in order to feel alive:

> Pain [...] energizes your nervous system, which God knows might be deadened by work or drugs or who knows what, and brings it alive so that sexuality can have an intensity. [...] Also, there's the whole thing of surviving. You flirt with danger and you survive – and that brings you to an incredible awareness of life and the value of life. People are very deadened, day by day, to their mortality and also to the intensity of life.[34]

In EXISTENZ, the players' nervous systems are directly energized through the umbilical cord connecting them to the game. Although the game does have a physical and even a painful aspect (to which I shall return later), its thrill is of a somewhat different kind than the masochist pleasures sought by the characters of both VIDEODROME and CRASH. You might say that they are the imagination made flesh rather than the flesh being subject to imaginative impositions. Or in Cronenberg's own words: 'It's really an attempt to fuse the fantasy and make it real, physical and organic. It's the game made flesh'.[35] But you might also argue that the games are a materialized metaphor of uninhibited desire. On the other hand, the game imposes certain restraints on the imaginative freedom – or the free will – of the players. When inside the game, the player assumes the part of a game character and as such he will have to do or say certain things in order to make the plot advance. If the character fails to live up to these rules and disregards the design of the game, the game will immediately pause and enter a sort of time loop. Only when the character reenters the correct dialogue or action path, will the plot continue.

This is, of course, completely in line with Rushdie's objections to computer games being true art, but Cronenberg tends to see these restrictions on the characters' free will in a more existentialist light. Although he is a firm believer in free will and auto-invention, in most of his films he has in fact explored the limits of this freedom of invention. Speaking of his film DEAD RINGERS (1988) which deals with identical twins who are both gynaecologists and who fall in love with the same women, he has stated that 'the whole concept of free will resists the idea of anything determining destiny. Freedom of choice rests on the premise of freedom from physical and material restrictions. But the twins' research suggests a fair amount of biological predestination. The twins just provide a basis to investigate that, not as an aberration but as cases in point of genetic power. There are religious and philosophical questions attached to this that make it even more disturbing in a society like ours. Do I like it? Like everybody else, I'm attached to the notion that I am free and that my will determines my own life, and maybe I'm wrong.'[36]

Although there are no identical twins in Cronenberg's other films, the case could be made that all his films are discussing the issue of biological predestination, i.e. the fact that we seem to be stuck within an organism which provides us with a certain gender and a certain body with certain functions ascribed to certain organs. But biological predetermination – whether real or imagined – is not the only restraint imposed on our free will. Other restraints may be imposed by some 'superior designer' or God. Cronenberg thus sees a strong link between his seemingly more mainstream Stephen King adaptation THE DEAD ZONE (1983) and all his other films about more or less mad scientists conducting more or less mad experiments. For in THE DEAD ZONE, God is 'the absentee scientist' who has been experimenting with the life of the film's protagonist Johnny Smith:

> Because many of the scientists in my early films are absent from the films themselves, although their influence remains, I think you could make a good case for saying that in THE DEAD ZONE, God is the scientist whose experiments are not always working out and that the Johnny Smith character is one of his failed experiments. [37]

In EXISTENZ, we are told about a game called THOU ART GOD: 'Thou the player art God, very spiritual, funny too. God, the artist, the mechanic.' The player is invited to assume the role of God and invent his or her own existence, within the game – and not only within this particular game. Although the promise of playing God may constitute the immediate attraction of the game, the player does not become God. What actually happens is that the player lays all his imagination and all his desires in the hands of a new God: the game designer – cf. how Allegra is referred to as 'the game goddess' or 'the demoness'.

But these restraints on the free will of the players may, on the other hand, be the true attraction of the game. For according to Cronenberg, 'we would love to have stabilities and we would love to have absolutes, and we have to invent them because they don't exist.'[38] And if we take a step further and move to the film itself, Cronenberg is, of course, the superior game designer, the absentee scientist or the God who has breathed life into the film's characters and mapped out their possibilities. And outside the film? Is our creativity also limited by some absentee director or game designer pulling the strings?

Although a quite destabilizing thought experiment, this may appear a much less original, much less radical, much less provocative – and also a considerably less Deleuzian – stance than the one taken by Cronenberg in his previous films. But the discussion of free will versus any kind of predestination is only one of the issues addressed by eXistenZ. In fact, eXistenZ is also a very strong statement against the Cartesian mind/body split, and in addition, it proceeds to investigate the issue of the new flesh as opposed to organisms on various levels. It is in these respects that eXistenZ is most interesting for a Deleuzian approach.

The complex Chinese box structure of the film in which what we thought to be reality is dissolved with every new disclosure of yet another game level, makes it very difficult not only to distinguish 'reality' from imagination but also to find a solid point from which to approach the film. All that is solid melts into imaginary game worlds. There truly is an element of psychosis involved, as Ted Pikul observes in the film. Or you might say that eXistenZ is a true materialization of what is referred to by Deleuze in *The Time-Image* as 'the powers of the false'. It could also be argued, however, that the hallucinatory states described by Cronenberg in videodrome are here taken further, resulting in a kind of a mental BwO where each element can shift place and be considered now reality now pure imagination.

In this respect, the game eXistenZ may be regarded as a (bio-)technological extension of the human nervous system which entails an auto-imputation of the physical organism to the extent that the human body in flesh and blood has lost much of its *raison d'être*. The players do not move physically through space while playing. And outside eXistenZ, we are led to understand that people no longer engage in purely physical games, like for instance sports. When the protagonists seek refuge in an abandoned ski resort, we are informed that 'nobody actually physically skis anymore.'

Physical exercise of the flesh has been replaced by the digitalized biotechnological transmission of repressed dreams and fears to a purely mental game world. 'I feel very vulnerable, disembodied,' Ted says after his first venture into the game world. When entering the mental world of the game, the player's physical organism is temporarily dissolved and substituted by a (potential) BwO. As hallucinatory characters inside the game, the players may have the immediate appearance of (more or less) normal human bodies, but they are, in fact, nothing but psychic energy floating through space, producing 'the real as an intensive magnitude starting at zero'. In Deleuzian terms, the game playing could therefore ideally be regarded as an egg before it stratifies into an organism, a subject, a signification. Only the game designers – and the players – tend to let the game world reproduce the outside world and its organisms. They are simply not ready to accept the challenge of the limitless possibilities offered. Or, to quote Allegra Geller in the film: 'People are programmed to accept so little but the possibilities are so great.' And the virtual world of eXistenZ (the game as well as the film) therefore looks surprisingly similar to the 'real' world as we know it.

As a souvenir of an almost forgotten past in which people actually engaged in physical exercise, Allegra uses a ski boot for a handbag. In this handbag the game goddess keeps her most cherished invention and the very heart of the game eXistenZ: a so-called gamepod which looks like some unknown human organ, a weird melange of a heart, a liver, a lung and a couple of female breasts. Through the fleshy umbilical cords inserted in their bioports, the players of eXistenZ are connected to this gamepod from which they download the design of the game. This may indeed sound very futuristic, but Cronenberg has taken his cue from already existing practices and research within the computer market:

> It seemed to me that what people are really doing in computer and video games is trying to get closer and closer to fusing themselves with the game. The idea that a game would plug right into your nervous system made perfect sense to me because putting on glasses and gloves is a crude attempt to fuse your nervous system with the game. So I went that little bit further... [39]

As Cronenberg explains to Rodley, 'Intel and all the chip makers are now experimenting with animal proteins as the basis for their chips. They cannot use metals any more – they have to get right down to the molecular and even atomic level. Imagine the market! People will want it – either on the entertainment or the health front. You have your little case full of different organs that have been designed specifically for game playing. Or organs for things we've never had before. You could have new sexual organs – which I play with metaphorically in the movie.'[40]

If physical games have been abandoned, physicality is still very much at the heart of the new games. The new bodily orifice, the bioport, is a source of both imaginary game pleasures and highly sensuous delights and pains of the flesh. On the one hand, the operation through which a bioport is 'fitted' into a player's spinal cord is described as extremely painful and quite dangerous. The only reason for going through this agony would be the promise of experiencing completely new sensations within the game world. On the other hand, we witness how the protagonists experience a strong erotic desire when touching, licking (or otherwise lubricating), and penetrating each others' bioports. The bioport is therefore also a new sex organ, and as such it constitutes a revolt against any biological determinism regarding gender. This artificial orifice may provide hitherto unknown sexual pleasures to male and female alike. It is a creative extension of the possibilities of desire offered by the organism.

But let us return to the heart of the matter, or should I say the heart of the mind, the gamepod. When touched by the director of the game, the pod seems to be breathing and animated by a life of its own. And in fact, it comes very close to being an organic living being. Not only can it fall sick – and contaminate the players – it is also made of actual organic flesh. The pod, which is produced in weird-looking factories, is grown from fertilized amphibian eggs stuffed with synthetic DNA. Its power source is the player himself, his body, his nervous system, his metabolism, his energy. If the player gets tired or run down, the gamepod – and hence the game – will not run properly. A by-product of the gamepod production process is an army of mutant amphibians – two-headed reptiles which have proven to provide quite delicious taste sensations. And the bones of these mutants can furthermore be used for producing organic guns which use human teeth for bullets.

All these instances of organic flesh-machine interfaces are, of course, still within the imaginary world of EXISTENZ, but they are also a further development of a theme already touched on by Cronenberg in VIDEODROME and THE FLY. Only now the metal of the machines, the guns, etc. of the previous films has been entirely substituted by flesh and bones which have been detached from the various organisms to which they belonged and directed towards quite new and creative uses. With their new bioport orifices, the players' bodies have only undergone a slight change, but the mutant amphibians and the organic gamepods point to a complete dissolution of the organism in favour of a Body without Organs in the most literal sense of the term.

But are these BwOs good BwOs in the Deleuzian sense? It would seem that Cronenberg draws a certain line between the human body and that of reptiles. The mutant amphibians appear to be good-natured creatures which do not mind their rather horrific bodily transformations. But at the same time, by way of the hesitant Ted Pikul – and a certain amount of irony – the film does not (initially, at least) fully embrace the bioports as something which everybody ought to have installed. Although Pikul is a cardboard character with whom it is almost impossible to identify either on a cognitive or on an emotive level, he is the most 'normal' character in the film. And he therefore comes to function as our guide into this bizarre world of games. We are thus meant to share Pikul's expressed fears of bodily transformations – but also to follow him when he eventually comes to think of the bioport as an exciting new orifice offering sexual pleasures he – and we – had never dreamt of.

In complete concordance with Deleuze and Guattari, Cronenberg seems to be issuing a warning: you should reach out for the BwO, seek to transgress your biologically determined organism, but you should never overdo it. To put it in another way, you should not seek to become an equivalent of the film's mutant amphibians. In Deleuze's and Guattari's words, you should, as already quoted, limit yourself to 'opening the body to connections that presuppose an entire assemblage, circuits, conjunctions, levels and thresholds, passages and distributions of intensity, and territories and deterritorializations measured with the craft of a surveyor'. And this is exactly what the game players do when investing their nervous systems, their metabolisms, and their desires in the game.

But if the physical or material organism should not be completely destroyed – which in this case would mean death to the players – there are other organisms in the film which function as undesirable obstructions to the free flow of desire. The enemies of eXistenZ are, as already mentioned, of two kinds. On the one hand, we have the various corporations which are eager to take over the game because they smell huge profits. On the other hand, there are the realist fanatics, fundamentalists who object to the potential dangers of the imaginary powers let loose by and within the games. This conflict between the game people on the one hand and the game's enemies on the other is of course just one more aspect of the game's dramatic plot line. At the same time, however, both kinds of enemies may also be seen as materializations of metaphorical organisms which are opposed both to the physical human body and to the (potential) BwO of the game worlds.

The large corporations in eXistenZ are quite similar to the ones appearing in previous Cronenberg films, not least SHIVERS, RABID, SCANNERS, and VIDEODROME. They are more or less fascist organisations which are ready to kill in order to take possession – and control – of a popular game. The potential profit is, of course, an important incentive for their behaviour, but they will also have an interest in designing particular paths for large sections of the population's imagination. If they are in charge of the most popular games and the most popular game designers, they will be able to control people's dreams and desires and make them stratify into specific patterns. In contrast, we have the realist fundamentalists. In Deleuzian terms, I suppose they could be qualified as 'people with trees planted in their heads'.

They want to uphold a certain version of 'reality' which is why they see the imagination discharged within the game worlds as an imminent danger to *status quo*. They therefore fight the game designers and players with just as violent and fascist means as those employed by the large corporations.

In the overall Chinese box structure of the film, it becomes extremely difficult to distinguish between the various enemy organisms. On one level, a character may be a realist, on another a representative of a large corporation. But in fact, it does not really matter which kind of organism we are talking about because any kind of organism will always be an enemy to the BwO experiments carried out by the so-called 'existentialist' players. If we try once more to step outside the film's own game, I guess Cronenberg would be pleased if we were to see those critics who persist in considering his films inferior horror stories as incarnations of just such fascist organisms which fear any transgression of established thought patterns.

But if we the spectators are also a kind of game players in so far as we choose to enter Cronenberg's filmic game design, would we also qualify as dangerous to those who seek to repress the imagination? Well, not necessarily, I suppose. Not unless we fully accept the challenge offered by eXistenZ – and Cronenberg's other films – and make the film be flesh, and revolutionary thought. Cronenberg is well aware that films – including his own – will always be an abstraction of the flesh:

> In cinema it's still a representation of the flesh, it's not the real flesh. It's an image, a reflection of the flesh, so it's still an abstraction [...], but we are able to make the translation ourselves. It's a creative thing to think that wine is blood and that cinema is the human body. [41]

But Cronenberg the designer would like us to open our bodies to the cinematic metaphor of the flesh which he offers on the screen. And he wants us to physically absorb these metaphors as if they were poured right into our nervous systems through some kind of fleshy bioport. But the film's design is meant to be transcended by our own imaginative thought. Through the flesh, he intends his films to reach our brains and make us question the virtual – but not necessarily actual – limits of our existence. In this sense, his cinematic experiments may be considered highly dangerous by all enemies of imagination.

'Viral film' – a poetics of the BwO?

A complete film-maker should be able to appeal to all facets of human existence, the sensual as well as the cerebral. If you do get this mixture together properly, you have a perfect example of healing the Cartesian schism. You have something that appeals to the intellect and to the viscera. If you mix them together you get a whole movie. [42]

This statement by Cronenberg recalls Deleuze's claim that 'Our belief can have no object but "the flesh"' and matches perfectly with the Deleuzian explorations of the relationship between 'cinema, body and brain, thought'. But I will argue that even in the way they address the spectator, Cronenberg's films may be said to converge with Deleuze's and Guattari's philosophy of the BwO.

Cronenberg uses the horror genre as a Deleuzian/Guattarian stratum from which he seeks out possible lines of flight. You may also say that he deconstructs the genre, but the important point here is that he makes it function as a kind of solid ground while experimenting with the BwO. And in doing so, he is in perfect keeping with the advice offered by Deleuze and Guattari to those who would be interested in reaching a BwO:

This is how it should be done: Lodge yourself on a stratum, experiment with the opportunities it offers, find an advantageous place on it, find potential movements of deterritorialization, possible lines of flight, experience them, produce flow conjunctions here and there, try out continuums of intensities segment by segment, have a small plot of new land at all times. It is through a meticulous relation with the strata that one succeeds in freeing lines of flight, causing conjugated flows to pass and escape and bringing forth continuous intensities for a BwO. [43]

It might be argued that the issue of the BwO would have been more aptly presented in a form which reflected the BwO's unbridled flow of intensity, i.e. an experimental, avant-garde form, but Cronenberg has deliberately chosen to 'lodge himself on a stratum', i.e. within an established genre, and 'experiment with the opportunities it offers'. If he had opted for an experimental form, he might not only have lost the vast majority of his audience, but he would also have risked missing the intensity produced by his incessant deterritorializations of the audience's expectations.

As would be clear from my above presentation of his work, Cronenberg is a highly ambiguous director. The ambiguity – or maybe even the ambivalence – of his work does not present itself as a flaw, however, but should rather be explained by the director's deliberate attempts at short-circuiting all rational thought. It might be argued, of course, that a philosophy which proposes to 'exterminate all rational thought' is not necessarily irrational in itself. In fact, Cronenberg's philosophy is not at all irrational, but in agreement with the main arguments of his thought, his aesthetic project would seem to be to circumvent the brains of his spectators in order to address the materiality of their bodies directly. In this sense, the extreme excesses of the flesh, the blood, and the detached organs which characterize the majority of his films would be well calculated shock effects intended to affect the spectator on an eminently visceral level. But the brain being part of the material body, this physical response is meant to entail thought. Cronenberg's films address the bodies of the spectators directly. There is simply no escape from the flesh. From the visceral imagery on the screen, the flesh imposes itself as a material effect upon the body of the spectator and leaves us no possibility of redemption. This experience is excruciatingly visceral in a way that cannot be accounted for by simply referring it to the realm of fantasy.

His films are rarely structured as linear narratives (cf. the complex structure of EXISTENZ), there is almost no causal necessity in the way the scenes are linked to one another, and it is usually quite impossible to identify empathically with his characters. Cronenberg's films defy the traditional narrative 'organism' and replace it by a narrative BwO in which 'plot lines explode in multiple, incompatible directions, following the delirious, paranoid logic of proliferating cancer cells, or of interfaces between biology and technology run amok'.[44]

Because there is no rational story line to divert our attention from the excesses of the flesh, the materiality of the cinematic metaphor – the film's sounds and images – affects the material body of the spectator directly. And just as telepathy is explained in SCANNERS as 'the direct linking of two nervous systems separated by space', you might say that the material flesh of the characters in Cronenberg's films connects directly to the body of the spectator in his seat. Only the incessant flow of intensity between screen and audience means that contrary to the nervous systems in SCANNERS, the metaphorical bodies on the screen and the spectators' material bodies are not separated by space. They become one flesh.

In this sense, Cronenberg's films can be compared to a BwO, for they 'cause intensities to pass; [they] produce and distribute them in a *spatium* that is itself intensive, lacking extension.' But they may also be compared to a virus, which is how Cronenberg conceives of them himself. He defines a viral film as something which 'embeds itself in your genetic structure, your chromosomal structure, and in that strange way becomes part of you even though it's not'. And in fact, by way of his formal strategy, his films do in a strange way enter our bodies and change them into something else. Watching a film by David Cronenberg does not mean that we will suddenly grow another arm or develop exotic new sex organs in strange places, but the virus will work its way through our bodies and force our minds to think what we thought to be unthinkable.

Although the viruses which Cronenberg is so eagerly spreading through his work are of course not lethal, it may be argued that they are dangerous because there is a philosophy behind them (to paraphrase one of the characters in VIDEODROME who is talking about the spreading of the subliminal Videodrome signal). In a Deleuzian sense, they are at once material and metaphorical stagings of a deterritorializing practice of the most radical kind. And as such they constitute a serious threat to any kind of established order. From the point of view of the organism – understood in the widest sense possible – they are truly horrifying; not as horror *fiction*, however, but because of their profoundly disturbing material invasion of the spectators' bodies, inflicting us with a virus which may make us desire to try out new and hitherto unknown facets of this game called reality:

> It's really a matter of self-replication, and the fact that a virus can't exist in a vacuum – it has to have a host, it has to embed itself in something. I mean viral film making sounds like film making as a disease, art as a disease, but also as something that embeds itself in your genetic structure, your chromosomal structure, and in that strange way becomes part of you even though it's not.[45]

Does this implicate that the films are alive? According to Cronenberg, it actually does, at least to a certain extent, for just like the virus, the viral film is 'in a strange way half-way between being alive and being dead', and he continues:

> I mean, viruses really are on the edge of being machinery that's alive. I think the images we create are like that too – they have the feeling of life, they have the semblance of life, and we're not sure whether it really is alive or not – is the communication, the life that's embedded in it still there, is it really there or is it just an illusion?[46]

Cronenberg is pleased to think that his films will change with each new viewer and 'shift with time, become re-perceived in another context'. This is true of any film, you may argue, but Cronenberg's visceral films may be more likely to shift with time than most other films precisely because they address the body of the viewer directly, which makes them just as unstable and ephemeral as the bodies which they represent. Cronenberg's films are engaged in a continuous and dynamic productive process with their spectators – the hallmark of a true work of art, according to Salman Rushdie. And just as the viewers are refused the possibility of 'subjectifying' through identification with the characters, Cronenberg's films will not ossify into any fixed significations. My own Deleuzian reading of his work does not hold any privilege either. It is 'just an idea' or 'just a game', a playful thought experiment.

Feature films by David Cronenberg:

SHIVERS (1975)
RABID (1976)
THE BROOD (1979)
SCANNERS (1980)
VIDEODROME (1982)
THE DEAD ZONE (1983)
THE FLY (1986)
DEAD RINGERS (1988)
NAKED LUNCH (1991)
M. BUTTERFLY (1993)
CRASH (1996)
eXistenZ (1999)

Section Two

Engaging in the Present

5   Micropolitics

A Political Philosophy from Marx and Beyond

Malene Busk

> It is true that philosophy cannot be separated from an anger against the epoch, but neither from a serenity it brings us.[1]

This article attempts to point out some main features of the specific political aspects of the philosophy of Gilles Deleuze. I will highlight two perspectives or levels related to 'the political Deleuze': firstly, his thematizing of the principal status of philosophy in relation to society when defining political philosophy as such, which is related to the concept of 'utopia'; and secondly some central aspects of his actual elaboration of concepts and portraits of epochal problems in his own 'micropolitics'. An important but somewhat 'quiet' impulse for the political Deleuze is a certain heritage from Karl Marx, though this heritage and its Deleuzian traits sometimes takes shape through a principal rejection of Marx's concepts. Following this line, I will try to trace in what sense Deleuze's work makes itself into a type of Marxism. Deleuze commented upon this feature even in his late authorship, while always distancing himself from any orthodox Marxism. This article will, therefore, pick out some themes from Marx, which can function as openings into Deleuze's positioning and definitions, as well as entering into the genuinely Deleuzian conceptual universe.

The epoch of capitalism today: from societies of discipline to societies of control

> You see, we don't believe in any political philosophy which is not centered around the analysis of capitalism and its developments.[2]

According to Deleuze, the years since since 1945 have shown various signs of crisis of one form of capitalist society as well as the discontinuous development and consolidation of a new form. The disappearing form, 'the society of discipline', was developed around 1800 when they replaced the autocratic forms of the so-called 'societies of sovereignty'.[3] Here, Deleuze is inspired by the works of Foucault, analyzing the development, function and change of the disciplinary institutions and how our lives are organized inside them. The societies of discipline are characterized by a series of well-defined institutions like the family, the school, the army, the factory, the hospital, the prison. They are all marked by discipline and hierarchy, tending to bifurcate into binary class- and power-relations with analogous function: man-wife, parents-children, teacher-pupils, owner-workers, doctor-patient etc. In the society of discipline, one defined compartment succeeds the other in the life of the individual: 'Now you are no longer in your family, you are in school, or in the army, at the factory, etc.' The individual becomes important as that special entity which can pass from one compartment to the other, an entity which in scale and profile matches the disciplinary, serial institutions.

We are now faced with important changes taking place in specific types of society, and in turn, this confronts us with institutions which are in crisis. The principal movements go from the closed to the open, from the solid to the gaseous, from acts of institutional discipline to communicative controlling. We are at the beginning of what Deleuze calls a 'society of control'. Deleuze's shift in 'paradigm' seems to follow the shift from modern industrial society to late- or post-modern information society. At the level of production, the factory is about to be replaced by the concern, heavy production is removed to third-world countries, while know-how, soft ware and service seem to dominate in the West. The masses in and out of the factories are replaced by a net of mobile, 'lonely fighters'. At the level of economy, the movements of capital measured by the solid gold bar are challenged by the virtual, gaseous currency-trade with money itself as primary object, and politically the national states are weakened and dissolving under the influence of the global network of market and communication.

The tendency for the individual life is likewise marked by a disintegration of stable measurements and an overlapping of hitherto separate entities. The family is becoming provisional and split, dissolving into mixed groups. We are supposed to undergo further education at work; work itself is often done while travelling or via the global network of communication in the home-office, mixed with other aspects of our lives. We can be sent home from hospital to self-dialysis or ambulant medication, thus reducing the number of beds on the wards. At the same time, convicted prisoners can serve a sentence at home, shackled with a control chip around the leg. These are visible signs of institutions in crisis, heading towards quite different ideas about how to organize a society. The human being in a society of control has to distribute, dole out, itself in a number of not very demarcated,

overlapping systems in order to satisfy the control of all areas simultaneously. Of course, this marks a liberation from the disciplinary repression
and the claustrophobia of successive closures, but at the same time it takes
away the possibilities of the small undisciplined (and somewhat subversive) 'free spaces' in between two institutional compartments or in the
breaking out from them, by striking, deserting, leaving home, etc. Today
one can hardly leave anymore, only fall through the net. We see experiments
in the US trying to bring homeless people back into society, not by giving
them a steady home, but by giving them an e-mail address, from where they
should communicate and fulfil the demands of control, in order 'to exist'
again socially.

   Pursuing these ideas with the aid of Deleuze, we could say that the individual is or was that which is 'breaking out': stories in books and movies often deal with the individual deserting, opening up the factory doors,
escaping from prison or the psychiatric hospital, and they could be seen as
signs of transition between the two types of societies. The system is cracking, it does not 'fit' anymore and has become the object of a critique which
unknowingly announces a new kind of system. This critique is nevertheless
born out of the society of 'individual-and-institution', and the break in these
stories thus always focuses on the self-realization of the *individual* through
the act of breaking away. This does not reflect the new discourse we are facing when our institutions are struck by crisis and are marginalized or re-
formed, particularly when the clear institutional confines are blurred and
the 'wall' to be broken has disappeared. As far as 'the individual' is bound
to the constructions of discipline, something 'post-individual' will be
shaped in the new western societies. Deleuze proposes the term *dividual*[4] to
indicate the form of human life living up to the demand that we divide and
distribute ourselves in many fast, simultaneous movements between new
open systems. The structure of society can no longer shape a life 'serially',
and instead we are marked by simultaneity: 'The human' as the dividual is
always busy with it all, and we are supposed to be so all life through, spun
into a net of and perpetually controlled by immediate communication. 'In a
society of control one is never finished with anything.'[5]

   The changes towards a society of control, for the individual as well as for
the collective, can partly be seen as liberations and reforms when compared
to the patterns of repression in the heavy industrial, disciplinary societies.
Deleuze does not deny these liberations, but wants to bring attention to the
new forms of repression which the new, more 'feed-back nervous' societies
of communication and control will produce, of which we are only getting
glimpses: 'There is no reason to ask which regime is the hardest or most tolerable, because it is within each of them that liberations and subjugations

are clashing. (...) There is no reason to fear or to hope, but to search for new weapons.'[6] I will try to see in what way political philosophy is contributing to this search in its own way, by examining its relation to society, or to the 'epoch', as Deleuze calls it.

If the definition of a political philosophy requires that it should attempt to analyse developments in contemporary society and in capitalism, this implies a rejection of a political idealism, since political ideas cannot be separated from the concrete societies within which they take place. In other words, there is no ideal sphere in which the politically Good can be calculated, and we are given no eternal system of speculative rights. Philosophy is thus emphatically placed in a milieu, an actual society, but the relation between them is nevertheless not an expression of a traditional Marxist partition between materialistic 'basis' and ideological 'superstructure'. Philosophy has neither an idealistic primacy over society nor a materialistic derivative character. It is another kind of relation Deleuze is looking for between philosophy and epoch; this possible alternative relation can, among others, be seen in the positive heritage from Marx and Spinoza.

The immanence of capital and of philosophy

Marxism has long been compromised by disappointing socialist experiments and the failing of 'the world revolution', by alternative forms of resistance which did not conform to Marxist models – women's lib, squatters etc. – and by its own dogmatism and tendency to reduce everything to an insensitive, political schematism. At several central points (like the idea of material basis vs. superstructure) this schematism ironically finds its sharpest critique in the late work of Marx himself.[7] And these are some of the aspects that one will be unable to track back in Deleuze's mode of being a 'Marxist'. Nevertheless, Deleuze acknowledges a heritage from Marx:

> What we find most interesting in Marx is his analysis of capitalism as an immanent system that's constantly overcoming its own limitations, and then coming up against them once more on a larger scale, because its fundamental limit is Capital itself.[8]

Capitalism regarded as an immanent system implies that in the analysis of the developments of capital, and the movements of the capitalist society, there is no reference to causes outside of the analysed system itself. Capitalism as an expanding, immanent system can neither be understood as arbitrary nor as the result of universals outside of capital, be those God, human nature or any type of contract.[9] The system expands by its own force. Therefore, capital is not a substance, a bag of money or a socio-economical tool, but a process: '[Capital] as value increasing its own value, does not only imply class relations, a certain social character, resting upon the existence of work as waged labour. It is a movement...'[10] Furthermore, Marx claims, 'capitalistic process of production (...) produces (...) not only goods, not only surplus value, it produces and reproduces the relation of capital itself'.[11]

'Capital' was Marx's name for that immanent dynamism he found as nothing less than the economical law of movement of the modern society. A movement has been started which has as its final end only the expansion of itself. Deleuze calls such a dynamism a process of de- and re-territorializing movements; like capital, this process is not about keeping but about moving even further, giving out the profit as soon as it is made, leaving the territories as soon as they are conquered. Deleuze is interested in exactly this aspect of Marx's concept of capitalism as an immanent, transgressive, self-reproducing movement.

In order to clarify the status of the relation between philosopy and the contemporary forms of capitalism, I will first give a brief sketch of Deleuze's definition of philosophy in general (not specified as political). This will demonstrate that the connection between philosophy and epoch is not that of a causal relation, but emerges out of their common immanent modus or presupposition. In *What is Philosophy?*[12] Deleuze and Guattari define philosophy as a discipline distinct from, for instance, wisdom or religion. They do so by presupposing that philosophical thought is taking place at a plane of immanence; they try to avoid installing transcendent universals to encompass and explain immanence; instead, they let thought produce open, local concepts which make up a whole landscape of interrelated, consistent concepts. Concepts of a given philosophy describe a plane, which can never itself be a concept, but is the background, landscape or space where they mutually determine each other as well as express the plane itself. Like this, a philosophy will draw its immanent, absolute intuition. Deleuze and Guattari thus define philosophical thought not as a meta-discipline but as a specific discipline, whose essence is to create complexes of concepts on a plane of immanence. A philosophy presupposing pure immanence means that it only has its own consistency and productivity with which to pose its new problems and experiment with new ways to conceive the world, since it cannot understand itself as a representation of a model 'plane behind the plane'. The presupposed (and thus pre-philosophical) plane is therefore a horizon that in itself is an infinite absolute movement, pushing its own limits, since it is not moving relative to anything, there being nothing over or behind it, nothing limiting or conditioning it. The concepts populating this immanence attempt to draw up its special movement as landmarks, flagging the significant, high-potented areas of the landscape as a movement of thought; following its ceaseless becomings, changes, connections, repetitions and differentiations.

This view of philosophy can now be connected to the epoch: 'Modern philosophy's link with capitalism, therefore, is of the same kind as that of ancient philosophy with Greece: *the connection of an absolute plane of immanence with a relative social milieu that also functions through immanence.'*[13] As absolute immanent thought, philosophy has a special relation to its society, beyond the alternative of trivial materialism vs. idealism. Ancient Greek philosophy was indeed inseparable from the Polis, but neither uncritical or subordinated to it, no more than philosophy in any way could be said to have created the Polis or to govern it. As a philosophy, Socratic dialectics could be born in the Greek Polis with its culture of 'agon' (the fight amongst equal rivals in olympiads, dramas, rethoric), differing from hierarchical societies founded upon religion or violence. Likewise, modern philosophy can exist in a worldly and immanent society of Western capitalism. Philosophies and their epochs are thus intimately connected qua immanence, but they differ radically qua nature. Whereas immanent capitalism is moving relatively to the profitable, 'capital as its own limit', in a relative social and material field of power, compromises, sufferings, resources, etc., philosophical thought is exchanging with its outside, with 'matter', in a more fundamental sense than things, goods or production units, moving infinitely on an absolute plane:

> Philosophy takes the relative deterritorialization of capital to the absolute;[14] it makes it pass over the plane of immanence as movement of the infinite and suppresses it as internal limit, *turns it back against itself so as to summon forth a new earth, a new people.*[15]

Here Deleuze is in his own way following Marx, since immanent capitalism is not to be criticized by a political philosophy through the means of ideal (transcendent) entities, but is itself indirectly carrying a critical potential. One should note that the special terminology of 'summon forth a new people' has as little to do with a vanguard[16] organizing the 'working class' or with the mobilization of the nationalistic 'Volk'. Rather, the term 'new people' suggests the possibility of existence, a horizon opening up; it is 'minoritarian', a point to which I will return in a later section.

Through the creation of concepts that are neither consensual nor representative philosophy can avoid habitual understandings, and instead expose unacceptable conditions as neither natural nor necessary. The epoch is shrouded in common sense about themes and non-themes, concerning the kind of lives there are to exist and how we are to understand ourselves; one might say that the epoch is confirming itself all the time, also in its self-analyses, corrections and expansions. When philosophy works as a construction of movement presenting movement, not as a set of answers, a critique can be made which challenges the doxas of the discourse of the epoch.[17] That philosophy for Deleuze thus is characterized by a critical anger against the epoch as well as a creative ability to form clear concepts by which to understand it, allows another common feature with Marx to be discerned. About his work *Grundrisse* Marx writes: 'It forms at the same time the presentation of the system and through the presentation a critique of it'.[18] In Deleuze we discover the doubling of presentation and critique through what is provided – the definition of the relation that political philosophy has with society, expressed in the autonomous philosophical concept. Strictly speaking, there is no uncritical conceptual apparatus. Those which are so and are thus non-philosophical and not genuine as concepts, are only able to measure parameters blindly sunken into the inner ratio of what they should measure. It is for this reason that they are not able to say anything new, but only make explicit the same old points.[19] On the contrary, a political philosophy should come into being by appropriating, thinking and creating concepts to conceive of precisely that fundamental 'law of movement' of our societies. With this special relation to its epoch it should distance itself from the shortsighted instrumentality of political science, journalism or marketing on the one side, and from the illusionary universalism of moral systems and abstract rights on the other. Because philosophy has immanent movement in common with capitalism, conceptualizing it in its own absolute movement so radically that also capitalism is deterritorialized, philosophical concepts can simultaneously be presenting and critiquing the epoch. But Deleuze has a further specification of this precise junction whereby philosophy turns political by both paralleling and going beyond its epoch.

The junction: utopia and revolution after Marx

> Actually, *utopia is what links* philosophy with its own epoch, with European capitalism, but also with the Greek city. In each case it is with utopia that philosophy becomes political and takes criticism of its own time to its highest point. Utopia does not split off from infinite movement: etymologically it stands for absolute deterritorialization but always at the critical point at which it is connected with the present relative milieu, and especially with the forces stifled by this milieu[20]

Utopia means 'no where' and has connotations both in the direction of unrealizable fantasies about religiously tinted 'exemplary societies' as well as of the 'realization' of so called scientific socialism, which departs from the communist utopia of Marx. H. J. Schanz describes how Marx was read 'with the expectation that he could provide the way to the concrete and obtainable utopia (...) That this was a gigantic overloading of Marx' theory and that this overloading in itself was contributory to a new form of distortion and deformation, there can no longer be any doubts about.'[21]

Characteristically, Deleuze's ideas of 'utopia' and 'revolution' are quite different, trying to deal with both the problems of traditional Marxism and contemporary capitalism. On the one hand the historical revolutions did go terribly wrong, failing to lead to Freedom. Thus confidence in socialist programmes has disappeared. On the other hand, global capitalism of today indisputable produces unacceptable social conditions that should meet more resistance than what is technocratizable within the frameworks of the nation states. Deleuze never went for a definitive 'solution' to the shifting problems of our societies. Resistance, however uncompromising it may be, is not about finding the 'End of history' in the eternal 'Good', what is a doubtful phantasm. Critique must proceed from an immanent starting point without a governing projection of the future (the end justifying the cruelty of the means) or a longing back to nostalgic idealizations of the past (the illusion of origin blocking new movements). As Deleuze and Guattari state, the no-where of Utopia is just as well a now-here.[22]

Whereas revolution normally designates a radical change of relative historical macroscopic patterns, Deleuze distinguishes between these historical revolutions (as the great American or the great Russian, 'failing in each their end of the West'), and the revolution as a *concept*, developing autonomously according to its own laws. Concepts are created by philosophy. Rather than belonging to the actual revolutions, the concept belongs to a certain *enthusiasm*, to the becoming-revolutionary of a people where a glimpse of the infinite is experienced in that which is right now and here. 'The event' is the special practice that the concept belongs to, 'calls out for', but does not control.[23] The now-here of the event is not a point on the chronological line of history – as this is always represented in the form of afterrationalization, from where the actions seem causal and continuous at a fact level. Now-here is a discontinuous experience, making a 'hole in time', standing out from the historical facts though having conditions in history. The phenomenon of May '68-enthusiasm is taken as an example of an event. Deleuze place the now-here of utopia in the critical point between the autonomy and absolute presupposition of thinking and a relative, actual milieu, that is, in casu between modern philosophy and western capitalism:

> Men's only hope lies in a revolutionary becoming; the only way of casting off their shame or responding to what is intolerable.[24]

The possible contribution of political philosophy to this chance, is to call out for the event of becoming, the now-here of enthusiasm in the relative social field. It will be 'looking for new weapons' by its simultaneous presentation and critique of the developments of contemporary capitalism, where new forms of power relations demand new forms of resistance. If communicative networks were about to tie us up in lifelong control, we might find a way out through the inventions of 'vacuoles of non-communication'.[25]

Philosophy can meet with its epoch and the social field of practice, power and resistance by way of two basic connections. Firstly it uses the very conditions against which the critique is turned, as for instance when philosophy shares the immanent movement of networks characterizing societies of control, but now in an absolute way. Secondly it proceeds from the events taking place in the individual and social field in order to create concepts, for instance when conceptualizing forces at work in our desires and beliefs. The movements of thought are, on the one hand, immanent and not determined by idealistic universals and, on the other hand, only in contact with, not determined by, material and historical circumstances. Talking about a heritage from Marx (immanent movement, presentation and critique), Deleuze's theoretical contribution as a political philosophy is concerned not to direct 'the way to concrete, obtainable utopia', but rather to make a philosophy which, in itself, presents a call out for a non-subordinate practice.

Spinoza's forces and the art of the encounter

Deleuze takes his inspiration from the 17th century philosopher, Baruch de Spinoza (1632-1677).[26] Philosopher Michael Hardt has shown how important elements of Deleuze's ideas on democracy, politics and theory are inspired by Spinoza's ethics and concept of force. As I will explain, not the least so in the creation of concepts which can do away with the more Hegelian aspects in Marx: contradiction, objective movement, historical subject.[27]

'The ethical task is to push the limit for what one is able to do to the utmost.'[28] This corresponds to Spinoza's ethical definition of a body: that a body is what it can do, that it is defined by its force. Spinoza was asking the question of politics and ethics with the body as a model: 'Everything a body can do is also its natural right.'[29] The natural right thus implies that the human being is free in relation to moral exterior concepts – these are always secondary, since no order is predetermined. One is only born with a certain force, not with a rationality or a citizenship. Natural right are thus posing a freedom from order, an abstract anarchistic condition, where the forces of the bodies are performed And even though 'we do not yet know what a body can do', the force of the human being is very small and partial amongst the innumerable bodies and forces of nature.

This state of nature is meanwhile proving intolerable to live in. Firstly we are determined by the force to be affected, to passive passions. The bodies have a force to feel and are most often filled by a 'sufferance under'; examples are hunger, hatred, fear, and since the encounters with other bodies according to natural right occur arbitrarily, the passions are mostly bad and sad. The result is anarchic violence, coincidental clashes: in brief a waste of forces. These states of nature therefore indicate but a minimum of force, which could be increased by meetings with other bodies in other ways. To make the natural state bearable to live in will then mean that the encounters are organized, that from natural right rather than the limitation or negation of it, we constitute a civil society: 'The civil state is the state of nature made livable; or, more precisely, it is the state of nature infused with the project of the increase of our power.'[30]

For Spinoza, there is no contradiction between natural right and the civil rights of reason, but according to him, we are not born with the latter. To discover and invent relations strenghtening joy, that is to become rational, is an apprenticeship of freedom. Anarchy is thus not to be overcome by order, but its freedom should be made positive. Instead of being just a freedom from order we will have to find a passage from here to a 'freedom to organisation'. 'The art of organizing relations and encounters' will be the fundament for a Spinozistic concept of democracy, understood as intensifying forces of activity and joyful passions rather than sad ones. This political scenario does not operate through self-restriction, limitation or moral victory over natural right, because it does not oppose democracy. This fact converges with Deleuze who, all the way through his authorship, fights the idea of negation or contradiction as a motive power and by so doing, maintains implacable in the face of Hegel. For Spinoza, it is not through negation that the societies are changing 'rationally', but through the forces of the bodies and souls, resistance and critique being positive or affirmative too in this sense.

The critical point is how to get from one moment, the contingently existing bodies and affects in their state of nature, to the next, exemplified by the democratic intensification of joyful affections by civil right. The *connection* itself to the concrete political constitution of a democracy is a process in the relative social field, in which new ways are invented to montage elements of jurisprudence, rather than 'universal rights', from the viewpoint of the users who make 'political assemblages'. And this is, as Hardt shows, the precarious point for Spinoza as well as Deleuze. As a consequence of the contingent, independent 'constitution' of natural right from where

Spinoza's ethics takes the body as a model, (not moral, religion or reason), the specification of this relation forms 'the limit of a "theory" of democracy, the point at which theory runs into a wall. Only social practice can break through this wall, by giving body to the process of political assemblage.'[31] Once again, we can see how Deleuze develops the anti-idealistic elements from Spinoza, from whom theory is not privileged in relation to the political practice; it is not 'bookish ideas' which are paving the road for practice. The concrete developments of forces and resistance against repressions belong to the social world of powers. Philosophy is not a power. The philosophical utopia of democratic organization of 'joyful encounters' is, therefore, only able to function as an experiment of 'the art of encounter', trying to encounter a practice.

Political trinities: from Marx to Deleuze

In the resumption of a political philosophy after Marx, Deleuze is abandoning central Marxian concepts and introducing radically new ones. Marx was operating from three mutually conditioning elements in his critical presentation. Society was defined by its contradictions; these would be expressed by the awakening of revolutionary consciousness. The agents for the revolutionary movement was a historically determined subject or class, namely, the proletariat. The following passage attempts to sketch Deleuze's new constructions by replacing this old trinity. Instead of a concept of contradiction he proposes 'lines of flight' or 'fluctuations of desire' as the grounds of society; instead of the concept of an awakening consciousness and a historical revolution he proposes the concept of 'war machines' as the contingent places where impulses for change are gathered and strengthened; and instead of the concept of class he refers to 'minorities' as the agents of movement. These concepts are formed under an inspiration from Spinoza's ideas that the political adopts the body as a model. Its power to be affected and affecting results in new terms of forces, lines and movements. Consequently, the 'normative' partitions that will appear here are not morally abstract, as in 'good versus bad', but rather, they are ethically concrete, as in 'joyful versus sad' affections, practices of intensification or diminishment of life.

From contradictions to lines of flight

'From the viewpoint of micropolitics, a society is defined by its lines of flight, which are molecular', state Deleuze and Guattari in A Thousand Plateaus.[32] In order to understand this statement it is necessary to see that they define societies in terms of segmentations, flows and power. Anthropologists have analyzed the so-called primitive societies without a state apparatus, political institutions, formalized diplomacies etc., by departing from considering how they were segmenting themselves, for example with respect to sex, status, religion, family, territory. But instead of opposing 'primitive segmentarity' to 'modern centralization', Deleuze and Guattari suggest that modern western societies perform another kind of very elaborate, 'hard' and formalized segmentarity, through the forces of classes, market segments, housing structures and gender patterns, instead of the softer, 'primitive' one. Having said this, society does not only consist of segmentations, be these the binary male-female pair or the linear hierarchies or the circular centre-peripheries. More important, perhaps, is the 'microscopic' or 'molecular' sphere, where meaning, grouping, economies, individuals or collectives are fluctuating, forming, dissolving and moving under and through the segments. This sphere is compared to 'quantum-fluctuations' with discontinuous jumps and the molecular ability to pass in and out of units that are separated on the macro-level. The fluctuations are hard to grasp; they are on the move, dissolving segmentations or working their way in between segment lines as well as contributing to the formations of new ones.

In between this couple and of another character, Deleuze finds 'centres of power', for example schools, banks, churches, state-institutions. They are seen as the central mediators between the two types of lines; on the one hand the macropolitical level of currency, gender, parties, classes, on the other hand fluxes of innumerable dynamisms as they work in a society. The centres of power do not control the segmentation. For example, it is not the banks which have 'decided' that the dollar segment exists and is strong; rather it is born of the fluctuations of currencies in the mass of economical transactions. The centres of power are not in control of these fluctuations, which form a 'zone of powerlessness' within them. Likewise the organisation of the banks and the stock-exchange, with their clearly defined tools, parameters, and spheres of influence are the 'zones of power' of these power centres: this is where they are actually exercizing concrete and recognizable power by translating or exchanging the fluctuations into segmentations: loans, currency-trade, balance, and interest. The centres of power are thus, for Deleuze, not defined as the ones 'ruling' society, but only as the mediators at the point of intersection between the visible segments of a macro level and the uncontrollable, less obvious lines of flight of a micro level.

The molecular level consists primarily of fluctuations in 'desire' and 'beliefs', quantifying the fluctuation into small assemblages: 'Beliefs and desires are the basis of every society'.[33] One could regard these two as synonyms of 'collective' and 'individual', but the new concepts express instead the transgression of both. 'Desire' is here not signifying a previous lack (negativity is for him completely unproductive and thus secondary), but a positive, complex drive (such as taking a walk or dance), whose nature conforms to the natural right of Spinoza. Doing so involves to use and to intensify force, mix up, change and 'erotically' combine, rather than to maintain and fortify an individual identity to which a desire as lack in its traditional sense will then be attributed. Furthermore, in Deleuze's definition, desire is always a 'smoothly' formed, assembled force, never an undifferentiated drift, a definition unfortunately sometimes forgotten when Deleuze's 'philosophy of desire' is discussed.[34] With respect to 'beliefs', these could be seen as the implicit, common presumptions which mark and transform themselves. Deleuze does not come up with political examples, but one could suggest our common belief in the value of money as one. And perhaps Wittgenstein's figure of the thread made out of many different fibres where none is continuous[35], here multiplied in all directions, can express the 'structure' of beliefs, which run discontinuously through different parts of society.

These micropolitical movements can displace focus in ways that throws new light on society and are unpredictable to the institutional analysis; actually they must have an effect at the macro-political level in order to mean something. For example, the developments in Eastern Europe around the fall of the Berlin Wall can be seen as the gatherings of different lines to an efficient line of flight, which in an uncontrollable manner is effecting the phase of segmentation of the project of the European Union: 'molecular escapes and movements would be nothing if they did not return to the molar organizations to reshuffle their segments, their binary distributions of sexes, classes, and parties.'[36]

The distinction between secondary segmentation (territorializing segment lines) and primary fluctuations (deterritorializing lines) turns analysis away from the established political (and personal) discourses and towards the minor movements.[37] But Deleuze's micropolitical concepts should not be mistaken for the usual idea about scale according to sphere of influence, from the individual as smallest unit to supranational institutions. The microscopical or molecular level as a concept of the ceaseless, uncontrollable movements in society is stretching through all the macropolitcal segmentations and thus has the same extension as them. The conceptual couple of 'individual and collective' has no force in the distinction between macro- and microlevel. At the macroscopic level we have both the individual and the collective as representations having stabilized as the pieces, which can be operated and manipulated, moving along the lines of segmentation, for example in medias, parties, citizenship... 'Representation' is characteristic for this level, be it as attributes attributed to an individual or collective norms and institutions. The microscopic level does neither operate by individual or collective representations, but by movements before, in between and beyond these, so the fluctuations of desire and beliefs can not be attributed to anybody, neither as the desire of the individual nor as expressions of the collective will. Trying to grasp social fluctuations outside of these is a struggle to avoid the representational way of thinking where effects are reflected as causes: for instance when the subject inevitably finds itself as condition for 'its desire', explaining nothing, only reproducing an illusion of the same. Thus the individual is not a basic unity for Deleuze, but rather an effect, just like the 'official' sphere of representational fixation of certain significative units.

From the party to war machines

A fluctuation can be intensified and effectuated in the form of an efficient 'machine'. As a second change of concept with respect to Marx, Deleuze talks about war machines as mechanisms opposing 'the State' in a broad sense. The sovereignty of the stateform is always coexisting and competing with a polymorph, diffuse form. Molecular lines are running in a number of directions with constantly changing energies, but when something starts to outline their course, when they are intensified and gain expressiveness, a war machine is made, rather like the nomads gathering for a deterritorializing attack on the city walls. State and 'nomadic' war machine are interacting as inside and outside, as the empire and the gang. The term 'machine' is marking a distance from connotations of vitalistic subjectivity, emphasizing the exteriority of the mechanism. War machines are inventions of the 'nomadic'. The nomad differs from the emigrant by never reterritorializing on a new place, but only 'inhabiting' deterritorialization itself, meaning that everytime he moves he stays where he is, namely on a movement. The nomad has absolute movement. If the war machine is a mechanism the existence of the nomad is effectuating it in space, as an event the philosopher can try to give a concept.

The concept of war machines is foremost an emancipatory figure. 'War' is connected less to destruction and more to a concentrated force, suspending usual boundaries and power relations. War machines make war without being a state, without having a territory, thus without defined front lines, confrontations, retreats. Rather than gaining and maintaining territories, deterritorializations have, at the starting point, nothing to do with the wars of states, even though the state can domesticize a war machine as an army. A war machine does not come about as the awakening of class consciousness about an objective determination, it is not the Hegelian breakdown of the system under its own contradictions, i.e. negation, but something new outside the state, emerging by its own means and without predecessors.

From class to minorities

As a third conceptual difference from Marx, the 'agents' performing subversive, political force is not understood as a historical class, but as minorities, not designating a numerical inferiority, but rather groups without a well-defined space-time in the social segmentation. Majority designates a normative model, as 'townsman, middle-class, male European', a majority regardless of the fact that 'he' is a numerical minority: nobody conforms restlessly to a model. 'The people', everybody, (or rather 'parts of everybody' and the groups we are making) is always about to make themselves and become other. This is also the definition of the minority: not model, but a becoming-other that has to be invented, as in cultural waves, youth gangs, green lobbyism. The PLO is mentioned as an example of a minoritarian, stateless, 'non-existing' people, emerging by creating a new social space-time, obtaining political reality. The minority usually wants to be majority, be a 'state', and be recognized. When 'the people' do become majority, this new model will still exist at another level from the people as varied and creative, and the two, therefore, do co-exist. Just as 'nobody' is a majority, 'the people' is for Deleuze always minoritarian and about to become (other).[38]

Deleuze is here describing resistance as an emancipatory, creative (not a negative) force, but is avoiding the doubtful idea of a historically determined subject of objective social change as is implied in the concept of 'class'. He is emphasizing the local, contingent assemblages of people who create a place to experience their significance, who negotiate a new jurisprudence and who create new social practices and possibilities.

While fluctuations are the grounds of society, they are not in themselves a 'utopian' category. They can become so in the form of the third type of lines, the absolute movement, or 'creative lines of flight'. The democratic 'encounters' of Spinoza are, when conceptualized by micropolitics, performing a fluctuation of desire in 'absolute becoming', intensifying force. With lines of flight as the one aspect of molecular fluctuations, the other aspect is their constant contribution to the emergence of segmentations. The duality of segmentation and fluctuation is now a trinity of lines: lines of macro-segmentation (like the dollar); micro-fluctuations from where the segments are emerging (mass of relative transactions); and finally the other potential of fluctuations, the absolute movement connecting and intensifying lines of flight in a creative process: here we find the Deleuzian warmachines, minoritarian becoming-revolutionary and utopia.

Fascism and desire

As we saw, the fluctuations can turn into static segmentarity as relative movements, the danger being that they are blocking and fixing our forces in stereotype, sad passions, and they can, as the other kind of movement, become intensified as absolute, creative movement. But Deleuze does not fail to see that at the level of intensifying lines of flight there are specific dangers, that is, that they can be intensified and reinforced 'negatively' as unlimited minimization of force, or destruction.

An urgent theme in French philosophy since 1945 has been the critique of totalitarianism. Meanwhile, Deleuze distinguishes between totalitarianism and fascism, and this distinction is informative in relation to his concepts about the macro- and micro-levels of politics, besides in itself being central as a portrait of fascism:

> Only microfascism provides an answer to the global question: Why does desire desire its own repression, how can it desire its own repression? The masses certainly do not passively submit to power; nor do they 'want' to be repressed, in a kind of masochistic hysteria; nor are they tricked by an idelogical lure.[39]

While the totalitarian state is characterized as state-conserving with a tendency to close in upon itself, the fascistic state is heading towards suicide. Fascism is destructivity that accelerates and does not stop at 'the enemy', but continues far into its own ranks. Whereas the totalitarian state will attempt to submit all other activities under the consolidation of power of the *macro-political* state apparatus, at no matter what cost, Deleuze regards fascism as a deterioration of *micro-political* fluxes towards self-destruction. The accelerating destructive micro-movements, – the anti-semitism, the humiliations and discipline of everyday life, the minor exclusions, the identifications with the group – did, in the case of Nazism, take over the state apparatus. This occurred to the extent that contrary to its conservative nature, the state came to serve dissolution and destruction, most particularly of itself. It was thus all the small fascisms simmering in the society of interwar Germany, as well as elsewhere in Europe, that gave Hitler such an enormous strenght and popularity, unlike for example a military *coup d'état*. The object for a great deal of the microanalyses of Horkheimer and Adorno from Critical Theory in Germany itself, was precisely the microfascisms sur-

rounding family, flag, and groups of youth culture, rather than the developments of the macro political institutionalization of fascism. 'How does
people become authoritarian?' was their counterpart to the question of how
desire can come to desire its own repression. The Nazi-machine of destruction did not hide that it was not only seeking the death of the enemy, but also
wanted the 'wedding and death' of the German people. The state-apparatus
became suicidal through microfascisms and the destruction penetrating
both the economy, prioritising weapons and the KZ-camps rather than food
production, and politics, continuing to send Germans to the front, while using the dwindling time to increase the 'production' of deaths in the camps.
Fascism is thus described as a kind of immanent movement like the ones of
capitalism, the fluxes of desire and the plane of philosophy, but now as
destructivity reproducing its conditions and constantly surpassing the limits of destruction.

Microfascisms are not to be done away with once and for all; they are getting no answer from the state or macropolitics since they are not directly accessible from their overcoded, hard segmentations. And worst of all, we are
creating them ourselves:

> Desire is never an undifferentiated instinctual energy, but itself the result from a
> highly developed, engineered setup rich in interactions: a whole supple segmentarity
> that processes molecular energies and potentially gives desire a fascist determina-
> tion. Leftist organizations will not be the last to secrete microfascism. It's too easy to
> be antifascist on the molar level, and not even see the fascist inside you, the fascist
> you yourself sustain and nourish and cherish with molecules both personal and col-
> lective.[40]

When Deleuze and Guattari are proposing that 'the ground of society is belief and desire' and thus is primarily to be understood at the level of
micropolitics, they do not deprive themselves of the possibility to take a position as to macropolitics, but they are acknowledging a certain impotency
in the macro-logical viewpoint with regard to these supple lines. Through
the conceptualization of fluctuations in beliefs and desire we are dealing
with the global question of our destructivity, making clear the importance
for Deleuze of the theme of anti-fascism.

The epochs of Marx and Deleuze

One could see Deleuze's new concepts as typical for the emergence of the
societies of control, as belonging to them. Like them he can operate with

gaslike networks, moving lines rather than essentialized units. Seeking independence from the categories of 'individual' and 'collective', he is emphasizing interactions crossing the segmentations in a non-deterministic
way, but also making developments more complex to grasp. The economic,
social, political and communicative fluctuations of the new system, the distributions of the 'dividual', the possibilities of creating adequate forms of resistance, 'seeking new weapons', and the ways in which human lives again
will be pressed, controlled and exposed in a new system, are phenomenas
which can be conceived by means of this micropolitics of lines, war machines and minorities.

The analytical apparatus of Marx on the other hand is sharing features
with the binary and serial structures of the disciplinary society, dealing with
the individual, the physical production and the class struggle. It is not quite
correct to say that Deleuze is the analyst of the society of control and communication, while Marx was the analyst of the society of discipline and production.[41] Rather, they are both creating their concepts in the actual world
while attempting to go beyond their milieu, seeking a new conceptual valid-
ity, and shedding new light over earlier societies and theories. This is how
Deleuze can reject central concepts of Marx while keeping others, when for
instance validating the basic problem as one of immanent capitalism, but
trying to understand its new forms. Marx emphasized that society and
economy are changing historically in ways that interact profoundly with
our 'selves' and our understanding and modes of life. Marx critically conceptualized the economical law of movement of the modern society as a
self-reproducing, blind 'rationality'. By his new focus on microscopic movements, Deleuze attempts to deepen an understanding of the work of the less
obvious machines and the new horizons of the life of the 'dividual'.

I have tried to show that Deleuze can be understood as a (post-) modern
heir to Marx on at least three fundamental points: firstly, that a political philosophy should be an analysis of capitalism as an immanent system; secondly, that the conceptual apparatus of such a philosophy at the same time
is both a presentation and a critique of the system; and thirdly that the positive impulse or utopia of the critique is emancipation understood as the occurrence in a micromovement of absolute becoming.[42] The key concepts of
micropolitics are, as we saw, divided into a trinity echoing a trinity in Marx,
but also rejecting and replacing the content of this: from contradicions, the
party and class to lines of flight, war machines and minorities.

The specific functions of the Deleuzian *political trinity* is rather informed
as a parallel construction to his own definition of the nature of the *philosophical trinity*: the creation of consistent *concepts*, sketching a fundamental plane
of immanence by mediation of the invention of conceptual personae. Poli-

tically, the fluctuations of desire and lines of flight are making a changing field or plane which 'grounds' societies. This could be seen as a micropolitical parallel to the presupposed plane of immanence 'grounding' a philosophy. The minorities, in their turn, are the 'actors' who can incarnate intense and creative lines of flight, in a parallel to how the conceptual personas give life to the concepts in a specific philosophy, as for instance 'Zarathustra's willing' does explicitly for Nietzsche or 'The Idiot knowing nothing' does implicitly for Descartes. And warmachines, finally, are the assemblages or microscopic segmentations in the fluctuations of desire – perhaps already microfascistic, perhaps as new social spaces – which the actors are giving life. Thus, one could say, they are describing the micropolitical parallel to the philosophical concept.

The concepts of the definition of philosophy are corresponding to those of social analysis and the definitions of both 'trinities' are strictly philosophical. The micropolitics Deleuze is presenting to us is a political philosophy with a remarkable inner consistency between the definition of philosophy, the definition of its character as political in relation to society and, finally, the specific working out of his own political concepts of society. Still, it would be wrong to say that 'the political Deleuze' is modelled after 'the ontological'. If there is any succession it is perhaps rather the other way around; the intuition of 'borderline-philosophical' anger and enthusiasm is a strong impulse in his thought all the way, be this on classical ontological problems, ethics, science or art.

Micropolitical critique and affirmation

As we have seen, a special trait in Deleuze's micropolitics is that the place of utopia and the functions of resistance are described within the same concepts as those comprehending the greatest micro- and macro-political dangers. In readings of Deleuze it can be tempting to place the static, the State, the consolidations of power as unambiguously confronting the emancipations of a 'smooth space' of deterritorializing and nomadic movement. But even though a great part of his sympathies are invested in the unpredictable forces of emancipatory change and creation that is described in the concept of 'lines of flight', it is also precisely these lines of flight and likewise, the positive concept of 'war machines', that can describe the greatest dangers: infinitely expanding fascism or infinitely expanding capitalism which are also warmachines. The Deleuzian concepts are thus not an apology for dissolution and anarchy, they are not a 'crusade of fragmentation' against 'the system' and they do not imply some 'pure force of desire'.

There is quite another subtle, double critique and constructivity at work which in a rather post-critical French milieu, are insisting on a critical emancipation, not to be abandoned to the mercy of the dangers of these emancipations themselves. The definition of new political concepts does not put any pure instances forwards as vehicles for a change of the unacceptable, since every model seems able to produce destructive and oppressive relations. Neither is it an emancipation from systems as such, but, as the inspiration from Spinoza showed, just as well an emancipation towards other types of 'open systems'. The investigation and affirmation of what we can do with consistency, conceptuality, and the rationality of encounters, are genuine elements of the micropolitcal philosophy of Deleuze; these are related to possibilities of creation, 'flight' and intensification. This affirmative aspect does not designate a resignation or retraditionalization on the grounds of status quo, but is more radical: Deleuze's philosophy intends to combine the anger against the epoch, against sufferings produced by our contemporary societies, with a creation of serene concepts on an absolute plane of immanence. To reach critically beyond the doxa as well as to express affirmatively the joy of intensifying forces on a plane of thought is Deleuze's philosophical ambition, within which he offers a variety of new concepts for the concrete, contingent and pragmatic practices of social reality to connect with – inviting encounters, but not controlling them. 'Radical pragmatism' is one of the paradoxical names of this thinking, expressing the challenge to invent new ways around conventional philosophical battles. Pragmatism with a radical implication of 'an absolute' is a paradox in the same manner as Deleuze's concept of 'transcendental empiricism' is.[43] Both formulations mark his attempt to point to a non-trivial issue: a creative, ontological passion of thought that distances itself by nature from the tendencies to reductionistic relativism of pragmatic communication and reductionistic positivism of empiricist experience, while still extracting and celebrating their immanent potential.

So, if Deleuze is the thinker providing us with concepts for the multiple, the moving, the immanent and the politically subversive, he is at the same time a philosopher cautiously providing us with the concepts to meet the dangers of precisely movement when it turns into unlimited destruction, of networks when they turn cynical and their control exhausting, and of immanent systems in the form of the global market of capital. The relation between the destructive and the creative war machines is like the relation between the relative immanence of capitalism and the absolute immanence of philosophy. For Deleuze, the critique of the first becomes the utopian movement of thought in the form of the second.

But philosophy is not a 'power', meaning that it does not mediate the exchange between fluctuations and segmentations; on the contrary, constructing concepts as real 'mental things', philosophy is itself creative, thus contributing to the world rather than just interpreting or representing it, but doing so in a 'virtual' or absolute way that does not directly push into the strategic zone of forces of the actual. In this respect Deleuze created the concepts of his micropolitics to make a 'simultaneous presentation and critique'. The utopia implied in such a critique is not to be formulated in a manifest, but should rather take place in, be performed by, philosophy itself, since this is the only place that is to its disposal. Philosophy and power-politics are operating in such different ways, in fields of a different nature, that they do not share their means or ends and cannot be reduced to one another. The philosopher is able to invent the philosophical 'actors' or conceptual personae, corresponding to his concepts, because they can act only within philosophy itself.[44] But he cannot invent minorities: they will be creating themselves in the concrete field and often in sufferings.[45] Therefore political philosophy has its strength in its utopian, absolute character and its necessary 'weakness' in its corresponding lack of power. The absoluteness of philosophy is in itself the attempt to present or express a utopian, creative movement, but it cannot do more than 'reach out for' the territory of relative social practice and call for new becomings.

6 Glamour and Glycerine

Surplus and Residual of the Network Society: From *Glamorama* to FIGHT CLUB

Patricia Pisters

> Perhaps the cinema is able to capture the movement of madness, precisely because it is not analytical and regressive, but explores a global field of coexistence.[1]

> In order to create soap, the yardstick of civilization, you must first render fat. And the best fat for making soap, because the salt balance is just right, comes from human bodies.[2]

David Fincher's film FIGHT CLUB (1999) and Bret Easton Ellis' novel *Glamorama* (1999) both deal with life at the end of the second millenium in which capitalism and media culture are determinant. In both works the main characters end up quite mad. At the end of FIGHT CLUB, 'Jack' and Tyler (Edward Norton and Brad Pitt) appear to be one single person: Tyler is Jack's schizophrenic double.[3] At the end of Brett Easton Ellis' *Glamorama*, the main character Victor Ward thinks he is victim of a conspiracy. He is constantly filmed, even in places he has not been and with people he does not know, until he becomes completely paranoid. One could see these denouements as rather forced narrative twists, especially in the case of FIGHT CLUB (in fact, many people were disappointed with this ending). However, as Deleuze and Guattari have argued in *Anti-Oedipus* and *A Thousand Plateaus*, the two volumes of *Capitalism and Schizophrenia*, schizophrenia and paranoia are the two dynamic poles of 'madness' in capitalism.[4] Inspired by FIGHT CLUB and *Glamorama*, I will explore the relevance of Deleuze and Guattari's views on capitalism and its madnesses for contemporary culture and society. Because their views largely have been written and received in the spirit of May '68, it is necessary to confront *Capitalism and Schizophrenia* with some of the major changes that have taken place over the last three decades.[5] It is necessary to determine which concepts from the Deleuzoguattarian toolbox are useful and in what way they can function in a productive way. Therefore, I will relate some of the ideas of Deleuze and Guattari on capitalism (the notions of surplus and residual) and schizophrenia (as opposed to paranoia) to Manuel Castells' massive study on the information age and what he calls the 'network society'. According to Castells, one of the biggest alterations in the network society is the increased importance of media culture. Audiovisual culture seems to have gone way beyond its (secondary) representative status. In his article 'Capital/Cinema' Jonathan Beller even goes as far as to argue that cinema is to our period what capital was to Marx.[6] So, the central issue that I will address on the following pages is the problem of the status of the audiovisual image in contemporary society in relation to capitalism.[7]

The network society in THE NET

Manuel Castells' *The Information Age* is widely recognized as one of the most extensive and valuable studies of society at the end of the second millenium.[8] In the first volume of his study, Castells elaborates on the rise of the network society. Let me first briefly recall a few concepts that characterize this network society. First of all, Castells emphasizes the idea of networks as the new organizational logic of the informational economy and society at large. As he states, networks have become the fundamental stuff of which new organizations are and will be made. Information technology plays a major role in all these networks: 'The network enterprise makes material the culture of informational/global economy: it transforms signals into commodities by processing knowledge.'[9] Keywords in these new organizational forms are global connectedness and local consistency. A further characteristic is that the logic of the network is more powerful than the powers in the network. Networks are fundamentally open structures that can grow in unpredictable ways.[10]

According to Castells, our highly technologically mediated network society has transformed our understanding of space and time. Instead of the traditional static conception of space as a 'space of place', we now experience space more as a process, a 'space of flows'.[11] While places are time-bounded, flows induce what Castells calls 'timeless time'. Timeless time is related to the selectivity of layers of time through informational networks and audiovisual media, which makes what we can live and relive instant and eternal presence instead of linear clock time. Furthermore, Castells relates this concept to time-space compression and the incredible speed of economical transactions ('the global casino'), to flextime work and to biological rhythms and life cycle changes through medical technology.[12] Spaces of flows and timeless time are characteristics of the informational networks that form contemporary society. The fundamental open structure of the network can cause dramatic reorganizations of power relationships, Castells argues: the power of flows takes precedence over the flows of power. Power holders are also relocated. In informational networks 'switches connecting the networks are multiple, the interoperating codes and switches between networks (...) are the privileged instruments of power. Thus, the switchers are the power holders. Since networks are multiple, the interoperating codes and switches between networks become the fundamental source in shaping, guiding, and misguiding societies.'[13]

If we consider cinema in a traditional way as a representation of what happens in real life, a very clear and clarifying example of these aspects of the network society can be seen in the film THE NET (Irwin Winkler, 1995). In this film, Sandra Bullock plays Angela Bennett, a young woman who works from her Los Angeles home as a computer virus-searcher for an IT company in San Francisco. During a holiday in Mexico, her purse (with her passport, credit cards and other personal belongings) is stolen, and she barely survives an attack on her life. When she recovers and goes back to her hotel, the receptionist tells her that according to the computer she has just checked out: there is no Angela Bennett in the hotel anymore. At the airport she finds out her social security number now matches with the name Ruth Marx. When she returns home, her house is for sale, and all her furniture has been moved out. In the police files Ruth Marx appears to be wanted for prostitution and drugs. Having no means to prove her identity, Angela has no other option than to go on the run and try to find out how the net operates against her.

It is easy to recognize in the plot of the film some aspects of Castells' network society. Although Angela Bennett still moves physically between different places, Mexico and the United States, which takes a certain amount of time, in the computer network, space and time have become flows and instants. She works in LA for a company in San Francisco that she has never actually visited, except through flows of information. Then she finds out she is not where she is supposed to be (she checked out of the hotel; her house has been sold). She is not even who she is supposed to be: her whole identity is erased or at least switched in no time. This is caused by a man who works for a criminal organization. He is a switcher, an example of Castells' power holder, who takes care of the informational misguidings that literally can delete one's whole identity. The organization this man works for produces an anti-virus program, The Gatekeeper. The organization deliberately messes up computer systems at airports and stock exchanges, in order to present themselves as the only safeguards of extremely valuable information and to force companies and organisations to buy their program. Because Angela has been sent information that can uncover The Gatekeeper's true intentions, economic reasons are behind Angela Bennett's erasure.

One could say of course that this is a Kafkaesque scenario that is not just related to the informational network society, but Castells' notions of time-less time and the power of flows (instead of slow bureaucratic flows of power) make this film an expression, in images and sounds, of the flipside of the network society. Another way of relating the space-time and power structures of the network society to this film is by looking at an important Deleuzian concept which I see at work here.

From discipline to control societies

In an interview with Antonio Negri in 1990, Deleuze speaks elaborately about the concept of *control societies*.[14] Here many of Castells' sociological ideas find their correspondence in political and philosophical terms. First of all, Deleuze (like Castells) emphasizes the role of capitalism, and the only universal thing there is in capitalism, that is, the market, 'the extraordinary generator of both wealth and misery'.[15] He then proposes an immanent analysis of capital in which he follows Marx: capitalism is an immanent sys-tem that constantly overcomes its own limits.

When he speaks of control societies, Deleuze draws on Foucault, who analysed disciplinary societies associated with the eighteenth, nineteenth and beginning of the twentieth century. Disciplinary societies operate by organizing major sites of confinement: family, school, military barracks, fac-tory, the hospital from time to time and sometimes prison. The guiding prin-ciple is to bring everything together and to give each thing its place and organize time. In short, the aim is to discipline society. According to Deleuze, disciplined societies have two poles: signatures standing for the individual and numbers or places in a register standing for their position in a mass. Money in a disciplinary society is related to moulded currencies containing gold as a numerical standard.

But societies and the way power is structured are changeable. And we have clearly moved into a new type of society which Deleuze labels as a con-trol society, where the confined spaces of the disciplinary society break down (or open). School, for instance, becomes continuing education; experi-ments with controlled home arrest instead of prison detention are frequent, and factory spaces become network businesses where it is no longer the aim to reach the highest possible production at the lowest possible wages but where ludicrous challenges and competition gain importance in a much less fixed way. Individuals become, what Deleuze calls, 'dividuals', no longer with a signature as individual marker, but linked to a digital code. And masses become samples, data or markets. Money is no longer related to a numerical standard, but to exchange rates, modulations depending on a calibration point that marks graduating values for various currencies. Deleuze compares discipline societies with moles. Control societies are more like snakes.

However, this does not mean that the disciplinary society has completely disappeared: prisons still exist and cheap labor in the third world that produces highly technological products for the global market. In Mexico, for instance, the working conditions resemble slavery; obligatory pregnancy tests for women, non-existent safety regulations and no labor unions demonstrate that cheap labor is still an important consideration as well. And in some sense institutions seem to reinforce themselves. At the beginning of the twenty-first century, the highest rate of people in prison ever has been reached in the United States, and the call for the return of family values is indeed loud. According to Michael Hardt, these developments indicate, however, that the disciplinary institutions are both in crisis and at the same time intensifying and extending over society as a whole, doing so outside the confinements of the institutions and into the society of control. Moreover, Hardt notices, the control society has become a global control society, led by a New Empire, the United States (as opposed to the older European Empires), who has become the power switchers that decide. [16]

Again we can recognize here elements of the network society: Castells' spaces of flows and timeless time are elements of the network society that can be related to the openness and snake-like movements of control society. In terms of power we could say that disciplinary societies know flows of power (the panopticum being a clearcut example), whereas in control societies we have to deal with the powers of flows that are no longer controllable but are present in all kind of different surveillance measurements: cameras, data surveillance and wiretapping. As Deleuze emphasizes, this is not to say that one society is better or worse than the other, but to find the structures of power and the possible weapons to resist too much concentrated power and especially to liberate desire, to think new things and experience new affects. [17] Coming back to THE NET, we could see this film as a representation or an example of the powers of flows in a control society (the new Empire) and the resistance of a single person in the net. And obviously it is necessary to know about the snake's coils in order to be able to resist its strangleholds. But, as I said at the beginning, cinema and other media are more than representations of the world. The omnipresence of cameras and computers is also an indication of the fact that the media are not only repre-

sentations nor even only control-instruments, but are also operating in another way in the network society.[18]

The culture of real virtuality: capital = cinema

As Castells reminds us, in the twentieth century, audiovisual culture took
historical revenge on the hierarchy of literary traditions: 'First with film and
radio, then with television, overwhelming the influence of written communication in the hearts and souls of most people. Indeed, this tension between
noble, alphabetic communication and sensorial, nonreflective communication underlies the intellectuals' frustration against the influence of television that still dominates social critiques of the masses.'[19] Castells has a
somewhat more complex view on media culture. Most interesting in respect
to audiovisual culture is his introduction of the idea of the 'culture of real
virtuality'. Castells explains this idea as follows:

> Perhaps the most important feature of multimedia is that they capture within their
> domain most cultural expressions, in all their diversity. Their advent is tantamount to
> ending the separation, and even the distinction, between audiovisual media and
> printed media, popular culture and learned culture, entertainment and information,
> education and persuasion. Every cultural expression, from the worst to the best, from
> the most elitist to the most popular, comes together in this digital universe that links
> up in a giant, a historical supertext, past, present, and future manifestations of the
> communicative mind. By doing so, they construct a new symbolic environment. They
> make virtuality our reality.[20]

According to Castells, reality, as experienced, has always been virtual because it is always perceived through symbols that frame practice with some
meaning that escapes their strict semantic definition. Therefore, the virtual
is also a real experience. The culture of real virtuality is a system 'in which
reality itself (that is, people's material/symbolic existence) is entirely captured, fully immersed in a virtual image setting, in the world of make believe, in which appearances are not just on the screen through which
experience is communicated, but they become the experience.'[21]

Again we can observe here a fundamental parallel between Castells' contemporary sociological observations and Deleuze's philosophical concepts.
Deleuze does not speak of the 'culture of real virtuality' as a (scientific) fact.
As a philosopher Deleuze speaks on a conceptual level of the virtual. Inspired by Bergson, he proposes to replace the classical real/virtual (in the
sense of unreal) opposition by the actual/virtual distinction. When he

makes this distinction between the actual and the virtual, however, Deleuze emphasizes, like Castells, that both the actual and the virtual are real. This does not mean that everything that is virtually contained in this world is or becomes actual. But to put it simply, the virtual (dreams, memories, imaginations, pure qualities of, for instance, light or color) is real insofar as it has an effect on us. In his two last texts, 'L'Immanence, une vie' and 'Le virtuel et l'actuel', Deleuze emphasizes that the virtual insists on the actual, and the actual influences the virtual.[22] In any case, with 'the culture of real virtuality' and the actual/virtual pair, both Castells and Deleuze assign an important role to cultural expressions: no longer is the virtual a by-product of society (as for example in traditional Marxist analysis), but it is at the heart of society, the centre of the system that can reposition society from within.[23]

We can see how Castells puts culture at the heart of society when he talks about 'the spirit of informationalism'.[24] This term is related to Max Weber's 'the spirit of capitalism' that he introduced in 1904. In the 'spirit of informationalism' capitalism is still operating as a dominant economic form, albeit in new, profoundly modified forms vis-à-vis the time of Weber's writing (changes that I just described in relation to the difference between disciplinary and control societies). As Castells states, in the spirit of informationalism the economic networks are glued together by a cultural dimension: culture is where many networks come together and depart again. Castells describes this culture as 'a culture of the ephemeral, strategic decision, patchworks of experiences and interests, rather than a charter of rights and obligations. It is a multi-faceted, virtual culture, as in the visual experiences created by computers in cyberspace by rearranging reality. The network enterprise learns to live within this virtual culture.'[25] It is not culture that is embedded in economy and capitalism, but it is economy (network enterprises) that is embedded in culture that has become capital itself.

As a philosopher, Deleuze has theorized the importance of cultural expressions as 'domains of thinking' in their own rights. In What is Philosophy? Deleuze and Guattari state that art thinks in percepts and affects, while philosophy thinks in concepts.[26] And in their own philosophical work, they often refer to writers (Kafka, Woolf), painters (Bacon) and filmmakers. Audiovisual culture seems to be even more important since Deleuze wrote two books on cinema.[27] In his article 'Capital/Cinema' Jonathan Beller elaborates on Deleuze's relationship to cinema. He argues that we might consider Cinema 1: The Movement-Image and Cinema 2: The Time-Image of equal importance for the twentieth century as Karl Marx's Capital was for the nineteenth century in that Deleuze's books develop concepts of capital as it colonizes the visual through and as cinema. Beller explains:

... the experiences of events in the cinema are, from the standpoint of capital, experiments about what can be done with the body by machines and by the circulation of capital. (...) If capital realizes itself as cinema, that is, if industrial capital gives way to the society of the spectacle, one might well imagine cinema, with respect to the body, geography, labor, raw material, and time, to have become the most radically deterritorializing force of capital itself. As production itself moves into the visual, the visceral, the sensual, the cultural, cinema emerges as a higher form of capital –.[28]

Beller makes an important claim here by establishing such an inextricable relation between capital and cinema that capital becomes an image: everything can be translated into (audio)visual terms: money is media.

It is true that in his cinema books, Deleuze has restricted himself to looking at the masterpieces of cinema, films by auteurs which he considers as machines that produce singular forms out of the flow of audiovisual material. In this respect, some elitist modernist thinking could be indeed attributed to Deleuze. If we now want to elaborate the role of cinema in political economy, it will be necessary to include also the non-masterpieces and other forms of media, like radio, television and tele- and cybercommunication. Very rightly, Beller proposes that we think of all human attention and consciousness as producers of value (and not just the masterpieces). In this way media culture can be analyzed for the multiple ways in which they have begun 'a global process of repaving the human sensorium, opening it up to the flow of ever-newer and more abstract commodities.'[29] Beller demonstrates that vision has become a form of work, and that technologies such as cinema and television are machines that replace the assembly line out of the space of the factory and put it into the home and the theater and the brain itself. In other words, he has demonstrated that not only, as Deleuze stated, 'the brain is the screen' but also the screen has become the brain.[30] Moreover, we can now see in which ways global organization has become so well organized as cinema/capital, whereby cinema must be considered in all its different media forms and is an immanent system, just like capital.

Glamorama: surplus and paranoia

One of the characteristics of cinematic/capitalist informational economy is that productivity comes with a residual. Manuel Castells talks about residuals such as energy supply, government regulation, education of the labour force and the whole category of services.[31] The residual is that which is left over, a remainder at the end of the usefulness of something. The word sounds rather negative and indeed that is the way it is used mostly. The word that Deleuze and Guattari employ to indicate 'that which is left over, a remainder' in capitalist culture is 'surplus'. This word has, however, a more positive connotation: excess over what is required, something extra, more value. In order to investigate these 'remainders' of contemporary culture, I would first want to look at some specific forms of surplus and residual that come from our audiovisual capitalist networks. Let me start with a simple thesis that I will then try to eleborate: stardom and glamour are the surplus values of audiovisually mediated capitalist culture. Both the media and the money are increasingly expanding, and so is its surplus value, glamour.

In the museum shop of the Museum of Modern Art in Paris, I recently found an interesting medicine cabinet. It contained nicely wrapped miracle drugs, produced by an art company called 'Jesus had a Sister Productions'. Besides pills to change your sexual preferences or skin color instantly, you could also buy 'Instant Fame Pills'. Success is guarantueed! Of course I bought the package, justifying it by the fact that I thought it was a nice metaphor for fame, glamour and stardom in our contemporary society: you can buy it, and it is as easy as swallowing a little pill. Money and media seem to be the only two conditions for stardom. Media-events such as *Big Brother* have provided the final proof of the influence of the camera on fame: if there are simply enough images of you around, fame will follow automatically.[32] Nominated for leaving the Dutch *Big Brother* house, resident Sabine became a true media-personality, a star who appeared regularly in many different media and signed autographs for her fans; and money will follow fame: all *Big Brother* residents found themselves being offered lucrative deals. And if you do not (yet) have access to the camera, you can always buy stardom; and fame will follow money. L'Oréal uses a whole series of stars (like Heather Locklear from *Melrose Place*, and Andy MacDowell from FOUR WEDDINGS AND A FUNERAL) to invite women to buy their products. The slogan 'Because I'm worth it. Aren't you?' implies that with the right commodities the surplus value of glamour will automatically endow us with radiance. In the same spirit gossip magazines present the recipe of makeup artist Sarah Monzani who unveils the secrets of Madonna's success with the help of Max Factor: the Madonna Factor, now available for all.

In the first half of this century, glamorous stardom was only available in and around the spotlights of Hollywood. Stars and glamour were far removed from daily life, Hollywood an unreachable 'dream factory'. Nevertheless, stars were influential in the daily life of many men and especially women. In her book *Star Gazing* Jackie Stacey reports the results of an elaborate empirical research on the influence of Hollywood stars on the life of ordinary British women in the Forties and Fifties.[33] Stars like Betty Grable, Rita Hayworth, Joan Crawford and many others were mainly fascinating because of the beautiful clothes they wore and the fantastic settings in which they moved. During and right after the war these dream images served an escapistic function.

Nevertheless, many also identified with the stars. Fans changed their identity and looks according to the example of their favorite star. With the increasing wealth in the Fifties, it became easier to actually take on the looks and lifestyle of a star: 'I favoured Lauren Bacall,' says one of the fans. 'My colouring was the same as hers, I wore my hair in a similar style and wore the same type of tailored clothes... matching shoes, gloves and handbag were a "must". (...) they were my "trademark" for years.'[34] In the Fifties, because of the growth of capitalist commodity culture, ordinary people could lead a more 'glamorous' life. But for a few decades Hollywood remained nevertheless covered with a distant utopian glow.

Everything changes with the arrival of MTV in the Eighties. Of course Hollywood is still attractive, as was clear from the hype around Leonardo di Caprio when he starred in TITANIC. But in the meantime many other types of stars have emerged. In her videoclip 'Vogue', Madonna pays a 1990s homage to the early Hollywood stars. At the same time she makes clear that in the age of MTV new stars have risen: models, pop musicians and actually everybody who would like to be star, provided that you wear the right clothes, strike the right pose (vogue) and let yourself be captured by a camera.

In his novel *Glamorama*, Bret Easton Ellis emphasizes the central role of MTV. Strikingly often he refers to this television station, the style programs, the videoclips and the clothes worn by the VJs and artists. The main character in the book is a model, Victor Ward. His average day consists of a photoshoot, a training session in the hippest sportschool of New York, a fashion show, an interview for MTV's House of Style, repetitions with his band and organizing a DJ for the opening night of a new club which he is setting up with a partner. In the meantime he calls on his Motorola cell phone about the guestlist for the club (in this way all 'real life' stars are mentioned in the book), cheats on his girlfriend (supermodel Chloe Byrnes) with the fiancee of his business partner, and courts a girl in Tower Records, who wears the perfect clothes and listens to the right music. In a humiliating way, Easton Ellis paints a portrait of modern society through the eyes of Victor Ward, in which Calvin Klein, Armani, Gap, DKNY and Dolce & Gabbana decide the looks; in which silicone breasts, sunglasses and cell phones are a 'must'; in which sushi and salads form dinner and Evian, diet Coke and (occasionally) champagne are the main beverages. Victor himself is very self-conscious about the poses he has to take in order for his beautiful abdomen to be just visible from beneath his Comme des Garçons t-shirt. The empty and cold relationships between all these glamourous people are portrayed with cutting satire. Sometimes there is a feeling that breaks through the shiny superstructure. For instance, there is the moment when Victor's girl-friend panics when she watches a tv-programme on the dangers of breast implants. The characters do not gain any sympathy by this, although it does make them vulnerable. Except for Victor, who lightly, luxuriously and lus-ciously continues his glamorous life.

This glamorous life lasts until the moment when he is offered a lot of money to find an old friend in Europe. Victor leaves for England and France and all of a sudden finds himself among a group of terrorists. Or is it just a movie in which Victor is playing? In the first half of the book, the glamorous surplus value of materialism has been uncovered as empty and cold but nevertheless also hip and cool. But in the second half of the book, the story changes into a nightmare in which it is no longer possible, neither for Victor nor for the reader, to distinguish between the real and the virtual. Every-where there are cameras, directors and paparazzi. This was also the case in the first half of the book, but gradually the distinction between Victor's real experiences become blurred with film scripts. He is constantly confronted with compromising photographs and videotapes. In the first half of the book he just denies, again and again, that he is the person in the image. He then just seemed to be a terrible superficial and irresponsibly narcissistic person who does not remember and does not care with whom he has spent time and where he has been. He just remembers what he was wearing.

But in the second half it all becomes much scarier: videotapes are now re-ally manipulated, and denial is futile. The manipulable image culture has blurred the borders between fact and fiction. Glamorous existence in the culture of real virtuality has turned into a violent movie. Glycerine tears have become panic attacks and violent bombs. And paranoia has become the unhealthy condition of life. At the end of the book, Victor finds himself in a sort of resthouse in Italy. He still feels like he is being filmed all the time. The only remaining stars are the ones in the sky. *Glamorama* witnesses the implication of the media in our 'culture of real virtuality' and the embeddedness of the network entreprises when the surplus value – glam-our through commodities and cameras – turns into a paranoid nightmare of manipulation and fascist violence through the camera's never ending sur-veillance.

Glycerine: FIGHT CLUB's residual and schizophrenia

With this violent and paranoid turn of *Glamorama*, Bret Easton Ellis seems to have emphasized what is hidden underneath the superficial beauty of sparkling stars and glamourous poses that come to us through the media. One of the 'real life' celebrities that Easton Ellis mentions is David Fincher. Fincher started out his career on MTV, where he directed among other things Madonna's clip 'Vogue'. With his latest film FIGHT CLUB, Fincher, too, seems to take a position against the superficiality of what is termed in this film, the 'IKEA-nesting instinct', Calvin Klein and other glamorous brands. Aesthetically, he demonstrates this beautifully at the beginning of the film, where main character Jack (Edward Norton) looks into an IKEA-catalogue, the computer designs his wishes and at the end of the scene, these furnish his actual appartment. This blend from catalogue to computer to actual home decoration again makes clear how close the virtual and the actual are related. However, Jack's apartment is rather empty and soulless.

The fact that Jack is not happy with his carefully composed and purchased life is made clear through his attacks of insomnia. He finds temporary relief by finding support as an illegal (because not actually sick) visitor to all kinds of self-help groups, which focus on everything from testicular and blood vessel cancer to the formation of brain parasites. But he finds his 'true self' (or his other self, as we will learn) when he meets Tyler Durden (Brad Pitt). Together they start a fight club that soon has branches in all major cities in the United States. Of course, the violence of the fights is a literal attack on beauty. Tyler and Jack look with contempt at Calvin Klein underwear ads and cherish their (self)mutilations as an act against glamour.[35] The most powerful symbol in the film, however, is fat, particularly body fat. At the beginning of the film, body fat was introduced when Jack, still in his job as damage reporter, has to investigate a burned-out car to see if it is worthwhile for the insurance company to recall the car, for later we learn that the cars are deliberately badly manufactured so money can be made from their repair. The seat in the car is covered in body fat, burned from the victim's body. In the spectator's mind, immediately a picture of a wealthy, fat man driving his expensive car pops up and is destroyed.

Later on, Tyler teaches Jack how to make soap and bombs. In order to do so they take the ultimate residual element of glamour-culture as the basic material for their products: they go to a liposuction clinic and steal liposuction fat. From that body fat they skim the glycerine from which they make both glycerine soap and nitroglycerine bombs. The soaps they sell to big department stores ('It was beautiful, we sold rich ladies their own fat asses').

The explosives are used to blow up creditcard company buildings and other symbols of capitalist network enterprises. In a very powerful way the residual (fat) is turned into surplus again (glycerine soap, glamour) and into the ultimate destructive weapon against surplus and the whole network society, nitroglycerine bombs.

At the end of the film Jack is Tyler, or Tyler is Jack.[36] This schizophrenic twist of the movie is no more than a simple consequence of the logic of the network society. Arguing from Castells' concept of the culture of real virtuality, it is just very logical that, as in Victor Ward's case, the virtual become just as real as the actual. The difference between Victor and Jack/Tyler is the difference between paranoia and schizophrenia. To understand this it is necessary to return to the work of Deleuze and Guattari and their immanent analysis of capitalism and the material and mental states it produces.

Immanence and micro-politics: capitalism and schizophrenia

As I said earlier, Deleuze and Guattari propose an immanent analysis of capitalist society, which carries in itself all the dangers and possibilities the system can possibly produce. The notion of surplus is precisely such a concept that is at work in an immanent analysis of capitalism. In *Anti-Oedipus* Deleuze and Guattari describe surplus value as follows:

> Instead of simply representing the relations of commodities, it enters now, so to say, into relations with itself. It differentiates itself as original value from itself as surplus-value.[37]

Furthermore, they state that surplus value (glycerine) is always absorbed, but also constantly injects anti-production (nitroglycerine) which they call schizophrenization. Capitalism calls for its dominant cultural and organizational forms at the same time as it produces its breakdown, which is a fundamentally schizophrenic process. It is this moment of coding, decoding and recoding that is so wonderfully made conscious in Jack and Tyler's actions throughout the film, animated as it is through schizo-flows. As Deleuze and Guattari put it:

> Our society produces schizos in the same way it produces Prell shampoo or Ford cars, the only difference being that the schizos are not saleable. (...) Yet it would be a serious error to consider the capitalist flows and the schizophrenic flows as identical, under the general theme of a decoding of the flows of desire. Their affinity is great, to be sure: everywhere capitalism sets in motion schizo-flows that animate 'our' arts and

'our' sciences, just as they congeal into the production of 'our own' sick, the schizo-phrenics.[38]

It may now seem that Deleuze and Guattari romanticise the clinical schizo-phrenic. In fact, they have indeed been regularly accused of that. However, they do not invite all of us to become pathological cases. Just as the term 'rhi-zome' is stolen from biology, 'schizophrenia' is taken from psychiatry, in fact from Lacan. But they differentiate schizophrenia as a process from schizophrenia as an entity or as a mental illness. Schizophrenia as a process operates in a broad sociohistorical field, rather than on a narrow psycho-logical scale.[39] As Eugene Holland argues in his *Introduction to Schizoanalysis*, at worst (when capitalism is unable to sanction the process of schizophrenia that it has itself produced) the result is clinical schizophrenia. At best, schizophrenia takes the form of a viable social practice and the joys of the unbridled, free-form of human interaction.[40] As such, schizophrenia is only one pole of the economic, cultural and libidinal dynamics of capital. The other pole is designated by the term paranoia: 'if we understand schizo-phrenia to designate unlimited semiosis, a radically fluid and extemporane-ous form of meaning, paranoia by contrast would designate an absolute system of belief where all meaning was permanently fixed and exhaustively defined by a supreme authority, figure-head, or god.'[41]

In their political philosophy, Deleuze and Guattari make a distinction be-tween molar movements (large segments in society, where the 'binary-ma-chine' divides the world into oppositions: private-public, man-woman, young-old, healthy-sick) and molecular movements (invisible micro-move-ments that affect, empower or disempower us, private thoughts and feel-ings, breaks with the system).[42] The difference between the molar and the molecular explains the difference between paranoia and schizophrenia. As Deleuze and Guattari put it:

> Paranoia and schizophrenia can be presented as the two extreme oscillations of a pen-dulum oscilating around the position of a socius as a full body and, at the limit, the body without organs, one of whose sides is occupied by the molar aggregates, and the other populated by molecular elements.[43]

In this respect it is significant that at the beginning of FIGHT CLUB, as we travel through Jack's brain, molecular processes are being visualized. There are other contemporary films that deal specifically with schizophrenia, such as David Lynch's LOST HIGHWAY (1997) and Spike Jonze's BEING JOHN MALKOVICH (1999); these also play with normally invisible mental move-ments.[44] By contrast, in *Glamorama* we always remain outsiders, looking at the molar surfaces. The emphasis on the revolutionary potential of molecu-lar schizophrenia is what Deleuze calls 'micropolitics'.

Both the molar and the molecular lines have their dangers: over-codification for the molar line (surveillance, fascism, Victor's paranoia) and microfascism and self-destruction for the molecular line (schizophrenia that becomes so destructive that it desires its own repression). The fact that all these lines can be operative correlates with the predicament that in a network society nothing is ever fixed. Everything moves in dynamic relations: cameras for fame can turn into surveillance and manipulative cameras, becoming sources of paranoia. *Glamorama* shows how the surplus value of capitalist media culture can become a source for paranoia, surveillance cameras being the ultimate meaning-imposing 'god'. Schizo-strategies can offer resistance to capitalism and release enormous personal and critical freedom[45], but it can also turn into fascism; and Richard Barbrook has demonstrated how the 'holy foolishness' of Deleuze and Guattari themselves can be subjected to this danger.[46]

It is precisely this ambiguity between freedom and fascism that is also clear in FIGHT CLUB. Tyler/Jack's schizo-strategies are clearly directed at releasing pressures from capitalist culture. When Tyler says things like 'the things you own end up owning you' and 'you are not your car or your credit card' he clearly aims at setting free new ways of living and making meaning. Also, the fights themselves are deterritorializing strategies of capitalist surplus value. Freedom, according to Deleuze also has a physical sense: ' "to detonate" an explosive, to use it for more powerful movements'.[47] This revolutionary potential is literally made visible in the images and sounds. But Fincher has also been accused of having made a fascist film. And indeed there are many elements in the film that relate to both molar and molecular forms of fascism: the black shirts of the men of Project Mayhem, the giving up of their names, except in death when they ritually start singing 'His name was Robert Paulsen'. It is at these moments where the problem of freedom turns into a problem of unfreedom that is also addressed in *Anti-Oedipus*: 'How could the masses be made to desire their own repression?' and to which Deleuze returns at many instants.[48]

In an article on freedom in the work of Deleuze and Guattari, Aden Events and Mani Haghighi (et al.) see this problem of unfreedom as the negative effect of the abundance of freedom, the impossibility to affirm and sustain freedom.[49] Moreover, they relate freedom to the deterritorializing of thought (thinking the unthought), the affirmation of pure chance (amor fati) and the power to decide, which is however not a power that we own:

> We are not the authors of our destiny. Even 'the gods themselves are subject to the ... sky-chance.' This is why theft is primary to thought: because 'another always thinks in me, another must also be thought.' The power of decision is realized in the thought

of these others. This is not a power that we own; it is not a power that can be owned. It is only available by theft. We must steal our freedom.[50]

This idea of 'another always thinking in me' might be another explanation of the schizophrenic resolution in FIGHT CLUB. Not only does the whole film present a process of schizophrenization, but also, in order to be free, Jack needed his other, Tyler, to think in him.[51] Still, the problem of freedom remains related to the problem of unfreedom and will always return as such.[52]

I have tried to argue that it is precisely this dangerous ambiguity of political lines and movements between freedom and unfreedom that we are confronting in the network society. Surplus and residuals are related to paranoia (at the level of society at large, the large segments) and schizophrenia (at the level of one's own body and mind, the micromovements). They can be both healthy (THE NET, the initial fight clubs) and unhealthy (*Glamorama*, the fascist elements in FIGHT CLUB). In any case these are elements of the network society that Castells as a sociologist of contemporary society does not talk about. An immanent and philosophical analysis of 'cinema and capital' as proposed by Deleuze and Guattari seems to be very appropriate for the evaluation of the media culture of real virtuality. Thinking itself seems to have become an 'art of the virtual', fundamentally related to cinema (and by extension all other media): 'cinema of thinking or the virtual as never seen before' as André Parente puts it.[53] Because of its richness of content and expression, cinema seems to be able to capture the broad socio-historical fields ('the global fields of co-existence') that constitute our contemporary madness. Cinema seems to be at the heart of the society of control, at the same time producing information, communication and control as well as an intelligence of the virtual that insist and subsist, and that can produce resistance.

To conclude, we may say that glycerine soap, glycerine tears and nitro-glycerine bombs are the slippery, snake-like and highly explosive surplus values and residual matter that we seem to take as our luggage into the new millenium in which audiovisual cultural products can still reflect and represent the network society (THE NET). But more importantly they are an integral part of it (*Glamorama*) and offer at the same time immanent possibilities of deterritorializing resistance and reterritorializing recodings (FIGHT CLUB). Culture, seen as a culture of real virtuality, has become 'a new regime for the production and circulation of economic value at a new level of economic practice as well as economic conceptualization'.[54] Cinema and other forms of media have become like capital, the principal form of thought and consciousness, the center of society that can shift in levels between virtual and actual and in which the virtual seems to gain ever growing importance.

They constitute the various levels we move through in order to help reposition ourselves and society from within.[55]

7   Is Bess a Bike?

Gender, Capitalism and the Politics of a BwO in Lars von Trier's BREAKING THE WAVES

Frans-Willem Korsten

A rosette of screens

'The Face is Christ' is one of those formulas through which Deleuze and Guattari produce a building block of their work.[1] The production of meaning is hooked on to a theoretical notion, 'face'. In its ideological form the face, such as Christ's face, is a model or a standard on the basis of which things are to be judged. In terms of its construction, operation, and effect, 'the face is a politics'.[2] To get away from this model, to change the politics of how meaning is made via that model, new faces have to be produced. In Lars von Trier's BREAKING THE WAVES (1996), we are presented with such a face, up front and close up. As the very first image of the film we see the face of Bess McNeill (Emily Watson). And in the course of the movie she will appear as an alternative to the 'man'/Christ. In this respect the film can be seen to act out a process of 'freed faciality'.[3]

Yet for me as a viewer, in freeing one face the film appeared to affirm the emprisonment of another one. I was not the only one who had ambiguous feelings while experiencing this film. The Internet collection of reviews and discussions on the film presents vehement adoration and rejection, and sometimes hilarious exchanges of arguments. The ambiguity seems to have one major source. While fleeing the model of man-Christ, Bess fuses with another model-face: that of the serving and abused woman. As Jonneke Bekkenkamp argues, the film unfortunately reproduces a hierarchical division that plays a major role in many forms of Christianity: the division between higher spiritual love and the lower instrumentalized body.[4] As that division is asymmetrically gendered, women are given the position of the embodied one, hence the servant, the one who has to give herself away for the sake of others. According to Bekkenkamp and many others, Bess fits into that pattern. More extremely put, some argued that the film is simply misogynist.[5]

Whereas I can underwrite important parts of the criticism of Bess as a sacrificial figure, I have three problems with it. The criticism restricts itself to
only one or two screens that are operative in the film – screen meaning one
'repertoire of representations by means of which our culture figures all of
those many varieties of "difference" through which social identity is inscribed'.[6] Considered rhetorically, in terms of its effect, there is never one
screen; effects connected to a film are at the center of a 'rosette' of screens.
Most specifically, in the case of BREAKING THE WAVES, everybody emphasizes
the screens of sexual politics and religion, without considering how the film
connects these to desire as it stands at the heart of capitalism, the system that
according to Deleuze and Guattari 'continually draws near to its limit,
which is a genuine schizophrenic limit'.[7] Secondly, the film is about judgment and about people who are trying to escape judgment. Most critics saw
this judgment as a religious matter only; they gave their verdict
unproblematically, whereas the film was trying to make (any) judgment a
topic of reflection. Thirdly, very few people paid careful attention to any actor other than the two major protagonists.

My thesis will be that the major issues the film explicitly addressed – religion and love – are not the film's main issue; in relation to capitalism they
are derivate issues. Within this context religion and love are redefined
through a rosette of screens that produce the film and that the film itself produces. To say it in other words, the film locates these themes simultaneoulsy
and differently within the rosette of screens. Let me first go into one distinct
aspect of religion which is faith. This aspect is most important for people
who want to 'free a face', who want to break away and enter unknown territories. It is an aspect that connects the film with medieval literature.[8]

A medieval intertext and the force of faith: Bess and the book

The camera work of Robby Müller in BREAKING THE WAVES suggests this is a
home movie, or a documentary. Recurringly, Bess is affirming the camera,
looking as if the figure behind the camera is someone she knows. The image
has a rough and grainy texture. The camera closely follows the movement of
the characters. During dialogues it swings from one face to another as if
there is only one camera actually present. Many people (particularly in
America) have complained that the film makes you feel nauseous. Sometimes there are jump cuts, sometimes it seems as if the cameraman forgot to
push the button. There are no tracking shots, no instances of panning. The

camera is never stable. Frequently, the focus lacks sharpness. Finally, there is the use of natural light. As Von Trier himself stated in an interview with Stig Björkman: 'The rough, documentary style in which I made the film, a style which actually annuls the film and contradicts it, has the effect that we accept the story as such.'[9] Indeed, all these features suggest immediacy and spontaneity, contradicting the notion of a directed film. [o]

In sharp contrast with the quasi-chaotic features, the film is carefully divided into a prologue, seven chapters and an epilogue, all indices to a book. At eight moments in the film we are offered an extended painterly and panoramic view of the landscape, shots actually made in cooperation with the artist Per Kirkeby.[11] During these moments there is extra-diegetic music, which is absent in the home movie/documentary sections. On the screen we see chapter headings, for instance: 'Chapter 1: Bess Gets Married'. The chapters imply that a story is being told in stages, and that these stages were planned by an author or director.[12] As indices to a book, chapters open up an intertextual field that contradicts the documentary style and connects the film to literature. In my case, one scene triggered such an intertextual reference particularly strongly. At the end of BREAKING THE WAVES, Bess's lover and husband Jan (Stellan Skarsgård), together with his comrades, give Bess a seaman's burial. After having dropped the body into the sea at night, they appear to have done the right thing at the right place because the next morning they can hear church bells ringing in the sky above them. This theme of the church bells appeared twice earlier. Jan's best friend Terry (Jean-Marc Barr) asks (after Bess and Jan's wedding) why the priest is not tolling the bells; the answer is that the church has not got any. Later, Jan asks the priest why the church does not have bells. Here the answer is that bells are not needed to worship God. Bess then playfully suggests that Jan go hang the bells in the tower. The implication is that Bess and Jan will be able to do so because they love each other and can have fun in the process. But Jan is involved in a nasty accident that will lead indirectly to Bess' death and her burial; a burial that is then festively framed by the bells at sea.

What was my reading of intertextual resonance? The hearing of bells at sea is a well known literary phenomenon in medieval literature. It made me think of the medieval story *Brandaan*. Between the film and this story a resonance occurred. A resonance that, in itself, would be of little use except that it allowed me to see the film's treatment of religion in a different light. Instead of focusing on the model of Christ or saintlike love, I was led to consider religion's ability to let people break away from their restraining contexts.[13] The story in *Brandaan* is as follows. Brendan is an abbot, who at the beginning of the story is safely at home, reading a book. The book tells him that there is another world beneath the one he knows, where night

starts when day starts in his world. Fantastic tales like this particular one ir-
ritate him beyond measure. He angrily throws the book in the flames of a
nearby fire. The book is destroyed, and as a consequence Brendan is pun-
ished by God. He is commanded by an angel to set out in a boat in order to
see the true wonders of the world and to describe them in order to repair the
damage done to the book. At the end of the journey, Brendan and his comrades are at sea and then hear church bells ringing from below as if there is a
city at the bottom of the sea. Brendan asks his writer whether he has written
down the event and whether there remains more to be seen. The writer answers that with this story the book is full and therefore finished. Brendan
goes home, where he is received like a saint. Soon thereafter he dies, and his
soul is carried away by the archangel Michael.

On the basis of this short summary of Brendan's story, the immediate allusion is clear: both BREAKING THE WAVES and *Brandaan* end with church
bells that toll where they should not be able to toll: in the middle of the sea.
As such, the bells indicate the existence of a world other than the one we
know. The bells are a metaphysical index, and in this respect they also point
to what in both texts motivates the action of the protagonists and the making of the text. That motivation concerns the relation between the fantastic
and the real. Brendan did not believe in the wonders of the world that were
described in the book, and he destroyed it. Bess is described by characters in
the film – in the beginning and at the end – as a kind of wonder in this world;
and she is destroyed as well. The link with *Brandaan* shows that one reason
for her destruction might be that Bess is 'too good to be true'. This formula is
also projected as a question towards the audience.

The most important parallel between the two texts concerns the element
of faith and also the title of chapter six in the film. In this chapter Bess starts
to do things that she previously could not even have imagined daring. What
makes that possible? The co-text of *Brandaan* offers an answer. Brendan's
voyage is based on the old Irish notion of the *peregrinatio pro Deo* (the pilgrimage for God). The idea was to choose voluntarily to live an isolated life.
The most respectable pilgrimage (the *potior peregrination*) consisted of leaving your land and delivering yourself to the currents of the sea to see where
they would bring you. Through this pilgrimage, the monks demonstrated
their willingness to live like the lowest, for they chose the same fate as heavy
criminals, who were also delivered to the sea in a boat. The powers of wind
and sea – God – would, or would not, take care of the fate of criminals and
monks. In comparison, Bess is both a saint and a criminal. Her willingness
to choose the lowest life is concretely enacted through her choice to prostitute herself. Her mother (Sandra Voe) warns her: 'Do you have any idea
what it's like to be cast out?' And a little later: 'It would kill you.' This does

not stop Bess. In the end she goes out to sea and delivers her fate into the hands of God, though she knows that this may mean her death. Her act is not just an act of self-destruction, as I will argue below. It is also an attempt to break free, to go beyond existing boundaries. And the one thing that allows her to be able to do this is faith.[14]

Bess's faith and consequent breaking through the boundaries of the world as she knew it have a formal analogy at the end of the film. The tolling church bells also act as a 'breaking through', and as a final variant of chapter-indication. The camera moves into the clouds, and there we see two huge bells tolling in the air, although it is not possible to see how they are suspended. In addition to being an allusion to a film that was also about an impossible love, Douglas Sirk's ALL THAT HEAVEN ALLOWS, the shot of the bells points emphatically to the fact that this film was not home-made but consciously directed. With the bells, like with the chapter headings, the home movie or documentary style is broken with. The final shot can be seen as a disruption – with the camera breaking through the clouds – of everything that was presented so far through the documentary style as true. But whereas the protagonist's breakthrough was fuelled by faith, the formal breakthrough seems to deconstruct it. I shall come back to that asymmetry at the end of this article. For now I conclude that not just the protagonist of the film, but also the structure of the film point to the probing of limits, of breaking through, discovering and deconstructing elements considered by Deleuze and Guattari as hall marks of capitalism. Indices to capitalism recur elsewhere and even more strongly.

Jesus: love as labor

In their reworking of the Oedipus complex, Deleuze and Guattari argue that Freud had it wrong at several levels but was right in: 'having determined the essence or nature of desire, no longer in relation to objects, aims or even sources (territories) but as an abstract, subjective essence – libido or sexuality'.[15] An analogy to this conception of desire is one aspect of the idea of love as it was propagated by Jesus: love as an abstract subjective essence that is not confined to one person, but that is free-floating and can be bestowed on anyone. The figure of Jesus and this free-floating conception of love is asymmetrically distributed over and incorporated into the figures of Jan and Bess.

Jan is Jesus-like in that he literally comes down from heaven; he is air-born and flown in by helicopter.[16] Like Jesus he loves the simple in mind:

Bess is considered to be either psychically ill or a simpleton. Yet Jan marries this seemingly simple-minded woman, respects her, loves her, and makes love to her. Furthermore, he is the spiritual leader of a group of men. He is rebellious against his employers and the ascetic orthodox church elders. He wears a kind of sheepskin coat. When one of his comrades seems to be dead, covered with oil after an explosion, he wipes the thick oil from his face and brings him back to life. And he himself is literally resurrected, first brought back to life after his hearts stops functioning during an operation and later resurrected because he has been lame and learns to walk again. Finally, after her first act of prostitution Bess compares herself to Mary Magdalene, further associating Jan with Jesus. Most importantly, Jan 'makes' love. In this context his so-called perversity still affirms the Jesus-index. When he is largely in coma, on the verge of dying, he asks Bess if she thinks that being on the verge of dying brings out the worst in people; later he scribbles down that he is 'evil in the head'. On the screen-plane of religion, Jan's isolation, his inability to do anything and his resulting perversity are an analogy to Jesus' retreat to the desert where he was tempted by the devil. Yet in the case of Jan the evil that comes out is not countered but worked through: it results in a continuation of Jan's 'making' love. More love needs to be made, be it a love that is called perverse: he asks Bess to go out, fuck other men, and tell him about it.

The mechanical, machine-like quality of this love-making is not an isolated feature. In the first half of the film, Jan's work on the oil platform only seems to function to qualify him as an outsider, or as a realistic detail that makes him life-like. Yet the scenes are structurally linked to the rest of the story. The men are drilling, trying to find new oil; Jan is the one who knows where to find it. The element of mechanical production is paramount here, and it is a process of production that knows no end. Even after Jan has been hospitalized, his men come to tell him where they will be moving next. A strong visual link between making oil and making love is made, again, via the theme of bells. When Jan has rescued his comrade from the oil, a huge iron bar swings down, and hits Jan on the head. The way in which it swings resembles exactly the swing of a clapper, hitting Jan's head as if it is the rim of a bell. As a result, Jan is immobilized and so is his production on the double plane of love and labor.

For Deleuze and Guattari desire is not the need to fill in a lack, but the positive search for and pleasure in 'variation and ramification'.[17] This is what Jan is about: he is the one who makes fun, who looks for the new, who in desiring moves on. This continuous desire needs a counterbalance:

> at the very heart of production, within the very production of this production, the
> body suffers from being organized in this way, from not having some other organiza-

tion, or no organization at all [...] The automata stop dead and set free the unorganized mass they once served to articulate. The full body without organs is the unproductive, the sterile, the unengendered, the unconsumable.[18]

Significantly, this is a rather apt description of Jan's state after his accident. Although the concept of the Body without Organs is not in any sense a real body, Jan's body is an index to it, since it is literally dis-organized, lame, unconsumable most significantly, in the sense that having sex is impossible. An unorganized mass is set free. In this case the sexual desire between Jan and Bess which was organized through their matrimony becomes disorganized. Having been set free, it results in what Dr. Richardson (Adrian Rawlins) and Bess' sister-in-law Dodo (Katrin Cartlidge) call perversity. Due to his inability to move, Jan now becomes a recording machine. As a recorder of connections instead of the producer of connections, Jan is a Body without Organs.

Bess' analogy to Jesus works out differently. Bess is pure or 'good' as Dodo describes it at the beginning or Dr. Richardson at the end. There is something in the face of Bess that makes her look like a child, which enforces her innocence.[19] She is the one who offers herself, for instance to Dr. Richardson with the words: 'You can have me now', as if she is a piece of holy bread to be swallowed. She thinks her sacrifice will save Jan, and in prostituting herself she becomes the scapegoat of the entire community. Finally, her body is taken away from the grave, just like the body of Jesus, and as the bells at the end appear to suggest, she is taken up into heaven. Most importantly, to all intents and purposes, her biological father does not exist in the film. Rather, Bess talks to her 'Father' whose servant she is, both metaphysically and literally as cleaner of the church. In the end when she knows she is going to be killed, she laments that 'Father' does not answer her; like Jesus, she feels forsaken by Him.

Unlike Jan, Bess does not make love; she gives it. As Dodo says at the wedding: 'Thank you for all you have given me.' So, there certainly is a strong, gendered asymmetry in giving and taking. That asymmetry is amplified in the title of the first chapter: 'Bess Gets Married'; the passive of 'Bess Marries'. Bess explicitly states that she has been waiting for Jan. These are all elements that confirm the criticism of the film for portraying Bess as the prototypical good wife. As Xandra Schutte says: 'Bess is good like all women have been good for centuries, that is how men for centuries have liked women to be good. Not word but body, speechless, sacrificing, masochistic and hysterical.'[20]

Yet like Jan, Bess produces a surplus: on the plane of meaning-production. Instead of making love, Bess makes meaning. For instance she desires so strongly that Jan return from the platform that she thinks his accident, which indeed brought him back home, is the effect of her desire. Later, Jan hallucinates that he is in a bus; he wonders what Bess is doing in 'this bus', and asks her to come to him, in the back. Accordingly, when Bess is in a real bus and a man walks to the back of the bus, she follows him and jerks him off, thus filling the hallucination of Jan with a 'real' meaning. In a conversation with Dodo, she finally confesses that whenever Jan is feeling a little bit better, it is because of her actions.

More abstractly, whereas Jan busied himself with concrete capitalist production and the making of love, Bess epitomizes capitalism's schizophrenia. According to Holland 'schizoanalysis takes schizophrenia – creative semiosis unlimited by fixed meaning – to be the fundamental tendency under capitalism'.[21] Capitalism has turned everything into a commodity that under new, contingent circumstances gets a new meaning; capitalism is defined by the production of a surplus. The 'schizo', in her shifting of codes, in the fluidity of her desire and meaning production is the capitalist figure *par excellence*, as Deleuze and Guattari have pointed out. The production of surplus may be useless, damaging, but it may also be creative, exploring, enriching. In the case of Bess, it is both. As a prostitute, Bess turns herself into a commodity with a double meaning: a negative one in which she is an instrument of others, and a positive one in which, in her view and later in others' views as well, she empowers herself and enables Jan to recover.

Considered in this way I see the theme of love (considered the central issue by many critics)[22] as not just something that may make us weep. Obviously, the film has a strong emotional impact. The entire crew wept on the set when Bess died, and large parts of the audience did the same, including myself. But since the theme of love is closely tied to capitalism's schizophrenia, its affective edge is not just private, personal and emotional. In fact, that edge becomes rather nasty when I consider the connections between love, capitalism and the family.

Communities: capitalism, terror, and the holy family

At first sight, the family is not the primary group in the film. A more foregrounded community is that of the church, exemplified by the collectivity of church elders. This old, traditional community is contrasted with the modern, loser community of oil platform laborers. These two stand in relation to the tiny community of Bess's family that consists of grandfather, mother, daughter and sister-in-law. Considering the latter in terms of the other two, there is a telling lack: where are the father and the son? Regarding the absent father, nothing is said. Regarding the absent son, he is revealed to be dead; his death triggered Bess's first attack of mental illness and her treatment in a clinic. This is why Dodo and Bess's mother are so afraid that Jan's accident will once again trigger Bess's psychosis. So, Bess's death is not the first one in this family; nor are the fear of Dodo and the mother accidental. Death and fear are intricately bound up with what holds these different communities together.

The different communities embody the simultaneity of different types of societies and economies that are distinguished by Deleuze and Guattari: savagery, despotism, capitalism and permanent revolution.[23] The element of savagery concerns the concentration of the village community on its own existence and the internal relations that hold the people of the village together. Such a concentration is evident in Bess's village from the film's beginning when the church elders despisingly ask her what the outsiders have ever brought that is of real value. By implication, anything of value has originated from within their own community, and from the relations of the people within it. In a savage society the social code determines what is of value and what is not.[24]

The regime of the church elders correlates in its orthodoxy with despotism. As church elders they represent the despot on top: God. To this god the subject-people are eternally indebted, without hope of ever having given enough. One owes God everything, always; one hovers in a permanent state of owing a debt of existence. There is one single thing that determines value in this system: orthodox belief in the letter of the Bible. Here Bess also breaks through, by breaking the code that women should be silent when she asks how one can love a word. In her mind one can only love a human being. Still, for this despotic God, Bess is a cleaner. It is not enough that she attends church on Sundays; she must return during the week to pay more. In the end Bess feels that she has to pay with the most comprehensive thing she has: her life. The debt is indeed one of existence.[25]

At the same time the regime of the church stands at the heart of capitalism with its propagation of asceticism. One needs to save first, to have money to buy something, and one needs to be a good subject first to be able to start to consume. Especially with regard to this latter aspect, the family plays a major role. The family becomes the factory through which subjects are produced. And at the heart of this factory, diffuse but definitely present, linger terror and death. (Fear of) biological death transforms, under capitalism, into (fear of) economic and social dysfunction. Will parents have enough food, a job that is, to secure the existence of their children? For the children this is experienced on a more psychological plane, in which (an economy of) parental love takes the place of money. If they lose their parents' love, particularly through some fault of their own, they will perish. This is why Deleuze and Guattari state that Freud's Oedipus model is not a universally valid psychological model, but a historically defined model: it is produced by and consequently affirms the condition of the family under capitalism.[26]

In this light the absent father and son can be understood, and the fact that the sister-in-law Dodo has remained part of the family. Deprived of means of income through the absent father and son, money has to be made; and the sister-in-law does just that. But in this context Bess is a disturbing factor: she does not bring in any money and her mental instability threatens the economic stability of the family. Here, we obtain a view of the terror that reigns in the family. That terror is contrasted and accentuated by the coming of Jan and his comrades who represent a society and economy of permanent revolution; this acquires a literal equivalent in the constant revolutions of their oil drilling machines. But they are also constantly on the move, staying here for a while and then starting elsewhere, moving from the platform to the shore. When they are on shore, they are constantly in cars moving to a party, or to a place where they can find mushrooms, or other entertainment. Theirs is a distinctly 'have fun' mentality, related to the aftermath of flower power via the popmusic from the Seventies.

The terror that grasps Bess stands out sharply in contrast to this fluid life style. Particularly telling is the scene that ends Chapter 2: 'Life with Jan'. When Jan has to go back to the platform, Bess is extremely frightened, she runs away, bangs with a iron rod on a digging machine, and Jan who has followed her does the same. Jan does not try to convince Bess by way of argument that he will return, but joins her aggression that started with fear and relieves her. Later on, Jan will come out of the helicopter and once more persuade Bess not forcefully, but by holding her. This stands in sharp contrast with the rigidity that Bess confronts in her mother. When Jan is away and Bess cannot get used to his absence, the mother follows her into her room and chastises her, commanding her to get used to Jan's absence and to behave. Bess' hysterical behavior leads immediately to the mother's consideration that perhaps it is best to put Bess away, in a clinic. That idea is more strongly expressed after Jan is sick at home and Bess begins to prostitute herself.

Jan's departure and absence and Bess's hysterical reaction to it demonstrate an intense fear of being left alone. Bess's family with the absent father, the absent son, and the – resulting? – stern mother embody the diffused but permanent terror that reign within the nuclear family of capitalist society. And Jan is of no comfort here. On the contrary, he acts as the destroyer of this 'holy' family. Not only does he not produce children, he is also not a good representation of the prohibiting father. In fact he forbids Bess nothing, but helps her to break away. And whereas his games at the beginning comfort Bess and are not really harmful to her position within society, his games become more destructive during his illness. Instead of reaffirming Bess's ties with her family or with the community, Jan turns into a destroyer of all these ties. And when the mother and Dr. Richardson are all too eager to get Bess in a clinic, and Jan unwillingly gives his permission, it is already too late. Bess has lost her fear of being (left) alone.

The fear that reigns within the family is controlled in BREAKING THE WAVES through the mother. She produces the voice that articulates the forbidding father and in accordance with this position refuses Bess any bodily comfort. In contrast to Bess's open, slightly comical and childish eyes, the mother's eyes are always threatening, except when Bess is dying. In looking at Bess, the mother embodies the gaze that produced Bess's subjectivity within the confines of the rigid ideology of the village. As articulation of the law, and as controlling organ of Bess's behavior, both voice and eyes play an important role. Since Bess always addresses God as 'Father', one might be tempted to say that God is a man, as all critics state. But the voice of that 'Father' is articulated by Bess. And when Bess speaks as God the Father, she speaks very much like her mother. The stern god that speaks to and via Bess, speaks like the parent that both stimulates and corrects her child. The accompanying stern eyes are those of the mother, most tellingly in a scene in chapter four. In that scene the mother sits still in the middle of the frame and looks as if she has condemned the 'silly' Bess. She will indeed suggest putting Bess in a clinic. Both the centrality of that look and the place of the mother in the middle resemble strongly one other remarkable pair of threatening eyes belonging to someone who also sits in the middle: Bess's murderer.

There are only two people with bulging eyes in the film: Bess's mother and Bess's murderer. When Bess goes to the ship which none of the other prostitutes dare to visit, there is a scene of actual terror. Bess is ordered by the man with the bulging eyes to fuck with his mate, but when Bess senses that something is wrong and asks to be permitted to leave, he attacks her with a knife. One could see this scene as the only scene that is actually terrifying. As I argued above, however, such terror is in fact inherent in Bess's life; it is a permanent possibility. Bess's mother is not her murderer. But she is someone who, as the spokeswoman of a much larger machinery, wants to do away with Bess. That machinery is embodied in the boys who start to insult Bess and treat her as a scapegoat by throwing mud and stones at her, but also in the figure of the medic, Dr. Richardson. Conversely, the murderer is not just a person who acts as an individual. He acts out what the entire community allows him to do.

Clearly Bess is excessive, and not simply according to the moral rules of the rigid community to which she belongs. Critical respondents to the film also described her behavior as excessive, whether they were conservative critics who considered her behavior pornographic and amoral, or feminist critics who viewed her behavior as too self-sacrificing. But Bess is also concretely fleeing, trying to escape; trying to flee the terror of the holy family, that unit from which she could be expelled always and at every moment according to the terms laid down by parental authority speaking in the name of an even higher authority: capitalist society at large. In more than one respect she functions like a 'counter-face':

> the face or body of the despot or god has something like a counterbody: the body of the tortured, or better, of the excluded. [...the scapegoat] incarnates that line of flight the signifying regime cannot tolerate...[27]

The question that remains implicit in this quotation is: what is the body, then, that the regime cannot tolerate? Let me turn to Bess as a body and as a BwO.

A Body without Organs or Hollywood resurrected

At the beginning of the film, when Jan and Bess are married, Dodo gives a speech. In it she explains that she had to learn to love Bess for what she is. Bess is so good, Dodo explains, that she would give anything to anyone who asked. Even if she has to give away someone else's bike. This had happened with Dodo's bike, given away by Bess to someone who needed it, as a result of which Dodo arrived late at work. This formula, that Bess would give anything, is reinvoked, though slightly altered, when Dodo is angry with Jan after his attempted suicide. Here Dodo says: 'You could get her to do anything you want to'. The resemblance in phrasing is also a resemblance in metaphorical imagery. Bess will start to resemble a bike in the sense that she gives herself away as a vehicle to anyone who wants to use her, and in that her operations become machine-like. For this reason Dodo at one time spits out that Bess has become the vehicle of Jan, acting out his perversities. As that vehicle, Bess is not so much experiencing things but recording them, and playing that record for Jan. As that recording machine, Bess is a BwO.

But how can Bess, as an individual, become a Body without Organs? Let me once more take a look at one definition of the BwO:

A BwO is made in such a way that it can be occupied, populated only by intensities. Only intensities pass and circulate. Still, the BwO is not a scene, a place, or even a support upon which something comes to pass. It has nothing to do with fantasy, there is nothing to interpret. The BwO causes intensities to pass; it produces and distributes them in a spatium that is itself intensive, lacking extension. It is not space, nor is it in space; it is matter that occupies space to a given degree – to the degree corresponding to the intensities produced.[28]

Formulated thus, one would have trouble considering Bess – an embodied individual – as a BwO. But in relation to film, it is relevant to consider that the BwO is not a fantasy, but a program: the 'motor program of experimentation. The BwO is what remains when you take everything away'.[29] So, let me consider Bess for the time being not as an index to an organic individual of flesh and blood, but as a motor program of experimentation. Then she becomes occupied, populated by intensities: those of herself, of the men who use her, and of the audience. She is the one who causes these intensities to pass; as a result of her experiment. For that is what she is performing, an experiment to see what will happen if she prostitutes herself; through experimenting Bess is trying to find out what will happen to her, and to Jan, with his body that is hard to separate from the machines that keep it alive.

As a BwO, the face of Bess is the primary *spatium*. It is her face with which the film starts. It is her dead face that we see in the last shot with Dodo, and in the last shot with Jan; not her body. In relation to her face the scenes of the landscapes can be understood. The film starts with her face, and every new episode afterwards is introduced with the scenery of a landscape. This structural alignment is meaningful.[30] Whereas the scenes with the landscapes seem to be odd fragments in a film that is entirely about human beings that are filmed close-up, it is precisely the 'close-upness' that treats the face as a landscape. Accordingly, the knit cap that Bess wears throughout the film is like a small mound of pebbles, covering her head; fusing her face with the Scottish landscape. Something happens in this landscape – a helicopter appears, a car finds its way up a mountain – just as something happens to Bess. Instead of being just beautiful intervals in the film, the landscapescenes (as the beginning of each new episode) point back to the beginning of the first episode: the one that starts with Bess' face. Like the landscapes, that face of Bess is the locus of happenings throughout the film.

This face, however, is not only that of an actress, but an index of a real woman with whom the audience is supposed or invited to identify. The major question here is whether we see Bess as a representative of 'women in general'. Bess as a BwO stands adverse to her being Bess, a woman with a body, and with organs that can be cut apart. One could argue that precisely

this cutting apart is the taking away of everything, turning her into a machine; or a concept. At the same time, rhizomatically, this cutting apart is
linked to what happens to women everywhere, every moment of the day, in
daily reality. This is what causes a considerable proportion of the feminist
criticism of the film. That criticism hinges on the asymmetry in gender relations, most specifically of who is being able to do something and who is not.
Very concretely, the camera in BREAKING THE WAVES is not gender neutral,
since it is allowed to follow Jan to a burial at the cemetery where only men
are allowed. And Bess is depicted as the one who desires to be desired; who
has been waiting for Jan, who starts to prostitute herself in order to tell him
about sex and love, in order to rescue him. Or as Cynthia Fuchs put it:
'You've seen women trapped like this in movies before.'[31]

Once more, I agree with this strand of criticism on the film. And yet. Let
me compare the body of another destroyed woman as analysed by Mieke
Bal in her article 'Body Politic'.[32] Bal studied one passage in the Bible's *Book
of Judges*. Here a woman has been thrown out of the house in order to satisfy
men who wanted to rape the woman's husband. Obviously, the motivation
for throwing the woman out in *Judges* and in BREAKING THE WAVES is different, but the result is the same: mutilation and death. However, the woman
in *Judges* crawls back to the front door of where she had been staying, and
then the husband opens the door and orders her to stand up. This order, according to Bal's analysis, demonstrates that the husband does not see his
wife, perhaps had never seen her from the start. This ignorance is then cru-
elly extended when he cuts her body in pieces to send it to the tribes of the
land in order to let them see what has happened. In BREAKING THE WAVES,
Jan has seen Bess from the very beginning, he has answered her face, and
partly thanks to that answer we could see Bess as more than a simpleton.
The instigation of Jan that sets Bess out to prostitute is partly cruel, partly
the extension of his taking her seriously and setting her free.

In this respect BREAKING THE WAVES can be seen to play out the discussion
that followed the appearance of Kathryn Bigelow's STRANGE DAYS (1995).[33]
In this film a man murders a prostitute in a horrible way, not unfamiliar in
Hollywood cinema. However, the important shift that Bigelow established,
as has been argued by Joan Smith, was that the audience experienced the
perspective of both victim and perpetrator. At the moment of death, all distance is cut short because via the main character Lenny Nero the audience is
virtually plugged into both the experiences of murderer and murdered. In
the responses to the film, male critics argued that female directors should
not produce such images. Joan Smith then comments:

> There is something illogical about this response, for it is precisely these women, the
> victims of serial rapists and killers, whose voices are silenced in real life and secondly

by the authors and directors who find their attackers endlessly fascinating. Men, it seems, can bump off as many women as they like in novels and on screen. What will not be tolerated is women speaking up for corpses.[34]

BREAKING THE WAVES does not allow for such a fascination with the murderer. But the fact remains that Bess is bumped off, whereas the suggestion is made that this is somehow right, since it served a purpose. One possible reading of the tolling bells at the end is that Bess's destruction was a solution to something, that her death is redeeming or that they suggest that Bess was right and everyone else wrong. No longer a home movie, no longer a documentary, no longer a book, we end up in Hollywood with its law that a story needs to end satisfactorily; if not happy in itself, then with the possibility of deriving a happy meaning from it. The film invests with hindsight the spiritual purity of a body that had become a vehicle. Utter cynicism is combined with the ideal of purity.[35]

And yet Terry, Jan's friend, has checked and double-checked on the radar whether there is anything out there to produce the sound of the bells. There is nothing. Considered thus, the sound of the bells is a final manifestation of capitalism's surplus of meaning. Through the bells, belief is shifted from the plane of naivity, where it was located at the beginning of Bess's story, to the plane of capitalism's schizophrenia with which Bess's story ends; we cannot know how these bells are suspended. Whereas suspended bells, or no bells at all, point to God as the anchor of faith, non-suspended bells point to a faith without such an anchor. The question with which the film started was: what of real value have the outsiders ever brought? This question suggests a standard, an anchor that grounds value and that consequently allows an univocal judgment. Through the end that is all changed into a political question in what Deleuze called a system of cruelty and combat: how would you like value to be made; and on what plane, and where and how far would you dare to go in establishing that value? The face of Bess is the locus of these latter questions. Instead of presenting a newly enforced image of religion and love, her face presents an image of combat. As Deleuze stated: 'Combat is not a judgment of God, but the way to have done with God and with judgment.'[36] And here the double operation of capitalism comes in. It is that which sentimentalizes old values, and that which compulsively brings new things into existence. Religion and love do not just relate to the first quality. Bringing new things into existence requires the faith to break away from old ones, and a love that replaces the restrictions of judgment. [37]

8   The Holy Fools

Revolutionary Elitism in Cyberspace

Richard Barbrook

> 'But I don't want to go among mad people,' Alice remarked.
> 'Oh, you can't help that,' said the [Cheshire] Cat: 'we're all mad
> here. I'm mad. You're mad.'
> 'How do you know I'm mad?' said Alice.
> 'You must be,' said the Cat, 'or you wouldn't have come here.'[1]

The lost utopia

The Net is haunted by the disappointed hopes of the Sixties. Because this
new technology symbolises another period of rapid change, many contemporary commentators look back to the stalled revolution of thirty years ago
to explain what is happening now. Most famously, the founders of *Wired* appropriated New Left rhetoric to promote their New Right policies for the
Net.[2] Within Europe, a long history of class-based politics and compulsive
theorising makes such ideological chicanery seem much more implausible.
However, this does not mean that Europeans are immune from embracing
digital elitism in the name of Sixties libertarianism. Ironically, this bizarre
union of opposites is most evident in writings inspired by Gilles Deleuze
and Félix Guattari.

Although these two philosophers were overt leftists during their life-
times, many of their contemporary followers support a form of aristocratic
anarchism which is eerily similar to Californian neo-liberalism. By doing so,
the Deleuzoguattarians have unwittingly exposed the fatal weaknesses
within what appears to be an impeccably emancipatory analysis of the Net.
Trapped within the precepts of their sacred creed, the disciples of Deleuze
and Guattari cannot even grasp why the spread of the Net really is such a
subversive phenomenon.

At the end of the century, the superficiality of postmodernism is no longer fashionable among radical intellectuals. Because the Soviet Union has

collapsed, the European avant-garde can return to its old obsession with Leninism. Instead, TJs look back to the libertarian spontaneity of May '68.[3]
Even after decades of reactionary rule, the folk memory of the Sixties still remains an inspiration for the present. The democratic ways of working, cultural experimentation and emancipatory lifestyles initiated in this period
survive – and even flourish – within the DIY culture of the Nineties.[4] However, belief in the overthrow of capitalism is no longer credible. Therefore,
contemporary European intellectuals have turned social transformation
into theoretical poetry – a revolutionary dreamtime for the imagination.

The cult of Deleuze and Guattari is a prime example of this aesthetization
of Sixties radicalism. Above all, their most famous book – *A Thousand Plateaus* – now provides the buzzwords and concepts for a specifically European understanding of the Net. In contrast with the USA, a vibrant techno-
culture has been flourishing across the continent for over two decades. Pio-
neered by computer-generated dance music, this digital aesthetic now em-
braces fashion, art, graphic design, publishing and video games. When it
emerged in Europe, the Net was at first seen as a place for social and cultural
experimentation rather than as a business opportunity. Unlike the Californian ideology, the writings of Deleuze and Guattari do seem to provide theoretical metaphors which describe the non-commercial aspects of the Net.
For instance, the rhizome metaphor captures how cyberspace is organised
as an open-ended, spontaneous and horizontal network. Their Body-without-Organs phrase can be used to romanticise cyber-sex. Deleuze and
Guattari's nomad myth reflects the mobility of contemporary Net users as
workers and tourists.

D&G now symbolises more than just Dolce & Gabbana. Within the rhizomes of the Net, the Deleuzoguattarians form their own subculture: the
techno-nomads. These adepts are united by specific 'signifying practices':
computer technologies, techno music, bizarre science, esoteric beliefs, illegal chemicals and cyberpunk novels. There even is a distinctive
Deleuzoguattarian language which is almost incomprehensible to the un-
initiated. Above all, these techno-nomads possess a radical optimism about
the future of the Net. While all that remains of hippie ideals in *Wired* is its
psychedelic layout, the European avant-garde – and its imitators – still
champions, the lost utopia of May '68 through the theoretical poetry of
Deleuze and Guattari. The revolution will be digitalised.

The politics of May '68

Far from deterring an audience educated in structuralism, the hermetic language and tortured syntax used within *A Thousand Plateaus* are seen as proofs of its analytical brilliance. However, this idiosyncratic Deleuzo-guattarian discourse is causing as much confusion as elucidation among their followers. For instance, the *Rhizome.com* web site blandly announces that: 'rhizome is...a figurative term...to describe non-hierarchical networks of all kinds'.[5] At no point does this web site explain either the political meaning of this peculiar concept or how its principles might be applied within the Net. On the contrary, rhizome is simply a hip European phrase borrowed to celebrate the disorganised nature of the New York cyber-arts scene.

Yet Deleuze and Guattari were not simply avant-garde art critics. The two philosophers were 'soixante-huitards' or supporters of the May '68 revolution.[6] Deleuze and Guattari championed the most radical expression of Sixties politics: *anarcho-communism*. As its name suggests, anarcho-communism stood for the destruction of both state power and market capitalism. Society would be reorganised as a direct democracy and as a gift economy. The appeal of anarcho-communism did not derive only from its abstract theory, but also from its concrete practice. During the Sixties, anarcho-communists led the search for radical solutions to the historically novel problems facing young people. With the arrival of consumer society, the traditional Left policy of unrestricted modernisation appeared to have reached its limits. Once almost everyone had annual rises in income and mass unemployment had disappeared, the problems of everyday life took on increasing importance, such as how to tackle restraints on sexual and cultural freedom.

Above all, many people now wanted a say in the decisions which affected them. They were no longer willing to accept leadership from above without some form of dialogue. Responding to these historically specific circumstances, young militants rediscovered and updated anarcho-communism not just as a theory, but also as a practice. Unlike their parents, parliamentary parties and trade unions, the New Left could articulate their contemporaries' demands for more participation. Instead of others deciding their lives for them, young people wanted to do things for themselves: '[Anarcho-]communism is not a new mode of production; it is the affirmation of a new community.'[7]

The romance of 'schizo-politics'

Like other gurus of the New Left, Deleuze and Guattari believed that the state itself was the source of all oppression. According to their foundation myth, the state and its allies had been using top-down tree-like structures to subjugate people ever since the dawn of agrarian civilisation. Described as a process of 'territorialization', they claimed that the media, psychoanalysis and language were the primary 'machinic assemblages' used by the state to control everyday life in the modern world. In contrast to Marxist analyses, Deleuze and Guattari believed that economics was only one manifestation of the state's primordial will to dominate all human activity.

Facing the transhistorical enemy of the state was a new opponent: the social movements. Deleuze and Guattari thought that the traditional style of left-wing politics was now obsolete. As part of the 'guaranteed' sector of the economy, private and public sector workers not only had been bought off by the system, but also had their desires manipulated by the family, the media, the dominant language and psychoanalysis. Like much of the post-'68 New Left, the two philosophers instead looked to social movements of youth, feminists, ecologists, homosexuals and immigrants to 'deterritorialise' the power of the state. As part of the 'non-guaranteed' sector, people in these movements were excluded from the system and were therefore supposedly eager to fight for the revolution.[8]

In *A Thousand Plateaus*, the nomads poetically symbolised the 'molecular' social movements which were making the anarcho-communist revolution against the 'molar' tyranny of political power. Far from trying to seize political power, nomads used their mobility to avoid the 'territorialised' control of the authoritarian state. Similarly, social movements formed a multiplicity of hippie tribes which were autonomous from all centralising and hierarchical tendencies, especially those supported by the mainstream Left. Along the 'lines of flight' mapped out by the New Left, the oppressed would escape from the control of the authoritarian state into autonomous rhizomes formed by the social movements. In *A Thousand Plateaus*, the rhizome became the poetic metaphor for this nomadic vision of direct democracy.

For Deleuze and Guattari, the overthrow of political power was only the beginning of the anarcho-communist revolution. They believed that political domination was only made possible through personal repression. The anarcho-communist revolution therefore had to liberate the libidinal energies of people from all forms of social control. The individual 'delirium' of schizophrenics prefigured the chaotic spirit of collective revolution. This meant that radicals not only had to detonate a social uprising, but also personally live out the cultural revolution. The New Left revolutionary was symbolised as the Body-without-Organs: a person who was no longer 'organised, signified, subjected' by the rationality of the state.[9] Such individuals were forerunners of the new type of human being who would emerge after the anarcho-communist revolution, that is, a hippie equivalent of Nietzsche's Superman. For Deleuze and Guattari, anarcho-communism was therefore not just the realisation of direct democracy and the gift economy. In their 'schizo-politics', the revolution would destroy bourgeois rationality so each individual could become a *holy fool*:

> [The Fool]...is the vagabond who exists on the fringe of organised society, going his own way, ignoring the rules and taboos with which men seek to contain him. He is the madman who carries within him the seeds of genius, the one who is despised by society yet who is the catalyst who will transform that society.[10]

The moment of community radio

Within the exuberant writings of the Deleuzoguattarians there is a curious yet revealing omission. They almost never mention Guattari's claim in the Eighties that the Minitel system was about to replace top-down mass media with bottom-up 'post-media'.[11] The reason for this absence must be found in the close similarity between Guattari's Minitel utopia and his earlier dreams about the revolutionary potential of community radio. Paradoxically, it is Guattari's anarcho-communist adventure within radio which provides the answer to why his contemporary disciples have developed such a curious affinity with the aristocratic ideology of *Wired*.

After May '68, many members of the New Left believed that producing alternative media was the most effective and fun way of putting their revolutionary theory into practice. In both Italy and France, the nationalised radio and television corporation had disseminated propaganda from the ruling conservative parties for decades. During the Seventies, New Left activists challenged this monopoly by setting up pirate radio stations. As the regulations against unlicensed broadcasting collapsed, thousands of 'free radios' emerged first in Italy and later in France. Although most were commercial, a minority were run by New Left activists.

According to Guattari, community radio stations were the only alternative to the domination of the airwaves by mindless 'disco radios'. He wanted radio broadcasting to be used to create an electronic form of direct democracy which could replace the corrupt system of representative democracy. Instead of elected politicians, people would directly express their own opinions on the programmes of the community radio stations. The community radio stations supposedly prefigured the imminent reorganisation of the whole of society around direct democracy after the anarcho-communist revolution. Even this ultra-left utopia did not go far enough for Guattari. The ultimate aim of a 'free radio' was the subversion of bourgeois rationality and repressive sexuality within everyday life. When people were able to express their own views over the airwaves, Guattari hoped that the 'delirium' of desire would be released within the population.[12]

In the early Eighties, Guattari was the leader of *Fréquence Libre*, a community radio station licenced to broadcast across Paris. However, it soon became obvious that turning Deleuzoguattarian theory into practice was impossible. Far from encouraging audience participation, the sectarian politics of the two philosophers actually discouraged people – including many on the Left – from getting involved in their community radio station. Guattari and his colleagues were more interested in lecturing the audience rather than engaging in discussions with them. This revolutionary elitism even extended the musical policies of the station. When some rappers approached *Fréquence Libre* about the possibility of making some programmes, the station refused to let any hip-hop crews on-air until their lyrics had been politically vetted! After they had alienated most of their potential activists and audience, Guattari's 'free radio' encountered growing difficulties in raising sufficient cash and recruiting enough volunteers to operate the station. Eventually, *Fréquence Libre* went bankrupt, and its frequency was sold to pay its debts. Guattari's attempts to turn theory into practice within the 'free radio' movement had ended in tragedy.[13]

From Stalin to Pol Pot

Techno-nomad TJs are attracted by the uncompromising theoretical radicalism expressed by Deleuze and Guattari. However, far from succumbing to an outside conspiracy, *Fréquence Libre* imploded because of the particular New Left politics which inspired *A Thousand Plateaus* and the other sacred texts. Unwilling to connect abstract theory with its practical application, the techno-nomads cannot see how Deleuze and Guattari's celebration of direct democracy was simultaneously a justification for intellectual elitism. This elitism was no accident. Because of their very different life experiences, many young people in the Sixties experienced a pronounced 'generation gap' between themselves and their parents. Feeling so isolated, they believed that society could only be changed by a revolutionary *vanguard* composed of themselves and their comrades. This is why many young radicals simultaneously believed in two contradictory concepts. Firstly, the revolution would create mass participation in running society. Secondly, the revolution could only be organised by a committed minority.[14]

The New Left militants were reliving an old problem in a new form. Back in the 1790s, Robespierre had argued that the democratic republic could only be created by a revolutionary dictatorship. During the 1917 Russian revolution, Lenin had advocated direct democracy while simultaneously instituting the totalitarian rule of the Bolsheviks. As their 'free radio' experience showed, Deleuze and Guattari never escaped from this fundamental contradiction of revolutionary politics. The absence of the Leninist party did not prevent the continuation of vanguard politics. As in other social movements, Fréquence Libre was dominated by a few charismatic individuals: the holy prophets of the anarcho-communist revolution.[15]

In Deleuze and Guattari's writings, this deep authoritarianism found its theoretical expression in their methodology of semiotic structuralism. Despite rejecting its 'wooden language', the two philosophers never really abandoned Stalinism in theory. Above all, they retained its most fundamental premise, namely, that the minds of the majority of the population were controlled by bourgeois ideologies.[16] During the Sixties, this elitist theory was updated through the addition of Lacanian structuralism by Louis Althusser, the chief philosopher of the French Communist party.[17] For Deleuze and Guattari, Althusser had explained why only a revolutionary minority supported the New Left. Brainwashed by the semiotic 'machinic assemblages' of the family, media, language and psychoanalysis, most people supposedly desired fascism rather than anarcho-communism. This authoritarian methodology clearly contradicted the libertarian rhetoric within Deleuze and Guattari's writings. But as the rappers who wanted to make a show for Fréquence Libre discovered, Deleuzoguattarian anarcho-communism even included the censorship of music. By adopting an Althusserian analysis, Deleuze and Guattari were tacitly privileging their own roles as intellectuals and the producers of semiotic systems. Just like their Stalinist elders, the two philosophers believed that only the vanguard of intellectuals had the right to lead the masses – without any formal consent from them – in the fight against capitalism.

For young militants, the problem was how this committed minority could make a revolution without ending up with totalitarianism. Some of the New Left thought that anarcho-communism expressed their desire to overthrow both political and economic oppression.[18] However, even this revolutionary form of politics still appeared to many as tainted by the bloody failure of the Russian revolution. Had not the experience of Stalin-

ism proved that any compromise with the process of modernity would inevitably lead to the reimposition of tyranny? Consequently, anarcho-
communist thinkers increasingly decided that just opposing the oppressive
features of economic development was not radical enough. Desiring a complete transformation of society, they rejected the transcendent 'grand narrative' of modernity altogether, especially those left-wing versions inspired
by Hegel and Marx. According to these ultra-leftists, the whole concept of
progress was a fraud designed to win acquiescence for the intensification of
capitalist domination. While the mainstream Left still wanted to complete
the process of modernisation, the New Left preferred to be leading a revolution against modernity.[19]

Once anarcho-communism was transformed into an ahistorical ideology,
the New Left's opposition to economic development soon developed into a
desire to abandon modernity altogether. Following the May '68 revolution,
support for rural guerrillas resisting American imperialism soon became
mixed up with hippie tribalism, concerns about environmental degradation
and nostalgia for a lost peasant past. Disillusioned with the economic progress championed by the parliamentary Left, many on the New Left synthe-
sised these different ideas into hatred of the mass urban society created by
modernity. For them, a truly libertarian revolution could only have one
goal, and that was the destruction of the city.[20]

Deleuze and Guattari enthusiastically joined this attack against the concept of historical progress. For them, the 'deterritorialisation' of urban society was the solution to the contradiction between participatory democracy
and revolutionary elitism haunting the New Left. If the centralised city
could be broken down into 'molecular rhizomes', direct democracy and the
gift economy would reappear as people formed themselves into small nomadic bands. According to Deleuze and Guattari, anarcho-communism
was not the 'end of history' as the material result of a long epoch of social development. On the contrary, the liberation of desire from semiotic oppression was a perpetual promise, an ethical stance which could be equally lived
by nomads in ancient times or social movements in the present. With
enough intensity of effort, anyone could overcome their hierarchical brain-
washing to become a fully liberated individual: the holy fool.[21]

As the experience of *Fréquence Libre* proved, however, this rhetoric of unlimited freedom contained a deep desire for ideological control by the New
Left vanguard. While the nomadic fantasies of *A Thousand Plateaus* were being composed, one revolutionary movement actually did carry out Deleuze
and Guattari's dream of destroying the city. Led by a vanguard of Paris-edu-
cated intellectuals, the Khmer Rouge overthrew an oppressive regime installed by the Americans. Rejecting the 'grand narrative' of economic

progress, Pol Pot and his organisation instead tried to construct a rural utopia. However, when the economy subsequently imploded, the regime em-
barked on ever more ferocious purges until the country was rescued by an
invasion from neighbouring Vietnam. Deleuze and Guattari had claimed
that the destruction of the city would create direct democracy and libidinal
ecstasy. Instead, the application of such anti-modernism in practice resulted
in tyranny and genocide. The 'line of flight' from Stalin had led to Pol Pot.[22]

The antinomies of the avant-garde

Ironically, the current popularity of Deleuze and Guattari comes from their
stubborn refusal to recognise the failure of the anti-modernist revolution.
Even when *Fréquence Libre* went bankrupt, Deleuze and Guattari never
questioned their 'schizo-politics'. Instead, they transformed the historically
specific politics of the New Left into theoretical poetry which existed outside history. The libidinal intensity of revolutionary failure was much pref-
erable to the limited achievements of parliamentary reformism.[23]

For 'cutting edge' TJs, it is now almost compulsory to sample from the
theoretical poetry of Deleuze and Guattari. Yet, this New Left revival is taking place in very different circumstances from the revolutionary Sixties.
However, the political irrelevance of Deleuze and Guattari does not dis-
credit their theoretical poetry among radical intellectuals. On the contrary,
the defeat of the New Left has enabled their disciples to complete the transformation of anarcho-communism from the hope of social revolution into
the symbol of personal authenticity, or what is an ethical-aesthetic rejection
of bourgeois society. Although defeated in reality, the ideals of May '68 can
be used to imagine a revolutionary dreamtime for the Net.

The aestheticisation of revolutionary politics is a revered tradition of the
European avant-garde. Back in the Twenties, the Surrealists perfected the
fusion of artistic creativity with social rebellion. Inspired by Lenin, this
avant-garde movement claimed that the consciousness of the majority of
the population was controlled by cultural mediocrity and puritan morality.
Therefore, radical intellectuals had the heroic task of freeing the people from
ideological domination. Their innovative art would undermine the repressive cultural norms of bourgeois society. Their bohemian way of living
would challenge the dull conformity of everyday life under capitalism. In
this interpretation of Leninism, cultural experimentation became the privileged expression of revolutionary politics. Whether from the tribal past or
the science-fiction future, any vision of a more authentic life should be used

to subvert the cultural philistinism of the bourgeois present. Innovative paintings, sculptures, photography, films and literature would be made '...in the service of the revolution'.[24]

The cult of Deleuze and Guattari is the latest manifestation of this European avant-garde tradition. The change in language disguises a continuity in practice. Just like its Surrealist predecessors, the contemporary avant-garde equates experimental art and bohemian lifestyles with social rebellion. Despite their involvement with radio and Minitel, Deleuze and Guattari hoped that the 'line of flight' from modernity would lead back to the tribal past. In contrast, their contemporary followers have no ambiguity about their relationship with modern technologies. Far from desiring the destruction of the city, radical intellectuals hope that the Deleuzoguattarian utopia will emerge from the hi-tech Net. Using intellectual alchemy, they transmute their gurus' anti-modernist scriptures into a philosophy of hyper-modernism.

This aestheticisation of May '68 is made much easier by the poetical style of Deleuze and Guattari. As in modernist painting, the 'realism' of the text has been superseded by a fascination with the formal techniques of theoretical production. For Deleuze and Guattari, theory was a piece of literature expressing authentic emotion rather than a tool for understanding social reality. Having failed in practice, New Left politics could live on as *theory-art*. Following this example, techno-nomad TJs sample Deleuzoguattarian discourse to produce left-field philosophy. But as is the case with Britpop bands, something is lost in these respectful homages to the past. In the sacred texts, the rational analysis of society had already been replaced by the literary celebration of irrational desires. The European avant-garde is now discarding the few remaining connections with practical politics. Using Deleuzoguattarian discourse, avant-garde intellectuals recreate the May '68 revolution as a theory-art project for the Net.

However, like the Leninist vanguard, the European avant-garde is haunted by the fatal contradiction between popular participation and intellectual elitism. In their theory-art, the techno-nomads use Deleuzoguattarian discourse to celebrate DIY culture. However, according to the sacred creed, most people – including members of the DIY culture – are brainwashed by semiotic 'machinic assemblages.' But when illuminated by the teachings of Deleuze and Guattari, radical intellectuals can amazingly cast off the mental shackles of bourgeois rationality and experience the redemption of ecstatic immanence. Although many are called, only few can become true disciples of the esoteric doctrine.

This elitism is a hallowed tradition of the European avant-garde. For decades, radical intellectuals have adopted dissident politics, aesthetics and morals to separate themselves from the majority of 'herd animals' whose minds are controlled by bourgeois ideologies.[25] Despite their revolutionary rhetoric, avant-garde intellectuals fantasised about themselves as an artistic aristocracy ruling the philistine masses. Following this elitist custom, the Deleuzoguattarians champion nomadic minorities from the 'non-guaranteed' social movements against the stupified majority from the 'guaranteed' sector. Once again, the revolution is the ethical-aesthetic illumination of a minority rather than the social liberation of all people.

Earlier in this century, this dream of an artistic aristocracy sometimes evolved into fascism. More often, the avant-garde supported totalitarian tendencies within the Left. Nowadays, cultural elitism can easily turn into implicit sympathy with neo-liberalism. The European avant-garde – and its imitators – could never openly support the free market fundamentalism of the Californian ideology. Despite this, as TJs cut 'n' mix, the distinctions between right and left libertarianism are blurring. On the one hand, the Californian ideologues claim that a heroic minority of cyber-entrepreneurs is emerging from the fierce competition of the electronic marketplace. On the other hand, the Deleuzoguattarians believe that this new elite consists of cool TJs and hip artists who release subversive 'assemblages of enunciation' into the Net. In both the Californian ideology and Deleuzoguattarian discourse, primitivism and futurism are combined to produce the apotheosis of individualism: the cyborg Nietzschean Superman:

> [...]the possibility to rear a master race, the future 'masters of the earth'; – a new tremendous aristocracy (...) in which (...) philosophical men of power and artist-tyrants will (...) work as artists on 'man' himself.[26]

The hi-tech gift economy

Following the collapse of the Soviet Union, the contemporary avant-garde had to substitute itself for the missing political vanguard. The techno-nomads therefore remix Leninism into Deleuzoguattarian discourse: subversive theory-art 'deterritorialises' the semiotic 'machinic assemblages' controlling the minds of the majority. Lenin is morphed into Nietzsche. In the late Nineties, revolutionary elitism can only be expressed in the words of May '68. Yet, important pioneers of the New Left were highly critical of this tradition of cultural elitism. For instance, the Situationists advocated transforming the social context of cultural production rather than the aesthetics of art. Instead of following the avant-garde elite, everyone should have the opportunity to express themselves.[27]

Above all, the Situationists looked for ways of living which were free from the corruptions of consumer capitalism. Despite their Hegelian modernism, they claimed that anarcho-communism had been prefigured by the potlatch: the gift economy of Polynesian tribes. Within these primitive societies, the circulation of gifts bound people together into tribes and encouraged cooperation between different tribes. This tribal gift economy demonstrated that individuals could successfully live together without needing either the state or the market. However, the Situationists believed that here could be no compromise between tribal authenticity and bourgeois alienation. After the social revolution, the potlatch would completely supplant the commodity.[28]

Following May '68, this purist vision of anarcho-communism inspired a generation of cultural activists. Emancipatory media supposedly could only be produced within the gift economy. During the late Seventies, pro-situ attitudes were further popularised by the punk movement. From then to the present-day, the 'cutting edge' of music has remained participatory. Crucially, every user of the Net is now also participating within a gift economy. Without even thinking about it, people continually circulate information between each other for free. They cooperate together without the direct mediation of either politics or money. Far from being the privilege of intellectuals, anarcho-communism is the mundane activity of ordinary people within cyberspace.

From the beginning, the gift economy has determined the technical and social structure of the Net. Although funded by the Pentagon, the Net could only be successfully developed by letting its users build the system for themselves. Within the academic community, the gift economy has long been the primary method of socialising labour. Funded by the state or by donations, scientists publicise their research results by 'giving papers' and by 'contributing articles'. Despite the dispersed nature of this educational gift economy, academics acquire intellectual respect from each other through citations in articles and other forms of public acknowledgement. The collaboration of many different scientists is only possible through the free distribution of information.[29]

From its earliest days, the free exchange of information has been firmly embedded within the technologies and social mores of cyberspace. Above all, the founders of the Net never bothered to protect intellectual property within computer-mediated communications. Far from wanting to enforce copyright, they tried to eliminate all barriers to the distribution of information. Within the commercial creative industries, advances in digital reproduction are feared for making the 'piracy' of copyright material ever easier.[30] In contrast, the academic gift economy welcomes technologies which im prove the availability of data. Users should always be able to obtain and manipulate information with the minimum of impediments. The design of the Net therefore assumes that intellectual property is technically and socially obsolete.

Even though the system has expanded far beyond the university, the Net remains predominantly a gift economy. From scientists through hobbyists to the general public, the charmed circle of users was slowly built up through the adhesion of many localised networks to an agreed set of protocols. Crucially, the common standards of the Net include social conventions as well as technical rules. The giving and receiving of information without payment is almost never questioned. Even selfish reasons encourage people to become anarcho-communists within cyberspace. By adding their own presence, every user contributes to the collective knowledge accessible to those already on-line. In return, each individual has potential access to all the information made available by others within the Net. Everyone takes far more out of the Net than they can ever give away as an individual.[31]

Despite the commercialisation of cyberspace, the self-interest ensures that the hi-tech gift economy continues to flourish. For most users, the Net is somewhere to work, play, love, learn and discuss with other people. Unrestricted by physical distance, they collaborate with each other without the direct mediation of money or politics. Unconcerned about copyright, they give and receive information without thought of payment. In the absence of states or markets to mediate social bonds, network communities are instead formed through the mutual obligations created by gifts of time and ideas.

The hi-tech gift economy is even at the forefront of software development. For instance, Bill Gates admits that Microsoft's biggest competitor in the provision of web servers comes from the Apache program.[32] Instead of being marketed by a commercial company, this program is *shareware*. Because its source code is not protected by copyright, Apache servers can be modified, amended and improved by anyone with the appropriate programming skills. Shareware programs are now beginning to threaten the core product of the Microsoft empire: the Windows operating system. Starting from the original software program by Linus Torvalds, a community of user-developers are together building their own non-proprietory operating system: Linux. For the first time, Windows has a real competitor.[33]

Beyond the avant-garde

The New Left anticipated the emergence of the hi-tech gift economy. People could collaborate with each other without needing either markets or states. However, the New Left had a purist vision of DIY culture. There could be no compromise between the authenticity of the potlatch and the alienation of the market. *Fréquence Libre* preserved its principles to the point of bankruptcy. Bored with the emotional emptiness of post-modernism, the techno-nomads are entranced by the uncompromising fervour of Deleuze and Guattari. However, as shown by *Fréquence Libre*, the rhetoric of mass participation often hides the rule of the enlightened few. The ethical-aesthetic commitment of anarcho-communism can only be lived by the artistic aristocracy. Yet, the antinomies of the avant-garde can no longer be avoided. The ideological passion of anarcho-communism is dulled by the banality of giving gifts within cyberspace. The theory of the artistic aristocracy cannot be based on the everyday activities of 'herd animals'.

Above all, anarcho-communism exists in a compromised form on the Net. Contrary to the ethical-aesthetic vision of the New Left, the boundaries between the different methods of working are not morally precise. Within the mixed economy of the Net, the gift economy and the commercial sector can only expand through mutual collaboration within cyberspace. The free circulation of information between users relies upon the capitalist production of computers, software and telecommunications. The profits of commercial Net companies depend upon increasing numbers of people participating within the hi-tech gift economy. Under threat from Microsoft, Netscape is now trying to realise the opportunities opened up by such interdependence. Lacking the resources to beat its monopolistic rival, the development of products for the shareware Linux operating system has become a top priority. Anarcho-communism is now sponsored by corporate capital.[34]

The purity of the digital DIY culture is also compromised by the political system. Because the dogmatic communism of Deleuze and Guattari has dated badly, their disciples instead emphasise their uncompromising anarchism. However, the state is not just the potential censor and regulator of the Net. Many people use the Net for political purposes, including lobbying their political representatives. State intervention will be needed to ensure everyone can access the Net. The cult of Deleuze and Guattari is threatened by the miscegenation of the hi-tech gift economy with the private and public sectors. Anarcho-communism symbolised moral integrity: the romance of artistic 'delirium' undermining the 'machinic assemblages' of bourgeois conformity. However, as Net access grows, more and more ordinary people are circulating free information across the Net. Far from having any belief in the revolutionary ideals of May '68, the overwhelming majority of people participate within the hi-tech gift economy for entirely pragmatic reasons. In the late Nineties, digital anarcho-communism is being built by hackers like Eric Raymond: 'a self-described neo-pagan (right-wing) libertarian who enjoys shooting semi-automatic weapons...'[35]

Threatened by the banalisation of the hi-tech gift economy, the European avant-garde is surreptiously embracing the capitalist fundamentalism of the Californian ideology. For this convergence to take place, Deleuze and Guattari's anathema against market competition must be skillfully abandoned. First, their adepts deny the wealth-creating powers of human labour. Then the work of living beings is subsumed within the mobility of dead matter. Finally, far from being condemned as a 'machinic assemblage' imposed from above, market competition is sanctified as the apotheosis of self-organising systems. As in the Californian ideology, this Deleuzo-guattarian heresy believes that the market is a chaotic force of nature which cannot be controlled by state intervention. Abandoning any residual connections with the Left, these TJs instead celebrate the new aristocracy of nomadic artists and entrepreneurs who surf the 'schizo-flows' of the information society. In this bizarre remix, anarcho-communism becomes identical with neo-liberalism.

As a consequence, the techno-nomads have to ignore the major social transformation catalysed by the new information technologies: the widespread adoption of a new method of working. Rejecting the 'economism' of the Left, many TJs have replaced the creativity of human labour on the Net with a digital vitalism inspired by Deleuze and Guattari's theory-art. Denying the ability of people to determine their own destinies, these techno-nomads believe that information technologies are the semiotic forces determining culture, consciousness and even the conception of existence. However, there is nothing inherently emancipatory in computer-mediated communications. These technologies can also serve the state and the market. The Net was originally invented for the transmission of orders from the military hierarchy. In the future, electronic commerce will play a significant economic role, and public services will increasingly be made available on-line.

At the same time, millions of people are spontaneously working together on the Net without needing coordination by either the state or the market. Instead of exchanging their labour for money, they give away their creations in return for free access to information produced by others. This circulation of gifts coexists with the exchange of commodities and funding from taxation. When they are on-line, people constantly pass from one form of social activity to another. For instance, in one session, a Net user could first shop using an e-commerce catalogue, then look for information on the local council's site and then contribute some thoughts to a list-server for fiction writers. Without even consciously having to think about it, this person would have been successively a consumer in a market, a citizen of a state and an anarcho-communist within a gift economy. The 'New Economy' of the Net is an advanced form of social democracy.[36]

The techno-nomads cannot comprehend the subversive impact of these everyday activities of Net users. As members of the avant-garde, they are looking for the intensity of ethical-aesthetic 'delirium' within the flows of vitalist matter. For them, there can be nothing particularly special about the mundane activities of Net users who aren't producing fashionable theory-art. Yet, at this particular historical moment, market competition is disappearing for entirely pragmatic reasons. While commodified information is closed and fixed, digital gifts are open and changeable. Instead of fixed divisions between producers and consumers, users are simultaneously creators on the Net. Obsessed with the immanence of semiotic flows, the Deleuzo-guattarians cannot appreciate the deep irony of this contingent moment in human history. This is the point in time when the old faith in the inevitable triumph of communism has completely lost all credibility. At this very moment, market competition is quietly 'withering away' within cyberspace.

Over the past few centuries, people within the industrialised countries have slowly improved their incomes and reduced their hours of work. Although still having little autonomy in their money-earning jobs, workers can now experience non-alienated labour within the hi-tech gift economy. From writing e-mails through making web sites to developing software, people do things for themselves without the direct mediation of the market and the state. As Net access spreads, the majority of the population are beginning to participate within cultural production. Unlike *Fréquence Libre*, the avant-garde can no longer decide who can – and cannot – join the hi-tech gift economy. The Net is too large for Microsoft to monopolise, let alone a small elite of radical intellectuals. Art can therefore cease being the symbol of moral superiority. When working people finally have enough time and resources, they can then concentrate upon '...art, love, play, etc., etc.; in short, everything which makes Man [and Woman] *happy*'.[37]

At such a historical moment, the European avant-garde is being made obsolete through the realisation of its own supposed principles. The techno-nomads celebrate digital DIY culture to distinguish themselves from the rest of society. Yet, far from being confined to a revolutionary minority, increasing numbers of ordinary people are now participating within the hi-tech gift economy. Rather than symbolising ethical-aesthetic purity, the circulation of gifts is a pragmatic way of working within cyberspace. Although it is impossible to predict the future of the hi-tech gift economy, one thing is almost certain. The intellectual elitism of Deleuzoguattarian discourse is being superseded by the emancipatory 'grand narrative' of modernity. As more and more 'herd animals' go on-line, radical intellectuals can no longer fantasise about becoming cyborg Supermen. As digital anarcho-communism becomes an everyday activity, there is no longer any need for the leadership of the cultural avant-garde. The time for the revolution of holy fools has passed. As has already happened within popular music, the most innovative and experimental culture will be created by people doing things for themselves. By participating within the hi-tech gift-economy, everyone can potentially become a wise citizen and a creative worker:

> [...] the word 'creation' will no longer be restricted to works of art but will signify a self-conscious activity, self-conceiving, reproducing for its own terms...and its own reality (body, desire, time, space), being its own creation.[38]

Respect is due to Andy Cameron, Armin Medosch, David Garcia, Fran Rayner, James Flint, John Armitage, John Barker, Luther Blissett, Michele Puccioni, *Mixmag*, nettime, Pit Schultz, Roya Jakoby and Simon Schaffer.

9   How to Endure Intensity

Towards a Sustainable Nomadic Subject

Rosi Braidotti

Introduction: 'eco-philosophy'

Deleuze's philosophy of becoming is neither the swinging of the pendulum of dialectical oppositions, nor is it the unfolding of an essence in a teleologically ordained process. His philosophy of becoming does not lead to the establishment of a supervising agency – be it the ego, the self or the bourgeois liberal definition of the individual. Rather, the Deleuzian becoming is the affirmation of the unalterably positive structure of difference, meant as a multiple and complex process of transformation and a flux of multiple becomings. Accordingly, the thinking subject is not the expression of in depth interiority, nor is it the enactment of transcendental models of reflexive consciousness.

The fact is that this model of subjectivity stresses complexities and multiplicity. However, it does not produce an infinitely regressing relativistic scheme. In this essay I will try to counteract the charge of relativism and moral nihilism that is often made against nomadic views of subjectivity. I would want to argue that there is much to be gained from Deleuze's radical philosophy of immanence, especially after all the dust and polemic about relativism have finally settled down. I am not proposing this in a spirit of philosophical corporatism, but rather out of a deep conviction that a qualitative leap is necessary for thinkers to emerge from the aporias and paradoxes that our historical condition imposes upon us.

Nomadic becoming is essentially an ethics of transformative forces. According to Gatens and Lloyd, it is an ethiology that defines Deleuze's project of philosophy as the imaginative reinvestment of reason and its application to social critique.[1] I also think that it is an aesthetic mode of absolute immersion of one's sensibility into the field of forces – music, colour, light, speed, temperature, intensity – which one is attempting to capture. Deleuze argues that painters make visible forces that previously were not, much as composers make us hear sounds that have never before been heard. Similarly, philosophers can make new concepts thinkable.[2] It comes down to a question of style, but style here is no mere rhetorical device but a set of material co-ordinates. Once these are assembled and composed in a sustainable and enduring manner that allows for the expression of the affectivity and the forces involved, these co-ordinates thus trigger the process of becoming.

In his discussion on the history of philosophy, Deleuze describes the study of classical philosophical texts as a set of portrait-studies – of landscapes as well as faces. By tending to each detail and nuance attentively, the apprentice learns gradually to *approach* the use of colours. Concepts are to philosophy what color is to painting. To learn how to approach them, however, one needs modesty, hard work and, ultimately, time. These are long-term endeavours. Moreover, the process of creativity/becoming is impersonal in that it requires the complete concentration of the author, be it the philosopher, writer, painter, filmmaker or composer, upon the field/territory s/he is immersed in. What is at stake is not the manipulation of a set of linguistic or narrative conventions; nor is it the cognitive penetration of an object or the appropriation of a theme; instead, the aim is to develop the ability to find orientation in a territory. Thinking here is the skill that consists in developing a compass of the cognitive, affective and ethical kind.

An exercise in cartographic bearings and orientation requires concentration upon the outside. In turn, this implies the abandonment of the self and of the century-old habits of inward-looking self-reflexivity. Quoting Spinoza but also *Zen and the Art of Archery*, Deleuze calls for an ascetic surrender of the self – of one's cherished but ultimately limited identity and the opening up of one's perceptive apparatus into a complex of multiple connections, sensations, perceptions and imaginings.[3] To create music, colours, concepts means to be able to render in a sustainable format this complexity of intense but impersonal affects, as well as being capable of sustaining the internally dissonant forces that structure these affects. The activity of thinking in this respect is closer to that of mindful breathing than it is to the exercise of the sterile protocols of institutional reason.

Whereas psychoanalytic theories of artistic creation play this back upon the holy Hegelian trinity of Lack, Law and power of the Signifier, an intensive or nomadic approach stresses the productive, rather than the regressive, structure of these forces. Shedding the mental habit that consists in Oedipalising the process of creation by indexing it indefinitely on an economy of guilt and unpayable ontological debts, what I find in rhizomatics is an overcoming of the dialectics of negativity. Nomadic, rhizomic thinking offers simultaneously a point of exit from the linguistic-semiotic, vicious circles of absence and negativity, as well as an empowerment of affective and unconscious forces as active, expressive, productive. At the heart of rhizomatics is a reading of the human as a positive, pleasure-prone machine capable of all sorts of empowering forces. It is just a question of establishing the most positive of possible connections and resonances.

A new philosophical concept, say an alternative view of subjectivity, or a new system of representation, a new sound or an alternative image produces a break-through in old mental habits. What is produced is a concept and affect that break through the established frame, illuminating a territory by providing orientation co-ordinates; made visible/thinkable/sayable/hearable are forces, passions and affects which were not perceived before. Thus, the question of creation is ultimately *technological*: it is about how. It is also *geological*: it is about where and in which territory. Ultimately, it is *ethical*: it is about where to set the limits and how to sustain the processes of change without hurting self or other. Resisting the aesthetics of nihilistic self-destruction is crucial also as a way of exiting the Romantic imaginary that still surrounds this debate in Europe. The issue about intensity is how to endure it, sustaining the altered states and the heightened intensity which the processes of becoming inevitably entail.

The concept of sustainability is no easy matter. I am of the generation that lost so many of its specimens to the dead-end experimentations of the narcotic, political, sexual or technological kind. Although it is true that we lost as many if not more of our members to the stultifying inertia of the *status quo* – a sort of generalized 'Stepford wives' syndrome – it is nonetheless the case that I have developed an acute awareness of how painful, dangerous and difficult changes are. They need to be dosed and timed carefully, according to one's threshold of sustainability. For the moment, let me stress then that the process of becoming is this trip across different fields of perception, different spatio-temporal co-ordinates. It is simultaneously a slowing-down of the rhythm of daily frenzy and an acceleration of awareness, self-knowledge and the senses. When dosed correctly it can lead to shifts in one's sense and orientation in the world – nothing as grandiose as Huxley's drug-induced hope of throwing open the doors of perception. Rather something more humble, like a quickening of one's perception, a being-there with and for other entities, forces, beings, so as to be transported fully into the magnificent chaos of life.

The notion of sustainability is not only an economic but also a social and ethical one. I see it as a positive answer to the crisis that accompanies the processes of transformation of late postmodernity. I think that postmodernity as a historical moment marks the decline of some of the fundamental premises of the Enlightenment, namely the progress of mankind through a self-regulatory and teleologically ordained use of reason and of scientific rationality allegedly aimed at the 'perfectibility' of Man. This liberatory project entails a view of subjectivity which excludes several 'boundary markers' also known as 'constitutive others': women, the ethnic or racialized others, and the natural environment are the three inter-connected facets of structural difference which simultaneously construct and are excluded in modernity. As such I have argued that they play an important – albeit specular- role in the definition of the norm, the norm-al, the norm-ative view of the subject. They represent a category of devalued otherness who historically have been perceived as different in the sense of being 'less than'.[4]

These structural 'others' re-emerge in postmodernity as the indicators, expressions or symptoms – some would say the 'cause' of the crisis – at a time when the project of modernity shows great strain, if not actual exhaustion. Deleuze and Guattari in their re-reading of 'capitalism and schizophrenia' bring the case against the pejorative relation to 'difference' to the point of implosion. They also propose powerful, affirmative and, in my opinion, highly necessary re-readings of subjectivity after the decline of naturalized and dialectically ordained humanistic paradigms. Significantly, Deleuze and Guattari express their new vision in terms of 'eco-philosophy'. This is to be understood primarily as a shift away from anthropo-centrism, towards a new emphasis on the inextricable entanglement of material, bio-cultural and symbolic forces. It is a bio-centered egalitarianism which Deleuze is bold enough to define as 'life-forces'.[5]

I think that the emphasis Deleuze and Guattari place on the embodied and embedded nature of the subject – through the notion of radical immanence – gives to their philosophy an eco-logical dimension. Knowledge claims rest on the immanent structure of subjectivity and must resist the gravitational pull towards abstract transcendentality. According to Deleuze and Guattari, we need to rethink the knowing subject in terms of affectivity, interrelationality, territories, resources, locations and forces. In so doing, we shall take our leave from the spatiotemporal continuum of classical humanism. Similarly, we need to move beyond the reductionism of social constructivism, which tends to underplay the continuity of the factors that provide the empirical foundations of the subject and which are mostly related to affectivity and especially memory and desire.

In post-structuralist thought the unity is posited in terms of time. A subject is a genealogical entity, possessing his/her own counter-memory, which in turn is an expression of degrees of affectivity and interconnectedness. Viewed spatially, the post-structuralist subject may appear as fragmented and disunited; on a temporal scale, however, its unity is that of a continuing power to recollect. The genealogical ties create a continuity of disconnected fragments; this is a discontinuous sense of time, which falls under Nietz-

sche's sense of the Dyonisiac as opposed to the Apollonian which, nevertheless, provides the grounds for unity in an otherwise dispersed self. Deleuze
documents this discontinuous sense of time with reference to classical philosophy. He borrows from the ancient Greeks the useful distinction between
the molar sense of linear, recorded time (*chronos*) and the molecular sense of
cyclical, discontinuous time (*aion*). The former is related to being/the mo-
lar/the masculine, the latter to becoming/the molecular/the feminine.

Becoming, temporality and endurance

A post-humanist and post-anthropocentric philosophy gives time a much
more central place in the structuring of the subject. Deleuze's 'nomadology'
as a philosophy of immanence rests on the idea of sustainability as a principle of containment and tolerable development of a subject's resources, understood environmentally, affectively and cognitively. A subject thus
constituted inhabits a time that is the active tense of continuous 'becoming'.
Deleuze defines the latter with reference to Bergson's concept of 'duration',
thus proposing the notion of the subject as an entity that lasts, that is to say,
that endures sustainable changes and transformation and enacts them
around him/herself in a community or collectivity. In this perspective, even
the Earth/Gaia is posited as a partner in a community which it still to come,
still to be constructed by subjects who will interact with the Earth differently. In some ways close to 'deep ecology', but radically anti-essentialistic
in their understanding, Deleuze and Guattari turn to Spinoza to find philosophical foundations for a vitalistic yet anti-essentialistic brand of immanence. We need to rethink continuities and totalities, but without reference
to humanistic or holistic world-views. As G. Lloyd put it, this subject's mind
is 'part of nature' and therefore is embedded, embodied and, in other
words, immanent and dynamic.[6]

The notion of time is crucial here. For Deleuze, the molar streamlined and
linear historical time of, for instance, emancipatory politics is both unavoid-
able and confining. The more effective time-span is the cyclical, dynamic
and molecular time of becoming. To use an example dear to my heart, at the
level of chronos, feminist women at this point in history have been legiti-
mated in their pursuit of 'molar' positions, claiming a woman-centred redefinition of their political subjectivity and identity. In this respect, they
cannot easily become 'molecular', maybe they cannot afford to undertake a
full-scale deconstruction of their sex-specific identity. The feminist engage-

ment with linear historical time, however, neither replaces nor encompasses women's relationship to the discontinuous time of becoming (aion).

It is to Deleuze's credit that he can see such a distinction in time sequences, but he fails to pursue it to its logical conclusion and thus envisage the genderisation of both time and history. He thus fails to see the scope of the theoretical horizon opened by sexual difference. In Kristeva's and Irigaray's work, the dyssymetry between the sexes stretches all the way to the most fundamental structures of being, including space and time. By comparison, Deleuze's theory of becoming and philosophy of time appear naively undifferentiated.

Feminists have argued that a complexified time-structure helps to clarify the tension and the paradox inherent in the feminist position. Thus, Irigaray rests on this analysis of the double structure of time to call for women's sense of their own genealogies, based on a bond of grateful recognition of the maternal as the site of origin. Kristeva, on the other hand, stresses the two-tiered level of time and argues for a distinction between the longer, linear model of history and the more discontinuous timing of personal genealogy and unconscious desire.[7] Kristeva couples this distinction with the analysis of various historical forms taken by feminist subjectivity: a form of which fits in with the linear historical time, whereas others are more attuned to cyclical patterns of repetition. By identifying the first kind with the Enlightenment belief in equality and the second with contemporary affirmations of difference, Kristeva sexualises historical sequences, developing a sense of women's own specific becoming. Although this way of associating certain forms of female subjectivity with certain moments of historical consciousness has been criticised for its Eurocentrism,[8] the associative procedure still marks a deep divergence from Deleuze's no less ethnocentric and considerably less feminist standpoint. There may, however, be a way of productively engaging Deleuze's sustainable subject with a more non-eurocentric, 'feminist' approach, by more profoundly articulating or bringing into deeper conceptual understanding what is meant by this sustainable subject and the way in which it becomes and endures in time.

The concept suggests a slice of living, sensible matter activated by a fundamental drive to life: a *potentia* (rather than *potestas* – by the will of God, not the secret encryption of the genetic code) and yet this subject is psychologically embedded in the corporeal materiality of the self. The enfleshed intensive or nomadic subject is rather an in-between: a folding-in of external influences and a simultaneous unfolding-outwards of affects. As a mobile entity in space and time, an enfleshed kind of memory (and this is a concept to which I will return), this subject is in-process yet capable too of lasting through sets of discontinuous variations, while remaining extraordinarily faithful to itself. This idea of the 'faithfulness' of the subject is central to the project of the 'sustainable self' that I want to defend here. This 'faithfulness to oneself' is not to be understood in the mode of the psychological or sentimental attachment to an 'identity' that often is little more than a social security number and a set of photo albums. Nor is it the mark of authenticity of a self that is a clearing house for narcissism and paranoia – the great pillars on which Western identity predicates itself – it is rather the faithfulness of duration, the expression of one's continuing belonging to certain dynamic spatiotemporal co-ordinates.

In a philosophy of temporally inscribed radical immanence, subjects differ. But they differ along materially embedded co-ordinates; they come in different mileage, temperatures and beats. One can and does change gears across these co-ordinates, but cannot claim all of them for all of the time. The latitudinal and longitudinal forces which structure the subject have limits of sustainability. By latitudinal forces Deleuze means the affects a subject is capable of following through its degrees of intensity or potentic, that is, the power to affect and to be affected. Longitude defines the span of the subject's extension, its speed and slowness.

Sustainable subjectivity re-inscribes the singularity of the self, while challenging the anthropocentrism of Western philosophies, understanding of the subject and of the attributes usually reserved for 'agency'. This sense of *limits* is extremely important to prevent nihilistic self-destruction. To be active, intensive-nomadic does *not* mean that one is limitless. That would indeed be the kind of delirious expression of megalomania that you find a lot in the cyber-freaks of today, ready and willing to 'dissolve the bodily self into the matrix' – as the fans of THE LAWN MOWER MAN (and THE MATRIX) will know. I want to argue instead that quite to the contrary, in order to make sense of this intensive, materially embedded vision of the subject, we need a sustainability threshold. The containment of the intensities or enfleshed passions and the limitation of their duration is a crucial pre-requisite which allows them to do their job. Their task consists in shooting through the humanistic frame of the subject, exploding it outwards. The dosage of the threshold of intensity is both crucial and inherent to the process of becoming.

What is this threshold, however – how does it get fixed? A radically immanent intensive body is an assemblage of forces, or flows, intensities and passions that solidify in space and consolidate in time within the singular configuration commonly known as an 'individual' self. It is worth stressing again that this intensive and dynamic entity is within the enumeration of an inner rationalist essence as opposed to being merely the unfolding of genetic information. The threshold is a portion of forces that is stable enough, at least spatiotemporally speaking, to sustain them and to undergo constant yet non-destructive fluxes of transformation. Mutation manifests but not into the nihilism of those contemporary narco-philosophers of today who celebrate 'altered states' for their own sake.[9] The threshold is a field of transformative affects whose availability for changes of intensity depends firstly on its ability to sustain the encounter with and the impact of other forces or affects. Moreover, the threshold comprises a radically materialist, anti-essentialist vitalism attuned to the technological era, and as such, cannot be further removed from the illusion of wilful multiplications of virtual embodiments of the contemporary techno-/teratological or cyborg imaginary.

In other words, Deleuze's enfleshed, vitalistic but not essentialistic vision of the subject is a self-sustainable one owing a great deal to the project of an ecology of the self. As I argued earlier, the rhythm, speed and sequencing of the affects as well as the selection of the forces are crucial to the process of becoming. It is the pattern of re-occurrence of these changes that marks the successive steps in the process, thus allowing for the actualization of forces that are apt to frame and thus express the singularity of the subject. This is a way of containing the excessive edges of the discourse about the techno-bodies of today, notably the denial of the materiality of the body itself in favour of fantasies of escape into the machine, while making sense of the powerful mutations that are taking place. Deleuze proposes a form of neo-materialism and a blend of vitalism that I find attuned to the technological era.

What I want to argue however is that thinking through the body and not in a flight from it means confronting the boundaries and limitations of a subject lying at the intersections with external, relational forces. Thinking through the body concerns assemblages. Encountering them is almost a matter for geography, leading to questions of orientations, points of entry and exit, and a constant un-folding. In this field of transformative forces, sustainability is a very concrete practice rather than the abstract ideal that some of our development and social-planning specialists often reduce it to. Sustainability is a basic concept about the embodied and embedded nature of the subject. The sensibility towards and availability for changes or transformation are directly proportional to the subject's ability to sustain the shifts without cracking. The border, the framing or containing practices are crucial to the whole operation, and one which aims at affirmative not dissipative processes of becoming, but joyful-becoming and *potentia* as radically ontological forces of empowerment.

G. Lloyd's remarkable studies of Spinoza and her collaborative effort with Gatens are helpful in explaining how such a vitalistic and positive vision of the subject is linked to an ethics of passion that aims at joy and not at destruction.[10] If it is the case that the composition of the forces that propel the subject, that is, the rhythm, speed and sequencing of the affects as well as the selection of the constitutive elements, are the key processes, then it is the orchestrated repetition and re-occurrence of these changes that marks the steps in the process of becoming even more intensive. In other words, the actualisation of a field of forces, argues Lloyd, is the *effect* of an adequate dosage, while it is also (and simultaneously) the prerequisite for sustaining those same forces. As Lloyd put it, 'the common notions of reason are grounded in imagination and conceived in joy'.[11] I would synthesise Lloyd and Deleuze into the concept of a sustainable self that aims at endurance.

The temporal dimension is linked to endurance, which is concerned with the state of lasting in time, and hence is connected to duration and self-perpetuation, with all the traces of Bergson implied. But endurance also has a spatial side associated with the space of the body as an enfleshed field of actualisation of passions or forces. It evolves affectivity and joyfully, with all the traces of Spinoza implied, as in the capacity for being affected by these forces, be these to the point of pain or extreme pleasure – which comes to the same – it means putting up with, tolerating hardship and physical pain.

Apart from providing the key to an ethiology of forces, endurance is also an ethical principle of affirmation of the positivity of the intensive subject and its joyful affirmation as *potentia*. Lloyd's reading of Deleuze's reading of Spinoza suggested to me the notion of *endurance* as a spatiotemporal compound which frames the boundaries of processes of becoming. This works by the power of transformation of negativity, transforming negative into positive passions through the power of an understanding that is no longer indexed upon a phallogocentric set of standards, but is rather unhinged and affective, imaginative, dynamic, complex. This sort of turning of the tide of negativity is the transformative process of achieving freedom, not through boundaries thrown awry, but through the awareness of our limits and of our bondage. This involves the freedom to affirm one's *potentia* or joy, requiring the encounters and mingling with other bodies, entities, beings and forces.

Becoming is an intransitive process. This does not comprise becoming anything in particular, but only what one is attracted to and capable of sustaining to life's edge but not over it, and hence exit Bataille. Even though not deprived of violence, becoming is deeply compassionate, forming an ethical and political sensibility that begins with the recognition of one's limitations as the necessary counterpart of one's forces or intensive encounters with multiple others. It has to do with the adequacy of one's intensity to the modes and time of its enactment. It can only be embodied and embedded, because it is interrelational and collective.

Reason, memory and imagination

Two notions support sustainability and make it work: memory and imagination.

Re-membering is about repetition or the retrieval of information. In the human subject, that information is stored throughout the physical and experiential density of the embodied self and not only in the 'black box' of the psyche. I find Deleuze's distinction between a 'majority' and a 'minority' memory very useful in illuminating the paradoxes and the riches of repetition as the engine of identity and coherence of the self.

First, is the notion of a 'minority' memory (mémoire) which is crucial to Deleuze's process of becoming. The phallogocentric subject, representing the majority of white, heterosexual, property-owning males, holds a large databank of centralised knowledge. He (and the gendering is absolutely *not* coincidental) holds the keys to the central memory of the system and has reduced the alternative or subjugated memories of the many minorities to the rank of a-signifying practices. Again, Freud's early psychoanalytic insights had caught a glimpse of two crucial notions: firstly, that processes of re-membering extended well beyond the rationalistic control of consciousness. In fact, consciousness is merely the tip of the iceberg of a far more complex set of resonances, echo and data processing which we commonly call 'memory'. Moreover, these processes of remembering are enfleshed; they encompass the embodied self as a whole and therefore rest on somatic layers that call for a specific form of (psycho) analysis.

According to Deleuze and Guattari, however, Freud immediately closes the very door that he had half-opened when he re-indexes this vitalistic and time-bound definition of the subject onto the necessity to conform to dominant sociocultural expectations about civilised adult human behaviour. Deleuze and Guattari argue that Lacan operates a sort of kidnapping of the subject from the solid, bodily or somatic grounds of Freudian psychoanalysis. This has the advantage of radicalising the politics of psychoanalysis by attacking conventional morality, expectations about bourgeois propriety and the reformist impact of American-dominated 'ego-psychology'. Lacan's approach also has the disadvantage, however, of introducing into the conceptual framework of the psychoanalytic subject a heavier dose of Hegelian dialectics, mostly through the idea of desire as lack and the role of negativity in the constitution of consciousness. This emerges as a major point of disagreement between Lacan and Deleuze, which I have outlined earlier.

In Deleuze's becomings, the Bergsonian continuous present is set in op-position to the tyranny of the past. This occurs not only in the history of phi-losophy but also in the psychoanalytic notion of remembering, repeating and working-through, that is, the retrieval of repressed psychic material. Via Bergson, Deleuze disengages memory from its indexicalising of a fixed identity, done so because predicated upon a majority-subject. The memory of the logocentric or 'molar' subject is a huge data-bank of centralised infor-mation, which is relayed through every aspect of His activities, the gender here being anything but coincidental.

The majority subject holds the key to the central memory of the system, thus reduced to an insignificant or rather 'a-signifying' role. The memories of the minorities, subjugated, marginal alternative 'counter-memories', as Foucault used to call them, engender empowering differences. In reaction to this centralised, monolithic memory, Deleuze activates a minority-memory, which is a power of remembering without *a priori* prepositional attachment to the centralised databank. This intensive, zigzagging, cyclical and messy type of remembering does not even aim at retrieving information in a linear manner. It simply intuitively endures. It functions rather as a deterritoria-lizing agency that dislodges the subject from his unified and centralised location. It disconnects the subject from his/her identification with logocentric consciousness, and it shifts the emphasis from Being to be-coming.

The minority-memory propels the process of becoming by liberating something akin to Foucault's 'counter-memory': a faculty that, instead of re-trieving in a linear order specific catalogue memories (les souvenirs), func-tions instead as a deterritorialising agency which dislodges the subject from his/her sense of unified and consolidated identity. It destabilises identity by opening up spaces where virtual possibilities can be actualised. It is a sort of empowerment of all that was not programmed within the dominant mem-ory. Minority-memory bears a close link to the idea of a traumatic event. A trauma is by definition an event that shatters the boundaries of the subject and blurs his/her sense of identity. Traumas cancel and even suppress the actual content of memories. As memory is the databank of one's identity, the struggle to remember or retrieve the embodied experiences that are too painful for immediate recollection is a formidable struggle. It also makes for no less formidable narratives.

Remembering in this mode requires composition, selection and dosage. The careful lay-out of empowering conditions allows for the actualisation of affirmative forces. Like a choreography of flows or intensities that retrieve adequate framing in order to compose into a form, intensive memories re-trieve empathy and cohesion between their constitutive elements. This takes the form of a constant quest for temporary moments when a balance can be sustained, before the forces dissolve again and move on. And on it goes, never equal to itself, but faithful enough to itself to endure and to pass on.

Of course, the question of the 'lived temporality' of the subject has wider implications. There is a genetic, even evolutionary side to it: the specific information contained in the organic layer of the individual is crucial to the unfolding of one's life span and the vicissitudes of one's organic existence. Deleuze refers to this question in a sort of zigzagging dialogue with G. Saint-Hilaire and Darwin, in terms of the 'animality' of the self.[12] The substratum of the radical immanence of the self which is a life has its own biological clock built-in; its duration is limited and only partially negotiable. The inner heat of life is portioned off and partitioned carefully. The 'I' that inhabits the specific portion of space and time within which it moves is not the owner of that life. Instead, s/he rents it on a time-basis. Memory is fluid and flowing, opening up the unexpected or virtual possibilities, transgressing these in that they work against the programmes of the dominant memory-system. This continuous memory is, however, not necessarily or inevitably linked to 'real' experience, or what I consider as one of the more radical conceptual attacks on the authority of 'experience' and the extent to which the appeal to experience both confirms and perpetuates the belief in steady and unitary identities.

Deleuze is more inclined to link memory to the second of the two notions I want to discuss in connection with immanence: imagination. The imagination plays a crucial role in enabling the whole process of becoming-minority. The imaginative, affective force of remembering, that which returns and is remembered/repeated, is the propelling force in this idea of becoming-intensive. When you remember in the intensive or minority-mode, you in fact open up spaces of movement and of deterritorialization that actualise virtual possibilities which had been frozen in the image of the past. Opening up these virtual spaces is a creative effort. When you re-member to become what you are, a subject-in-becoming, you actually reinvent yourself on the basis of what you hope you could become with a little help from your friends.

It is crucial in fact to see to what an extent processes of becoming are collective, intersubjective and not individual or isolated. 'Others' are the integral element of one's successive becomings. Again, my quarrel here is with any notion of the subject that would imply an ethics of individual responsibility in the bourgeois liberal model. A Deleuzian feminist approach would rather favour the destitution of the sovereign subject altogether and consequently the overcoming of the dualism Self/Other, Sameness/Difference which that vision of the subject engenders. Subjects are fields of forces that aim at duration and joyful self-realisation and which, in order to fulfil them, need to negotiate their way across the pitfalls of negativity that phallogocentric culture is going to throw in the way of the fulfilment of their intrinsic positivity. As far as I am concerned, then, exit Hegel and Lacan to give the stage to Spinoza and Nietzsche as they are re-read with Deleuze.

Remembering in this nomadic mode is the active reinvention of a self that is joyfully discontinuous as opposed to being mournfully consistent or as programmed by phallogocentric culture. The tense that best expresses the power of the imagination is the future perfect: 'I will have been free'. Quoting Virginia Woolf Deleuze also says: 'It will have been a childhood, though not necessarily my childhood.' What occurs here is a shifting away from the reassuming platitudes of the past to the openings hinted at by the future perfect. This is the tense of a virtual sense of potential. Memories need the imagination to empower the actualisation of virtual possibilities in the subject. They allow the subject to differ from oneself as much as possible while remaining faithful to oneself and enduring. Thus, a Deleuzian feminism seeks not to pursue Hegelian or Lacanian identities, based on the need for a phallogocentric position, however equal or unequal; rather, if such a feminism as a mode of becoming is to be articulated, then it is to do so through a becoming as breathing gender, as shifting pressure points, as molecular transformations of gender itself. What takes place, then, is a radical challenge to any notion of a self that plays itself out in a matrix of having and/or lacking, self and Other as psychoanalytic or transcendental categories. Indeed, a personalised overthrowing of the internal simulacra of the self constitutes a kind of imaginative recollection of the self which is more about repetition, and less about forgetting to forget, or what could be paraphrased as Freud's definition of neurotic symptoms.

The imaginative force of this operation is central to what I would consider as a vitalist, yet anti-essentialist theory of desire. Desire is the propelling and compelling force that is attracted to self-affirmation and to the transformation of negative into positive passions. The desire not to preserve, but to change. A deep yearning for transformation or a process of affirmation is to enact the different steps of this process of becoming. In order to do so, one has to work on conceptual co-ordinates. These are not elaborated by voluntaristic self-naming, but rather through processes of careful revisitations and retakes which can be compared to filmic shots. These are ways of describing the figures of nomadic yearning.

Empathy and compassion are key features of this nomadic yearning for in-depth transformation. The space of becoming is a space of affinity and correlation of elements, between compatible and mutually attractive forces:

a space of sympathy between the constitutive elements of the process. Proximity or intellectual sympathy is both a topological and qualitative notion through both geography or meteorology and ethical temperature. It is an affective framing for the becoming of subjects as sensible or intelligent matter. The affectivity of the imagination is the motor for these encounters and of the conceptual creativity they trigger off. It is a transformative force that propels multiple, heterogeneous 'becomings' of the subject.

The notion of 'figurations' – as opposed to 'metaphors' – emerges as crucial to Deleuze's use of the imagination as a concept. Figurations bring into representation that which the system had declared off-limits. There are situated practices that require the awareness of the limitations as well as the specificity of one's locations. They illuminate all the aspects of one's subjectivity which the phallogocentric regime does not want us to become. Brian Massumi refers to this process as the actualisation of philosophical monstrosity.[13] In this kind of philosophical teratology or transgression, a shift of paradigm does occur towards a positive appraisal of monstrous differences (deviances or anomalies) not as an end in themselves, but as steps in a process of recomposition of the co-ordinates of subjectivity in techno-culture. Though this is neither a romantic valorisation of otherness *per se*, nor is it a move towards political and cultural decadence. It is rather an attempt to disengage the process of becoming from the classical *topos* of the dichotomy self-other. It is also a direct engagement with the issue of how to disengage the notion of 'difference' from its hegemonic and negative implications.

There is something extremely familiar and almost self-evident about these processes of transformation of the self through an other who triggers processes of metamorphosis of the self. That is precisely the point: this theory of radical immanence is very simple at heart, and it is intuitively accessible. What happens is really a relocation of the function of the subject through the joining of memory and the imagination into propelling a vital force that aims at transformation. As a rigorous reader of Spinoza, Deleuze suggests a positive and equal relationship between reason and the imagination. Overthrowing the traditional hierarchy of intellectual and mental faculties, which had discriminated against the imaginative and the oniric, Deleuze locates the potentia of affirmation firmly on the side of the imagination. In doing so, he produces a new theory of desire.

Shame and ethical transformation

Deleuze speaks openly of the 'shame' of being human. He does so in relation to Primo Levi and the issue of the Holocaust which marks the fundamental moral bankruptcy of European civilisation. In this respect, Deleuze can be compared to Bauman in that he takes the Holocaust as a point of no return and is committed to elaborating an ethics that faces up to the complexities engendered by the historicity of Europe's genocide.[14] Contrary to Bauman, however, Deleuze connects this ethical failure of European culture to the historical decline of an Enlightenment-inspired faith in humanism. It is in response to this failure that he formulates an alternative ethics.

The sense of shame about being human does not encompass only the macro-events of our culture, such as the Holocaust of the Jews, fascism, colonialism, the economic exploitation of the many by the few, it applies just as easily to the micro-instances of life on this planet. It also covers most effectively the practice of philosophy and the much-discussed 'role of the intellectuals'. A very modest man himself, with an extremely low profile in the media, Deleuze carefully avoided the circus of self-promotional activities that mark intellectual life in the West at the end of the millennium. He explicitly criticised the intrusion of the media and its 'star-system' into the work of research and study which should remain the philosopher's main task. Deleuze kept his low-status job at the University of Paris VIII to the end of his life and never enjoyed the benefits of fame and wealth which so many of his peers indulged in. Notably, he steered clear of the Trans-Atlantic academic exchange market, a major cash nexus which established so many originally marginal French philosophers in well-endowed chairs in the USA, particularly in California. I think that Deleuze both practised and preached an ascetic style which conceptually expresses his rejection of a morality of negative passions, such as guilt, envy, resentment and anger, and his commitment to positive passions, namely affirmation, desire, sympathy, connection. His asceticism, as Goodchild astutely observed, takes the form of a critique of the thinker as the judge (or the priest) of reason and affirms instead the potency of creativity and interconnections.[15]

Examples of the micro-instances of reactive or negative morality are all the self-aggrandising gestures that mark social, professional and institutional life. Narcissism and paranoia are the two pillars on which most social institutions are erected. In ethical terms, this means that institutions generate, instill and reward the reproduction of negative passions upon their Oedipally subjugated participants. Deleuze surveys the circus of narcissistic performances and the inevitable cycles of competition and hatred which

propel academic, institutional and social life with the distance and the compassion of someone who simultaneously knows that this negativity affects
him/her, too, but also knows that s/he has nothing at stake. I think it important to clarify this paradoxical position, which in my opinion holds the key
to the materialist and posthumanistic ethics which Deleuze proposes.

I find this one of the most striking and also most touching aspects of
Deleuze's philosophical practice: his capacity to call himself out of the game
of potestas (negativity), while partaking in it, as if he had no stakes in it, as if
he were already part of the ratrace. This capacity to disconnect from the
paranoid-narcissistic-self-nexus so as to activate a more affirmative set of
passions enacts simultaneously an act of withdrawal (a minus) and of addition (a plus). The subject subtracts him/her-self from the reactive affects by
stepping out of the negativity circuit. By virtue of this, s/he transcends
negativity, thereby generating and making room for more affirmative
forces. In other words, what the subject ultimately calls off is the cycle of
repetition of the negative passions which mostly structure social and institutional life by declaring a priori that s/he has no stake in that kind of game.

I think that the ethical moment, however, is not so much the ascetic withdrawal from the world of negativity/potestas with its quick, short-term,
hit-and-run successes. It rather rests in the act of transcending the negativity
itself, transforming it into something positive. This transformation is only
possible, however, if one does not sit in judgement either upon oneself or
upon others, but rather recognises within oneself the difficulties involved in
not giving into the paranoid-narcissistic-self nexus. In fact, it is only at the
point of utter destitution of one's 'self' that the activity of transformation of
negativity can actually be undertaken. This effort requires endurance, pain
and time, calling for creativity, in so far as one needs to provide precisely
what one does not immediately dispose of, namely, positive passions. These
have to be created. The conditions which allow for this creation must be immanent and therefore depend upon external circumstances, as well as an internal disposition of self-irony, a non-tragic sense of one's failings. One has
to think the unthinkable and imagine the unimaginable, that is to say con-
template the unedifying spectacle of one's Lack(s) and then – over and
against centuries of established logocentric philosophy which compel us to
fill the Lack by rationalistic over-compensation – have the courage to sit on
the verge of the abyss, look into it and let other forces come to the rescue.
The best part of the exercise is that they inevitably do.

In other words, there is no judgmental, self-imposed distance here, but
rather an active effort to reconnect oneself to the game of social exchanges,
after one has subtracted oneself from their more destructive interrelational
effects. The ethical moment consists in overcoming the slight sense of

shame, the ethical nausea which marks the recognition of the intrinsically negative structure of one's passions. In other words, the ethical act consists in relinquishing the paranoid-narcissistic-self-nexus and installing instead an open-ended, interrelational self instead. Left to itself, in fact, the sense of shame about humanity can breed very negative effects such as misanthropy, fear and anger. This would defeat the purpose of this materialist ethics by re-instating negative passions. It is the empowerment of the positive side that marks the ethical moment of transformation, the reversal of the negative dialectics and its eternal repetitions, and the transcendence of one's starving ego. What matters most is the process by which the transformation takes place, which is neither painless nor self-evident. As Villanelle, the endlessly self-transforming but self-repeating narrator of Jeannette Winterson's *The Passion* puts it: 'you lose you play, you win you play, you play'.[16]

Whatever gets you through the day

Crucial to the ethics of affirmation is the transformation of negative into positive passion through the concept of limit. For Spinoza this limit is built into his affective redefinition of reason, in that affectivity is that which activates an embodied subject, empowering him/her to interact with others. This acceleration of one's existential speed or increase of one's affective temperature is the dynamic process of becoming. Because of this, it follows for both Spinoza and Deleuze that a subject can think/understand/do no more than one's embodied, physical spatiotemporal co-ordinates are capable of. Potentia has built into it its own limits. Alternatively, what bodies are capable of doing – or not – is biologically, physically, psychically, historically, sexually, emotionally specific, and by this I mean it is partial. Ultimately, the thresholds of sustainable becomings are also their limit. Thus: 'I can't take any more' is an ethical-energetic statement, not the assertion of a defeat. Learning to recognise thresholds as borders or limits is crucial to the work of the understanding.

Deleuze has an almost mathematical definition of the limit, as that which one never really reaches. In his ABÉCEDAIRE Deleuze discusses with Claire Parnet the question of the limit in terms of addiction. Reminiscing on his own early alcoholism, Deleuze notes that the limit or frame for the kind of alterations that are induced by alcohol is to be set with reference not so much to the last glass, because that is the glass that is going to kill you. What matters instead is the 'second-to-last' glass – the one that is going to allow you to survive, to last, to endure – and consequently also to go on drinking again. A true addict always stops at the second-to-last glass once removed and, therefore, from the fatal sip, or shot. A death-bound person, however, usually shoots straight for the last one, without any desire to repeat the experience or start again tomorrow. In fact, there is no opening towards the future in the unfolding of the death-drive: time folds in upon itself and creates a black hole into which the subject dissolves.

In *A Thousand Plateaus*, Deleuze and Guattari speak out clearly against the unsustainable lows of transformation induced by drug consumption. Before we go on to misread this as moralistic, we would do well to remember that both 'mind-expansion' and 'mood-enhancement' drugs are something that neither Deleuze nor Guattari are a priori against. What they are against is the addiction to drugs, which tips over the threshold of tolerance of the organism. Addiction is not an opening up, but a narrowing-down of the field of possible becomings. It locks the subject up in a black hole of inner fragmentation without encounters with others. The black hole is the point beyond which the line of flight of becoming implodes and disintegrates.

I want to stress that Deleuze's position on the thresholds of sustainability attempts to strike a new position that would coincide neither with the 'laissez-faire' ideology, nor with the repression and moralism (which for me are synonymous). A Spinozist-nomadic notion of the limit, of 'not going too far', is a far cry from mainstream culture's appeal to moderation and savvy management of one's health. This renewed appeal to the individual's management of his/her bodily resources, health potential and life-capital is the distinctive feature of contemporary neo-liberalism. As Jackie Stacey has critically noted, it results in a misappropriation of the notion of 'responsibility' and a mistranslation of the term into styles of self-management based on 'prevention' and the pursuit of 'a healthy life-style'.[17] This cultural obsession with healthy, clean, functional bodies is the corollary of the proliferation of the monstrous, gothic imaginary. Both entail social, cultural and bodily practices which are simultaneous but in open contradiction to one another.

That Deleuze is on the side of the new monsters is quite obvious. What is equally clear to me, however, is that he is not doing so in any facile manner. E. Grosz pointed out this dimension of Deleuze's thought in terms of the pursuit of what she calls 'health'.[18] In contrast to normalising and homologising practices and understandings of this notion in general culture, 'health' expresses the body's capacity to continue entering relations and experience affects. It banks on and actively promotes a future. It is enduring and sustainable: it does go on. To stop is to encounter the state of termination of one's intensity. Given that intensity is the body's fundamental capacity to express its joy, positivity and desire – to put a stop to it marks the death of desire. I think it is the purity of these states of intensity that often makes them implode into the black hole of contained, ego-indexed forces, which are likely to hurt the bodily entity. This is where drug users, alcoholics, anorexics and workaholics implode and self-destroy.

The ethics of sustainability that I find in Deleuze's nomadic thought combines a flair for and a commitment to change with a critique of excess for its own sake. I specifically see a rejection of the metaphors of excess as in the work of Bataille and other early sensualist, psychoanalytically inspired writers. I would be equally critical of the notion of 'pushing to the edge', such as has been practised in various brands of counter-cultural movements since the 1960s. There has been an ideology of excess on the far left of the political spectrum, which has merged with the global culture of 'sex, drugs and rock n' roll'. Thus, in stressing the notion of sustainability, I want to refocus the debate around the need for embodied and embedded perspectives, not the fantasy of boundlessness. I also want to reiterate the importance and positivity of *transformative* experimentations, which construct differences without going too far. Vitality and transgression need not necessitate self-destruction.

This is not supposed to fall back, however, into easy moralising or mainstream appeals to moderation. Quite on the contrary, I think that 'whatever gets you through the day' – whatever help and support one needs to get on with it – is just fine. The sharp pang at the back of your head, which Martin Amis captures with such cruel accuracy; the diabolical thumping ache in the belly, which makes Kathy Acker run; or whatever shot of adrenaline one needs in order to go, to get going.[19] I believe that one of the most persistent and unhelpful fictions that is being told about 'life' is its alleged self-evidence and its implicit worth. Centuries of Christian indoctrination have left a deep mark here. The secularisation of life that follows has confined into the container-category of 'sin' or 'nihilism' phenomena which are of daily significance to my culture and society: disaffection of all kinds; addictions of the legal type in the form of coffee, cigarettes, alcohol, over-work and achievement; and of the illegal kind; suicide, especially youthsuicide; birth control and the choice of sexual practices and sexual identities; the agony of long-term diseases; life-support systems in hospitals and outside; depression and burn-out syndromes.

In contrast to the mixture of apathy and hypocrisy that marks the habits of thought that sacralise 'life', I would like to cross-refer to a somewhat more 'darker' but more lucid tradition of thought that does not start from the assumption of the inherent, self-evident and intrinsic worth of 'life'. I think that one has to 'jump-start' into life each and every day; the electromagnetic charge needs to be renewed constantly. There is nothing natural or given about it. As a consequence, I find that the non-evidence of 'getting on with it' generates another relevant question: 'What is the point?' I do not mean this in the plaintive or narcissistic mode, but rather as the necessary moment of stasis that precedes action. The question mark that both prefaces and frames the possibility of ethical agency. When Primo Levi, who asked that question *all* his life, and struggled to answer it all his life, actually failed to find the motivation for raising the question once more, suicide followed. That gesture, however, was not the sign of moral defeat or a lowering of one's standards. On the contrary, it expresses one's determination *not* to accept life at an impoverished or diminished level of intensity.

Commenting on Primo Levi's and Virginia Woolf's suicides, Deleuze – who also chose this way to terminate his own existence – put it very clearly: you can suppress your own life, in its specific and radically immanent form and still affirm the potency of life, especially in cases where deteriorating health or social conditions may seriously hinder your power to affirm and to joyfully endure. This is no Christian affirmation of Life nor transcendental delegation of the meaning and value system to categories higher than the embodied self. Quite on the contrary, it is the intelligence of radically immanent flesh that states with every single breath that the life in you is not marked by any signifier, and it most certainly does not bear your name. André Colombat in his comment on Deleuze's death links the act of suppressing one's failing body, as in suicide or euthanasia, to an ethics of assertion of the joyfulness and positivity of life, which necessarily translates into the refusal to lead a degraded existence.[20] Philip Goodchild quotes Deleuze most effectively on this point: 'Since destructive forces are always exchanged among people, it is much better to destroy oneself under agreeable conditions than to destroy others.'[21]

Because of this ethics of affirmation and positivity, a Deleuzian approach suggests that 'whatever gets you through the day', whatever life-support, mood-enhancement system one is dependent on, is not to be the object of moral indictment, but rather a neutral term of reference: a mere prop in the process of becoming. Of course 'whatever gets you through the day' may become the preface to minor dependencies, to legal or illegal forms of mood-enhancement systems. Whatever facilitates the release of adrenaline, including high levels of physical exercise; workaholism or the standard assemblage: 'writing/books/the friendly purr of the pc/e-mails/music/concentration/think think think'. We all have the patterns of dependency that we deserve. Even the standard line of assemblage described above, however, can sure take hell-bent deviations towards excessive snacks (anorexia/bulimia variable), or drinks (alcoholism variable) or any other 'fix' (the narcotics variable). The boundaries between these and the other, 'normalised' life-support systems, however, is merely one of degrees, not of kind.

If life is *not* a self-evident category, if 'what's the point?' is an ethically viable question, then whatever gets you through the day is an equally viable option, a suitable way of handling the problem, as well as an adequate exemplification of the question. I am absolutely non-moralistic about this. All I want to emphasise is that what is affirmed, asserted and empowered in the ethics of sustainable subjects is the positivity of potentia itself. What is empowered is the singularity of the forces that compose the specific spatiotemporal grid of immanence which composes one's life. This life is an assemblage, a set of points in space and time, a quilt of retrieved material. It is the project that makes for the uniqueness of one's life, not any deeply seated essence. Life as a project that aims at affirming the intensity and positivity of desire rests on the materialist foundation of the enfleshed subject.

Bio-ethics

By stressing this biological aspect, Deleuze is simultaneously addressing the issue of contemporary biology and also disagreeing with the neo-determinism of social biologists and evolutionary psychologists. In some ways, Deleuze disagrees with a great many molecular biologists as to the actual vision of the subject which they endorse. By interpreting contemporary biology with reference to the 'enchanted materialism' of empirical philosophies of immanence, Deleuze attempts to disengage biology from the structural functionalism of DNA-driven linearity and to veer it instead towards the zigzagging patterns of nomadic becoming.

Elizabeth Grosz, a careful reader of Deleuze, has recently stressed the importance for feminists of rethinking the biological structure of the human. This call for a return to the body reiterates the rejection of social constructivism which, as I noted earlier, is crucial to feminist theory in the third millennium. In her recent work on Darwin, Grosz sets the agenda as follows: 'What are the virtualities, the potentialities, within biological existence that enable cultural, social and historical forces to work with and actively transform that existence?'[22] I find this appeal to be invested by the kind of radical immanence and the 'enchanted enfleshed materialism' that both Irigaray and Deleuze defend, in parallel but analogous ways.

This approach is made explicit in Keith Ansell Pearson's work on Deleuze's vitalistic philosophy. By reading Nietzsche and Darwin with

Deleuze, Pearson emphasises the continuum of becomings as well as the transmutation of values that is implied in Deleuze's concept of 'life'. In so doing, Pearson uses Deleuze's insights to 'begin to map non-human becomings of life'.[23] Combining in a skilful manner biology and technology, Pearson envisages a 'trans-human' space of pure, processual metamorphoses that asserts the infinite powers of a life that does not require the supervision of the human mind in order to endure.

The life in 'me' does not, indeed, bear my name; 'I' does not own it; 'I' is only passing through. In a culture saturated by egotism, 'I' is more often than not a hindrance to the project of affirming and empowering the unstoppable and triumphant return of the impersonality – or rather the a-personality – of becomings, or eternal returns. These becomings do not privilege anthropocentric subjects, but rather emphasise assemblages of all heterogeneous kinds. Animals, insects, machines are as many fields of forces or territories of becoming. Beyond the subject/object distinction that supports the paranoid-narcissistic empire of the Ego-life as eternal becomings goes on, regardless and relentless.

This enchanted, anti-essentialist, high-tech vitalism, however, echoes the ideas of Irigaray about the subject as a bodily human entity, sensitive flesh framed by the skin. I find it significant that Irigaray turns to Judaism, notably to the philosophy of Levinas, to expand on this notion. In the reading of Levinas, Luce Irigaray writes an apology of the caress as a mode of approaching the other – the erotic, respectful touching of the other's skin is distinctly posed as the basis for an ethics of sexual difference.[24] This respectful contemplation of the contained boundaries of another's life – his skincloud, enfleshed existence – is also a response to the philosophy of excess in Bataille. This cruel and violent attempt to break beyond the enclosed space of the embodied self leads him to theorise both the inevitability of violence and the desirability of a transcendence which requires – ontologically – the consumption of another's body.

As in Bataille's unreconstructed phallogocentrism, another's body is preferentially the body of the other, of woman as 'other-of-the-same' – the specular, necessary and necessarily devalorised other – Bataille's theory of transcendence is also an apology of female sacrifice. Deleuze takes his distance from both Irigaray's sexual difference ethics and from Bataille's notion of transcendence. What he proposes instead is a radically immanent concept of the subject as dynamic becoming, where the bodily self is analysed according to the concrete forces or material variables that compose it and sustain it.

I would want to argue therefore that Irigaray's emphasis on the 'enchanted materialism' of feminine morphology constitutes a parallel project

to the nomadic, anti-foundationalism of Deleuze. The ethics of sexual difference and the ethics of sustainable nomadic subjectivity are two faces of the
same coin: that of an enfleshed, immanent subject-in-becoming, for whom
life is embodied, embedded and eroticized. To present them as mutually incompatible is not doing justice to either. I think that a parallel reading of
Irigaray's ethics of sexual difference and Deleuze's sustainable nomadic
ethics can be mutually illuminating, but I will not pursue this parallel reading further here.[25]

The 'life' that is empowered is not the uniqueness of life as in the Christian dogma; nor is it the equally unchallenged scientific belief in the powers
of biology. It is staggering to note to what an extent our understanding of
the human subject is still tied up with a sense of the body as a container, or as
an envelope. Containing a divinely-ordained soul, or an equally despotic
genetic code. Governed by the black-box of innately sovereign reason, or by
a rationally regulated libido that knows what's right for you. So much humanistic convention, packaged as human essence. In opposition to this, I
would argue with Deleuze that the singularity rests in the *project* that ani-
mates one's becoming, i.e. in the minority consciousness that unfolds and
expresses itself through multiple becomings.

The subject-in-becoming is the one for whom 'what's the point?' is an all-
important question. A high-intensity subject is also animated by unparalleled levels of vulnerability. With nomadic patterns also comes a fundamental fragility. Processes without foundations need to be handled with care;
potentia requires great levels of containment in the mode of framing. In
Viroid Life, Ansell Pearson comments in a very illuminating manner on the
distinction between personal and impersonal death in Deleuze's philosophy of becoming. The paradox of affirming life as potentia, energy, even in
and through the suppression of the specific slice of life that 'I' inhabits is a
way of pushing anti-humanism to the point of implosion. It dissolves death
into ever-shifting processual changes, and thus disintegrates the ego, with
its capital of narcissism, paranoia and negativity. Death from the specific
and highly restricted viewpoint of the ego is of no significance whatsoever:

> A positive, dynamical and processual conception of death, which would release it
> from an anthropomorphic desire for death (for stasis, for being), speaking instead
> only of a death that desires (a death that is desire, where desire is construed along the
> lines of a machine or a machinic assemblage), can only be arrived at by freeing the be-
> coming of death from both mechanism and finalism. (...) This is to posit the world as a
> 'monster of energy' without beginning and without end, a Dionysian world of 'eter-
> nal' self-creation and 'eternal' self-destruction, moving from the simple to the com-
> plex and then back again to the simple out of abundance: cold/hot/hot/cold,
> 'beyond' satiety, disgust, and weariness, a world of becoming that never attains 'be-

ing', never reaching a final death. For death (becoming) lives on itself; it is its own food and excrement.[26]

Death need not be the 'unproductive black hole'[27], but rather a point in a creative synthesis of flows, energies and becomings. In her critique of the vulgarity or commonness of Freud's notion of the death-drive, Olkowski underlines the extent to which psychoanalysis indexes the Ego to powers of desexualisation and emptying out of unconscious libidinal forces.[28] In opposition to this, Deleuze proposes endless contractions and expansions/duration and extensity in processual becomings or qualitative differentiations.

I prefer to refer to this process in terms of sustainability, and I would like to stress the idea of continuity which it entails – it does assume faith in a future and also a sense of responsibility for 'passing on' to future generations a world that is liveable and worth living in. A present that endures is a sustainable model of the future. Hence the importance of stopping at the second-last drink/smoke/shot. 'Enough' or 'not going too far' expresses the necessity of framing, not the commonsense morality of the mainstream cultural orthodoxy. 'Enough' designs a cartography of sustainability. This ethics of stopping before going too far is collectively decided; it is variable in each and everyone; it is action-orientated; it is affirmative of potentia; it banks on empowerment but invites compassion for those who cannot sustain it ('we don't need another hero', as Barbara Krueger would put it) and also asserts unrelenting hatred of the moralists.

I would like to develop this notion of sustainability into an ethics of differential sustainable subjects. I would like to propose a *public* discussion on these issues right across some of the problematic social issues of today: drugs, addictions of all kind, youth suicide, Aids prevention and sex education, euthanasia, anorexia/bulimia, abortion, the burn-out and stress related to post-industrial life styles. I would like this agenda to be taken seriously. As important at this stage is for me to challenge any claim by any conceptual, theoretical or philosophical school to the monopoly over issues of ethics and moral values. Whether in the neo-liberal brand of cosmopolitanism defended by Nussbaum, or in the neo-Kantian mode that is so prevalent in feminist theory today, such claims to moral superiority or rectitude are simply untenable, as well as internally contradictory.[29]

I want to plead instead for a less moralistic and conceptually more rigorous agenda that combines a broader approach with a serious commitment to think *alongside* contemporary culture and not against its grain. 'Whatever gets you through the day' as the melancholy refrain of 'fin de siècle' covers the depression of suburban opulence, as much as the despair of homeless life in the streets. Both the centre and the periphery are shot through by profoundly destabilising, perverse power-relations which engender equally sombre social relations. It seems to me that a critical agenda for the next millennium, both in feminist theory and in mainstream social philosophy, cannot fail to address these issues. We need to talk about the simultaneity of opposite social and cultural effects, and to address them in a non-moralistic manner. 'Whatever gets you through the day' need not be the manifesto for self-destruction that it is often made to be. It can merely help us frame a threshold of sustainable patterns of transformative changes, of becomings as modes and moods of empowerment.

Section Three

Micropolitical Becoming:
Duration and Change

10 Against the Doxa

Politics of Immanence and Becoming-Minoritarian

Paola Marrati

> [T]he struggle with chaos is only the instrument of a more profound struggle against opinion, for the misfortune of people comes from opinion.[1]

Most essays on Deleuze's politics focus, rightly, on the books he wrote with Guattari during the seventies: *Anti-Oedipus: Capitalism and Schizophrenia*, *Kafka: Toward a Minor Literature* and *A Thousand Plateaus: Capitalism and Schizophrenia*.[2] These explicitly political texts elaborate an analysis of capitalism rather different from all the Marxist trends in French post-war thought.[3] Written with May 1968 as the backdrop, they are also clearly engaged in formulating a new politics. 'Micro-politics', as well as all the related notions, is a concept *co-signed* Deleuze and Guattari.

I would like to argue in this chapter that some political concepts developed by Deleuze and Guattari are nevertheless closely linked to a major issue in Deleuze's thought as early as *Nietzsche and Philosophy* and *Difference and Repetition*.[4] I do not mean thereby to deny the importance and novelty of the books produced by Deleuze and Guattari, but rather to emphasize the political implications of Deleuze's previous works. For a long time, these implications went largely unnoticed in the French political and intellectual scene of the period. In 1972, Foucault significantly opened up his dialogue with Deleuze on intellectuals and power by relating the surprise of a Maoist militant about Deleuze's political engagement:

> A Maoist once said to me: 'I can easily understand Sartre's purpose in siding with us; I can understand his goals and his involvement in politics; I can partially understand your position, since you have always been concerned with the problem of confinement. But Deleuze is an enigma.' I was shocked by this statement because your position has always seemed particularly clear to me.[5]

The evidence Foucault referred to does not seem to be, even today, broadly acknowledged.[6] In the following pages, I will try to show how the concepts of 'majority' and 'becoming-minoritarian', as developed by Deleuze and Guattari, relate to a central issue of Deleuze's thought from its outset. The concept of 'majority' as it is discussed in *A Thousand Plateaus*, provides a critique of representation which is the background to this politics of becoming that Deleuze and Guattari are at once describing and calling for. In *Difference and Repetition*, as it is well known, Deleuze criticizes of the ontological category of representation as that which neutralises both true difference and true repetition. It has been less often noticed that the critique of representation in this work, already contains explicitly political aims. I would like to argue that these political aims are inherent in Deleuze's philosophical project of breaking with the powers of *doxa* and that, therefore, the encounter with Guattari was not for Deleuze the discovery of the realm of politics. It was instead a *new experiment* in politics, in a politics without representation, where it would not make sense to separate Gilles-Félix.[7]

I will proceed in three steps: first, I will begin with a discussion of the critique of representation implied in the concept of 'majority' as analysed by Deleuze and Guattari in *A Thousand Plateaus*. Second, I will argue that the concept of 'becoming-minoritarian' puts forward a form of universality that is antagonistic to any representative politics; and finally, I will return to *Difference and Repetition* in order to emphasise the political aims inherent in Deleuze's philosophical critique of representation.

Deleuze and Guattari: majority as empty representation

Etienne Balibar recently noted that the political reflection of Deleuze and Guattari stands entirely under the sign of antifascism, which implies that fascism is still today a genuine danger, an undeniable political threat.[8] This analysis of Deleuze and Guattari is pertinent especially when one considers that for them, the problem is not so much that of an eventual return of the historical forms of fascism that we have known, even if such an eventuality cannot be excluded, but instead, that of diffuse forms of microfascism that traverse our societies and do not need to be found grouped together in a Fascist State for them to be dangerous.

But if Balibar is right in underscoring the central role that the analysis of micro-fascisms plays in *Anti-Oedipus* and *A Thousand Plateaus*, this is so because this analysis demonstrates in an exemplary manner mechanisms of the constitution of identity that have a much wider relevance. Against the backdrop of the fascist danger, the dangers of all identity politics receive their distinctive profile. Parliamentary and representative democracies are not sheltered from these dangers. In any case, what is unsheltered is one of the fundamental elements of their functioning: the very notion of majority.

What Deleuze and Guattari question are not only the factual distortions that occur now and then, or even often, in the constitution of this or that majority. For these empirical distortions do not affect the concept of majority and its representative value, they only testify to a particular democratic dysfunctioning that can always be corrected. According to Deleuze and Guattari, the problem is not one of *fact* but one of *right* (i.e., the *quaestio juris*): it is the constitution of the majority and its functioning *as such* that exclude from the outset the possibility that the majority can have some representative value.

But why can a majority never have a genuine representative value? The first reason put forward by Deleuze and Guattari is that the concept of majority is not primarily defined by quantitative criteria. In order to establish a majority, one does not begin by counting: a majority is never just the expression of the 'greatest number', the product of a calculation. On the contrary, it is the product of a state of power and domination and of a given balance of forces, which defines a *standard measure*. First and foremost, the majority is a *constant*, a *model* determining what is, independent of relative quantities, what is majoritarian and what is minoritarian. Let us take up an illuminating example from *A Thousand Plateaus*:

> Let us suppose that the constant or standard is the average adult-white-heterosexual-European-male-speaking a standard language (Joyce's or Ezra Pound's Ulysses). It is obvious that 'man' holds the majority, even if he is less numerous than mosquitoes, children, women, blacks, homosexuals etc. That is because he appears twice, once in the constant and again in the variable from which the constant is extracted. Majority assumes a state of power and domination, not the other way round. Majority assumes the standard measure, not the other way round.[9]

A given balance of forces produces a majoritarian model as a norm, that which Deleuze and Guattari call a majoritarian 'fact'. This 'fact' constitutes a homogeneous system in which the minorities are sub-groups. And it is within such a homogeneous system that we have the choice of representative politics:

> This is evident in all the operations, electoral or otherwise, where we are given a choice, but on the condition that your choice conform to the limits of the constant (you mustn't choose to change society...).[10]

According to this first argument, the majority has no real representative value because the choice of the representative politics cannot but confirm a given state of domination. The representation cannot but confirm the relationship between existing forces. But this first argument only draws its force from a second and more radical one. Within the first argument one could, in fact, still imagine that another majoritarian model, more open to differences, would be capable of representing 'the greatest number'. One could still imagine a majoritarian model that would take into account certain minorities: women, blacks, homosexuals, etc. But whatever the progress made in the recognition of minorities' rights and 'multicultural politics', these progressions will never settle the issue of the representative value of the majority.[11] The reason for this is simple. The majority represents literally *no one*. It is a *model* of the construction and attribution of identities; as such, it is necessarily an *empty model*. In order to understand this second argument, which is by no means self-evident, let us see how Deleuze and Guattari describe the constitution of the majoritarian standard.

In the analyses of different social formations carried out in *A Thousand Plateaus*, Deleuze and Guattari emphasise the importance of what they call 'faciality' (*visagéité*).[12] The state of actual domination – and the production of the majority that corresponds to it – takes the form of the constitution of a face (*visage*). Or, more precisely, what is at stake is the *unity* of a face. This unity is anything but personal. It is neither human nor animal. The face is produced in humanity, but it is produced by a necessity that does not apply to human beings 'in general'.[13] What is this necessity? It is that of producing a model of identity and normality in relation to which deviations can subsequently be detected. One must first construe the norm in order then to exclude – or tolerate – its deviations. That production proceeds according to successive binary choices. In a first step, we are dealing with the construction of a face starting out from singular traits; concrete faces, following the choice of the order 'this is an *x or* a *y*'. For instance, one might be a man *or* a woman, an adult *or* a child, a rich person *or* a poor one, etc. In a second step, once the unity of the face is constituted, the machine of binarization proceeds to a selection. It judges whether or not a given face conforms to the standard. This is a choice of the type 'yes-no': the rejected faces, the faces which do not conform to a first selection, will be submitted to successive binary selections. For instance, what is neither a man nor a woman would be classified as a transvestite. In sum, the constitution of the face proceeds first as a 'computation (*ordination*) of normalities' and then as a 'deviance detector'.[14]

According to Deleuze and Guattari, the constitution of identity (or the attribution of normality) always takes place prior to all eventual discrimination and, in a sense, makes discrimination possible, or even calls it forth. There would be no 'good' politics of identity to be opposed to 'bad' ones. European racisms are no aberrations; they follow the logic of that very same construction of identity. They are not strategies of exclusion from without, they are strategies of constitution from within:

European racism as the white man's claim has never operated by exclusion, or by the designation of someone as the Other: it is instead in primitive societies that the stranger is grasped as an 'other' (...). From the viewpoint of racism, there is no exterior, there are no people on the outside. There are only people who should be like us and whose crime is not to be. (...) Racism never detects the particles of the other; it propagates waves of sameness until those who resist identification have been wiped out. Its cruelty is equaled only by its incompetence and naïveté.[15]

Once again, Deleuze and Guattari's point is not to put different political regimes on the same level. Parliamentary democracies, fascisms or situations in which racism becomes a politics of the state are not equivalent.[16] The degrees of tolerance with respect to those who resist identification can be enormous, and their political importance, needless to say, is fundamental. What is at stake for Deleuze and Guattari is to show how a specific identity standard is constructed and what are its intrinsic dangers. In this context, it is impossible to discuss all the consequences of such a concept of identity. I will limit myself to the issue of representation.

It is only on the basis of this analysis of the face that we can understand why, according to Deleuze and Guattari, no majority will ever be able to represent the people. In *A Thousand Plateaus*, the production of the face that we have just described corresponds exactly to the production of the majority. The face is the abstract standard, the majoritarian model according to which a system is constituted and wherein a majority, as well as minorities, are identified. But as we have seen, the normative model, produced as a grid of identification, is in itself *empty*. The face, the majoritarian 'fact', represents literally *no one*. The problem is not that minorities are excluded. As we have already said, this could be changed. The problem is rather that not even the majority can be truly represented by the standard of the face:

For the majority, insofar as it is analytically included in the abstract standard, is never anybody, it is always Nobody – Ulysses – (...). There is a majoritarian 'fact', but it is the analytic fact of Nobody (...).[17]

This analysis of the majoritarian fact as the production of a necessarily empty standard is a critique of representation. But one must note that the critique of representation is not a critique of the universal. Or, in any event, representation and universality do not coincide. The face is not a universal. It is not even the universal of the White Man: as a standard, as a majoritarian model, the unity of the face is empty, just as the 'majority is Nobody'. What is in question is not the production of a universal but the production of an abstract and empty model, one which analytically comprehends the majority, independent of any relation to quantity. This model produces the 'majoritarian' as a constant and homogeneous system and minorities as subsystems. As a consequence, it represents neither the 'majority' nor the 'minorities'.

The emptiness of the majoritarian model of which Deleuze and Guattari speak is not a *universal* emptiness. It is not the emptiness that is necessary to democracy, an emptiness that prevents each particular historical figure from coinciding with the universal, and from occupying its place in a non-contingent manner.[18] The problem of the majoritarian model is not, according to Deleuze and Guattari, that a dominant group imposes its identity as universal. The problem of the majoritarian model is that it produces norms of identification which impose themselves on the whole world and yet represent no one. The major identity is just as much constructed and imposed by a state of domination as the identities that are minor. The majoritarian model oppresses men *and* women, heterosexuals *and* homosexuals, albeit to different degrees. The consequence of this critique of the majority model is not the revindication of a 'minority politics'. As we have seen, as groups minorities form part of the system. They are produced by the construction of identity. The politics of Deleuze and Guattari is a politics of the *becoming-minoritarian*. And as we shall see later, that is something completely different from any minority politics. Moreover, it is precisely this becoming-minoritarian that reintroduces the universal into *A Thousand Plateaus*.

According to Deleuze and Guattari, there is indeed a universal, and a universal in the strict sense of the term, since this concerns everybody. But it is a paradoxical universal of de-identification. The majoritarian 'fact' is the real (but empty) product of a state of domination. Deleuze and Guattari oppose to this 'fact' a 'universal minoritarian consciousness' that is not of the order of power (*pouvoir*) and domination and that has no other content, no other identity, than a potential (*puissance*) of becoming.[19] It would be futile to oppose a counter-power to power and to actual domination, just as much as it would be vain to replace the model of the White Man with another identitarian model, even if it be that of a minority. The only possible politics, in Deleuze and Guattari's perspective, is a politics of resistance, a politics of a universal becoming-minoritarian that does not aim to 'win the power'. But before analysing some consequences of this politics of becoming, we must clarify its contents.

Becoming-minoritarian as universal consciousness

What does the concept of 'becoming' mean? Why is any becoming a becoming-minoritarian? And why does becoming matter to politics? The examples given by Deleuze and Guattari are not always easy to grasp: becoming-animal, becoming-molecule, -music or -vegetal go along with more 'human' becomings like becoming-woman, -black, -Jewish, -child, etc. What do all these different forms of becoming have in common? One initial response to this question would be that any becoming is a movement of de-identification. The first thing to underscore when we speak about becoming—in fact, its most easily determinable feature—is that which it is not: becoming is not imitating. Let us take the example of becoming-animal, which is a highly political becoming according to Deleuze and Guattari.[20] It is worth keeping in mind that the same could be said about any becoming. Becoming-animal does not consist in 'acting like' an animal. But the becoming-animal neither is an organic transformation that would result in 'being' an animal. The becoming is neither of the order of being nor of the order of *mimesis*—assuming one could distinguish the two. On the contrary, it is that which escapes this 'false alternative'. One only becomes insofar as one subtracts oneself from all identification as well as from all imitation. Nevertheless, becoming is perfectly *real*.

But what kind of reality is at stake here? According to Deleuze and Guattari, the reality of becoming is a purely immanent one: what is real is becoming itself, regardless of the reality of the supposedly fixed terms of departure and arrival:

> The becoming-animal of the human being is real, even if the animal the human being becomes is not. This is the point to clarify: that a becoming lacks a subject distinct from itself; but also that it has no term, since its term in turn exists only as taken up in another becoming of which it is the subject, and which coexists, forms a block, with the first.[21]

A useful way of clarifying this point is to take into account the concept of 'external relation'. First elaborated by Deleuze in his *Empiricism and Subjectivity*,[22] this concept plays an important role in all his later work, including *A Thousand Plateaus*. According to Deleuze, the empiricist tradition (from Hume to Russell and Whitehead) produces a new theory of relation that constitutes its own contribution to philosophy. Empiricism is not founded on the abstract principle that 'any knowledge orginates in sensibility'. On the contrary, it substitutes abstract principles by the idea of experimentation in/of life (*expérimentation de vie*), and the theory of 'external relations' is a

crucial issue of this experiment. For the empiricists, relations are not dependent on the terms they relate. Let us take for example: 'The glass is on the
table.' This relation is not determined by the properties of either 'the glass'
or 'the table'. It is not interior to one of the terms, which would then be its
subject, nor to both elements taken together. A relation can change even if
the properties of its terms do not change. Thus, according to Deleuze, empiricism traces a geography of relation that contests the priority of the verb
'to be'. Instead of judgements of attribution and existence, the empiricists
develop a logic of conjunctions. And this logic, far from being a principle, is
a protest of life (*protestation vitale*) against any principle.[23] It is the very logic
of becoming where what happens does not depend on fixed essences or
properties but on the open field of encounters that allow for new relations to
be established and new experiments in life to take shape. From this point of
view, we can understand that the becoming-animal of a man is a relation
that does not depend on any given quality of either man or animal. It is on
the contrary a relation, or an encounter, that creates a new 'line of flight' that
has a direction of its own and in which both man and animal are
deterritorialized.

   If becoming is a 'nonlocalizable relation', a shared deterritorialization,
this implies not only an encounter between at least two terms, but also the
coexistence of two asymmetrical movements. This is a crucial point concerning Deleuze and Guattari's politics. According to them, all sorts of becoming – be these human or inhuman, becoming-child, woman, black,
becoming-animal, music, vegetal, molecule or, finally, imperceptible – are
becoming-minoritarian and thus *political*. The shared deterritorialization and
the asymmetrical movements implied by becoming must be understood in
relation to the analysis of the majority as an empty standard.

   Where the majoritarian and empty model, which presupposes a state of
domination, has as its function to assign fixed places and identities, the
becomings-minoritarian are the processes through which one deserts these
places and undoes these identities. This is why there are all sorts of
becomings, but never a becoming-Man.[24] There is no becoming-Man for at
least two reasons. First, because Man, as an empty model, is literally *nobody*.
Furthermore, because Man, as an empty model, refers to a state of domination whereas becoming does not remain in any state at all and does not aim
at power. This is a point to which I will return. Put otherwise – in terms that
would no longer be Deleuzian – if Man is a figure, becoming is a de-figuration.

   So far, we have assessed why becoming always implies a double movement and why it has no term since this exists only as taken up in another becoming. 'Man' is always the 'subject' of a becoming precisely where he or

she lets himself or herself be taken up by a becoming-minoritarian which subtracts him or her from his or her major identity. Becoming is always a process of de-identification and de-figuration. But such a process does not come about all by itself: it needs an encounter. A minority, whatever its nature, is the trigger of the becoming, its 'active medium.' Provided – and this is crucial – that the 'minority' in question becomes something else in turn. For the becoming-minoritarian is certainly not to be confused with the belonging to a minority. Belonging to a minority as a state could mean being bound to an identitarian model that is at least as strong as that of the face of Man. The 'molar identities' (in the terminology of *A Thousand Plateaus*) are no less heavy to carry when they are those of a minority as a fixed state. Also the minorities have to become, to undo their forms and functions, to desert their assigned places:

> In a way, the subject in a becoming is always 'man', but only when he enters a becoming-minoritairian that rends him from his major identity (...). Conversely, if Jews themselves must become-Jewish, if women must become-woman, if children must become-child, if blacks must become-black, it is because only a minority is capable of serving as active-medium of becoming, but under such conditions that it ceases to be a definable aggregate in relation to the majority. (...) There is no subject of the becoming except as a deterritorialised variable of the majority; there is no medium of becoming except as a deterritorialised variable of a minority. We can be thrown into a becoming by anything at all, by the most unexpected, most insignificant of things. You don't deviate from the majority unless there is a little detail that starts to swell and carries you off. It is because the hero of Focus, the average American, needs glasses that give his nose a vaguely Semitic air, it is 'because of the glasses' that he is thrown into this strange adventure of the becoming-Jewish of the non-Jew. Anything at all can do the job, but it always turns out to be a political affair.[25]

Now the becoming-minoritarian, in its flight from the face, has an immanent end. When the becomings do not disintegrate (which can always happen), when they link up with each other, they are propelled into an *imperceptible and impersonal becoming* which is the 'immanent end' of all becomings. The becoming-imperceptible propels the flight from the grid of dominant identifications up to the point where one is no longer recognisable, when one is just like 'everybody else' (*tout le monde*). The 'man of becoming', according to Deleuze and Guattari, must go unnoticed; there must be nothing special to be perceived from the outside.[26] But becoming-everybody (*devenir tout le monde*) is not just a matter of being unrecognisable, of being like 'everybody else'. Deleuze and Guattari are playing here with the different possible meanings allowed by the French expression 'tout le monde'. Thus *devenir tout le monde* also entails a becoming *of everybody*, a *becoming-everything* and a *becoming of the world itself*:

> If it is so difficult to be like everybody else, it is because it is an affair of becoming. Not everybody becomes everybody (and everything: tout le monde), makes a becoming of everybody/everything. (...) For everybody/everything is the molar aggregate, but becoming everybody/everything is another affair, one that brings into play the cosmos with its molecular components. Becoming everybody/everything (*tout le monde*) is to world (*faire monde*), to make a world (*faire un monde*).[27]

This becoming imperceptible entails a becoming of everybody and of the world that turns the abstract emptiness of the face in the direction of an 'universal minoritarian consciousness'. Deleuze and Guattari oppose the figure of an *universal minoritarian consciousness* that, in principle, concerns everybody to the majoritarian 'fact' that itself is the product of a state of domination, but is the analytic fact of *nobody*. Universality is neither on the side of a representative majority – the majoritarian standard measure is empty – nor on the side of minority groups as such. No minority can pretend to represent the universal for the good reason that there cannot be a *representation* of the universal. According to Deleuze and Guattari, the only legitimate claim to universality is a universal becoming-minoritarian where what is universally shared is nothing but becoming itself.

The micropolitics Deleuze and Guattari are calling for is the very opposite of *any* political strategy of power: 'how to win the majority' is 'a totally secondary problem'. It is important to emphasise that Deleuze and Guattari are not just criticising parliamentary democracies in the name of a radical revolution. 'How to win the revolution' is not a better question to ask than 'how to win the majority'. What matters is not power (*pouvoir*), but becoming, and becoming requires a potential (*puissance*), an active micropolitics, and this is the opposite of any strategy of domination.

Politics is active resistance. Does this mean that micropolitics is one more utopian politics? Here, utopia is a misleading concept. If we want to use the word, we should say that it is an *immanent* utopia, and this deployment of terms makes a difference.[28] Because what is at stake in becoming are *immanent forms of life*. Politics – be it revolutionary – usually thinks, like History, in terms of past and future, means and ends, but immanent becoming has its own temporality which is indifferent to past and future, which 'passes between the two'.[29]

Resistance to power, resistance to the present, to the intolerable, to shame and servitude has no messianic dimension, no teleological *telos*. Its aim is a *becoming of the world* as a possibility of inventing new forms of life, different modes of existence. The search for these new possibilities of life is not submitted to the future of any perfect State or revolution. Becomings, as we already said, are perfectly real in themselves, whenever and wherever they occur.

This concept of politics as 'resistance' and the consequences it entails should be discussed further on different levels.[30] For my present concern, I will limit myself to one aspect of resistance: resistance to *opinion*. If Deleuze's thought has from the outset political aims and implications, as Foucault suggested, it is precisely because he understands philosophy as a struggle against opinion. And it is in this very struggle against the power of opinion that Deleuze's ontological and *political* critique of representation finds its justification.

Representation as the power of opinion (difference and repetition): How to be a minoritarian Platonist?

On one major point Deleuze has always been a strict Platonist. From *Nietzsche and Philosophy* and *Difference and Repetition* through to *What is Philosophy?*, he claims that the very aim of the philosophical project is to break with *doxa*. Philosophy struggles against any form of opinion, which does not mean that it always succeeds. On the contrary, philosophy more often fails to be faithful to its own project. This is why, as Deleuze states in *Difference and Repetition*, 'where to begin in philosophy has always – rightly – been regarded as a very delicate problem'.[31] The problem of beginning is precisely the problem of breaking with opinion. Beginning, for philosophy, would then mean eliminating all presuppositions.

If the question of beginning is thus as old as philosophy, its modern form is inaugurated by Descartes' Cogito. Descartes presents the Cogito as a definition that does not rely on any given concept. This is, for instance, the well-known argument in the Second Meditation where Descartes does not want to define man as a rational animal because such a definition explicitly presupposes the concepts of rationality and animality. This Cartesian gesture has been repeated by Kant, Hegel, Husserl and Heidegger. However differently they determine the 'beginning', they were also searching to free philosophy from any pre-given presupposition.

Now, the problem, according to Deleuze, is that in setting aside *objective* presuppositions philosophy does not escape from another kind of presupposition which is as dangerous as it is implicit – that of *subjective* presuppositions. By 'objective presuppositions' Deleuze means *concepts* explicitly presupposed by another pre-given concept. These conceptual presuppositions are easy to recognise and, as a consequence, easy to eliminate. But in philosophy we not only deal with concepts, we also deal with all sorts of *implicit* presuppositions contained in *opinions* rather than concepts. These implicit and preconceptual presuppositions are what Deleuze calls *subjective* presuppositions.

The *cogito* does not refer us back to the concepts of the animal and the rational, but instead to a supposedly universal and pre-conceptual knowledge. It presumes that everyone knows, without concepts, what is meant by 'self', 'thinking' and 'being'. The cogito appears as a true beginning, but in fact it has referred all its presuppositions back to subjective opinions. Getting rid of given concepts is not enough for philosophy to break with doxa. The powers of opinion come back in the form of subjective presuppositions. The same holds true, according to Deleuze, for Kant, Hegel or even Heidegger, who constantly invokes a pre-ontological understanding of being.

What is important to notice is that subjective presuppositions take the form of *representation*. The form of a subjective or implicit presupposition is always: 'Everybody knows...', 'No one can deny...'. For Descartes, everyone knows in a pre-philosophical manner what it means to be or to think. For Heidegger, everyone knows, in a pre-ontological manner, what Being means. Now, according to Deleuze, '*Everybody knows, no one can deny* is the form of representation and the discourse of the representative'.[32]

In the first chapter of *Difference and Repetition* ('Difference in itself'), Deleuze already presented a critique of representation as that which allows philosophy to subordinate difference to identity in the context of a discussion of Aristotelian categories. I cannot follow this line of argumentation here. That would lead us to discuss the question of Deleuze's ontology of univocity of being as opposed to an ontology of analogy, which is not my topic in this context.[33] In the chapter I am discussing here (chapter 3, 'The Image of Thought'), Deleuze's concern is the nature of thought (or, more precisely, as we'll see, the absence of such a 'nature') and the task of philosophy. In this context, representation is the target of a critique which is both philosophical and political. Representation is a dangerous category that conveys an image of thought cut off from its own power (*puissance*) and inclined towards a dubious orthodoxy.

The true philosopher looks for a new beginning, he does not want to rely on any traditional knowledge. He trusts only his good will and his natural capacity for thought. Thus, he takes the side of the individual man against the too cultivated man, 'the pedant', perverted by the generalities of the culture of his time.[34] He takes the side of the 'idiot', as Deleuze puts it. But the philosopher is not idiot enough. He is endowed with too much good will and too much common sense. He can put aside any pre-given concept and any traditional knowledge, but he trusts the powers of opinion too easily. Certainly not any particular opinion, but their very form, the form of representation. Which is worse.

According to Deleuze, the philosopher should indeed take the side of the 'idiot'. But the side of a Russian idiot, the idiot of Dostojevski, or of Shestov. The philosopher who wants to begin should break with the discourse of representation:

> Such protest does not take place in the name of aristocratic prejudices: it is not a question of saying what few think and knowing what it means to think. On the contrary, it is a question of someone – if only one – with the necessary modesty not managing to know what everybody knows, and modestly denying what everybody is supposed to recognise. *Someone who neither allows himself to be represented, nor wishes to represent anything.* Not an individual endowed with good will and a natural capacity for thought, but an individual full of ill will who does not manage to think, either naturally or conceptually. Only such an individual is without presuppositions. [35]

When the philosopher assumes (as universally recognisable) general presuppositions as to what is meant by thinking, being or self, he seems to be disinterested or interested only in 'pure knowledge'. He does not seem to take the side of any established value. But he accepts the very form of representation, and this *form* is anything but innocent because it also has a *matter*. The 'matter' Deleuze speaks of is the assumption that thought is the natural exercise of a faculty. Which implies that thought, as well as the thinker, are naturally oriented toward the truth:

> Thought has a natural affinity with the true under the double aspect of a good will on the part of the thinker (*bonne volonté du penseur*) and an upright nature on the part of thought (*nature droite de la pensée*).[36]

According to Deleuze, the most general form of representation is thus founded in common sense understood as upright nature and good will. Philosophy has as its implicit presupposition a pre-philosophical and natural image of thought, borrowed from pure common sense.

I would like to recall here only two major features of this image of thought which Deleuze extensively analyses. The image of thought, grounded in common sense, is nevertheless a philosophical assumption in the measure that it produces a *transcendental* model of what it means to think. But this very transcendental model is a model of *orthodoxy*. Indeed, the concept that the representation of thought as a natural exercise which is naturally in affinity with the truth is not a *fact*. The affinity of thought with the truth and, as a consequence, the assumption that error is its only danger, are stated as a *philosophical principle*. Whatever the difficulty of 'translating this principal into fact' may be. The observation that men usually do not think, or think only rarely, that thought is threatened more by meanness and madness than by error, would not be sufficient to shake the presupposition of an upright nature of thought. The image of thought, and it is in this that it is philosophical, institutes a redistribution of the empirical and the transcendental, of the rightful and the effective (*du droit et du fait*). There is a transcendental model implied in the image: the model of *recognition*. To think is to recognise.

According to Deleuze, to make of recognition (*récognition*) the transcendental model for thought is an act presenting two major disadvantages. As a speculative model of what thinking means, recognition is 'insignificant'. There are, of course, acts of recognition taking place all the time, but nothing which is truly at stake in thought takes place in the 'recognition' of an object. However, the model of recognition ceases to be insignificant, thereby becoming dangerous as soon as we consider 'the ends it serves'. If to think is to recognise, then that which is recognised is at once an object and the values attributed to it. It is in this sense that for Deleuze, the image of thought, with the transcendental model it produces, is necessarily a dogmatic image and an orthodoxy: 'The form of recognition has never sanctioned anything but the recognisable and the recognised; form will never inspire anything but conformities.'[37] The image of thought permanently prevents philosophy from achieving its most intimate vocation – that of breaking with the *doxa* and with common sense. Philosophy will limit itself to suspending all particular *doxa*, but so as to retain the essential, so as to universalise it and make of it a transcendental model.

The image of thought encloses philosophy in an orthodoxy, condemning it to the reduplication of that opinion and of that common sense with which it wished to break. The problem of beginning, of the search for that starting point from which thought might be born to itself in separating itself from any and all objective presupposition, will be without solution for Deleuze as long as the image which imprisons thought does not undergo a radical critique. This radical critique should have 'the power of a *new politics* which would overturn the image of thought'.[38] This new politics cannot be merely the matter of thinking or of thought. In *Difference and Repetition*, Deleuze opposes to the orthodox image of a thought which would develop naturally the idea that we think only when something in the world forces us to think. Like becoming, thought is only put into motion by means of an encounter:

> Do not count upon thought to ensure the relative necessity of what it thinks. Rather count upon the contingency of an encounter with that which forces thought to raise up and educate the absolute necessity of an act of thought or a passion to think. (...)

> Something in the world forces us to think. This something is an object not of recognition, but of a fundamental *encounter*. [39]

The critique of the concept of representation is not an exception to what Deleuze states in *Difference and Repetition* in regard to the necessity of an encounter. In themselves, concepts are nothing but possibilities and cannot independently engender a true act of thinking. They lack 'the claws of absolute necessity'. This necessity must come from without. In the exchange with Foucault that we cited earlier, 'Intellectuals and Power', Deleuze underscores that the critique of representation effected on the 'theoretical' level had lacked, and was awaiting, its 'practical' translation. He thus credits Foucault with having been the first to 'teach us the indignity of speaking for others'[40] and the necessity of others speaking for themselves. The political involvement of Deleuze in the GIP (*Groupe d'information sur les prisons*),[41] created by Foucault, is precisely such an attempt of not being a 'representative intellectual', but of helping 'others speak for themselves'.

For Deleuze, the 'claw of necessity' took the shape of the political events of the Seventies and remained inscribed in his thought. He re-elaborated again and again, both in his own texts and those written with Guattari, the theme of the 'indignity of speaking for others'. But the abandonment of the pretension of speaking for others, and the refusal of all representative discourse, cannot be conducted under the sign of a solipsism. The philosopher does not break with the powers of opinion in the solitude of his own thought.

In commenting upon Artaud's formula, 'to write for the illiterate – to speak for the aphasic, to think for the acephalous,' Deleuze and Guattari explore what is meant by such a 'for' once all forms of representation have been excluded.[42] It certainly cannot mean to write in their place or name, nor even for their benefit. To write 'for' someone or something signifies rather the event of being taken up into the double movement of a becoming wherein the philosopher finds his or her 'zones of indiscernibility' with the illiterate and headless, with a dying animal, where he becomes a non-philosopher in the hope that even the headless and the animals will become, in their turn, something else:

> The agony of a rat or the slaughter of a calf remains present in thought not through pity but as the zone of exchange between man and animal in which something of one passes into the other. This is the constitutive relationship with nonphilosophy. Becoming is always double, and it is this double becoming that constitutes the people to come and the new earth. The philosopher must become nonphilosopher so that nonphilosophy becomes the earth and people of philosophy.[43]

The philosopher represents no-one, but he thinks only because he is haunted by a people which is lacking (*le peuple qui manque*), a people 'oppressed, bastardized and irredeemably minor'. What is more, he shares with the people the effort of creating and resisting the present. Resisting and creating amounts to a single act. To break the power of opinion, one must resist. Resistance, however, is an active power (*puissance*), it is the creation of the new:

> The artist or the philosopher is quite incapable of creating a people, each can only summon it with all his strength. A people can only be created in abominable sufferings, and it cannot be concerned any more with art or philosophy. But books of philosophy and works of art also contain their sum of unimaginable sufferings that forewarn the advent of a people. They have resistance in common – their resistance to death, to servitude, to the intolerable, to shame, and to the present.[44]

The Platonic stand of Deleuze, his desire for philosophy to break with any given opinion, does not lead him to share Plato's dream of a Philosopher-King. Philosophy, and philosophers, have no key to build the perfect state. But they struggle against the power of opinions that oppresses everybody, even if to dramatically different degrees. Philosophy is (should be?) on the side of the oppressed people. Whatever this side may be according to different geographical and historical situations. No national, social, 'ethnic' or even sexual identity should be too strong to prevent philosophy from struggling against dangerous opinions and 'common' sense.

11 SCHINDLER'S LIST and the Facing of History

The Return of the Promised Land

Sasha Vojkovic

Deleuze and Guattari versus Spielberg

By changing the original title of Thomas Keneally's novel *Schindler's Ark* into SCHINDLER'S LIST, Steven Spielberg's film announces a shift from the Genesis narrative as a pretext to the story about the 'chosen people' from the Exodus.[1] Noah's act of salvation of the species from the collective doom brought down by the wrath of God gives way to the story of Moses liberating the chosen people from slavery and leading them on their passage towards the Promised Land. Spielberg's play with the notion of land or territory as it is related to the mythical pretext is complex and involves more than the opposition between the safe territory, such as Schindler's factory described by the workers as the 'haven', and the territory of death such as the Plaszow labor camp or, worse yet, Auschwitz. As we learn from the film, there is a third option to be attained, and it lies in that territory in between, the Promised Land. This third option, as I will explain, which carries with it the theological hope of returning to Jerusalem, is a reminder that deportation and diaspora, as they emerge and evolve in the biblical narratives, are constitutive of Jewish identity.

In this respect, I would suggest the film problematizes the Jewish subject as exemplary of an ethnic group existing without/on an impossible territory; hence, 'giving a face' to this subject is in the first instance bound up with the myth of the origin of land. The 'territoriality' of the subject can be traced via the structuring of the narrative; SCHINDLER'S LIST stages a return to the promised land by structuring the events in such a way as to build up the expectation for the arrival of the Messiah who is to save the chosen people. In such a narrativization of redemption, utopia is achieved, and the irreconcilable is reconciled. By appropriating a version of Jewish redemption, Spielberg constructs an allegory – the story of countless individual deaths becomes enveloped in a promise of salvation. The promise of salvation entails the notion of a home as a memory of the past, projected into the future, but also the arrival at a Promised Land and a reacquisition of a long-lost territory. This infers that such a movement of reterritorialization is bound up with the affirmation of Jewish identity, and conversely, that there is a Jewish specificity affirmed in a semiotic system which governs this movement of reterritorialization.[2]

In *A Thousand Plateaus*, Deleuze and Guattari take precisely this structure that governs the movement of reterritorialization as a basis to theorize a specific regime of signs. More precisely, their fourth regime of signs, the so-called 'postsignifying system' is elaborated as an allegory of the history of the Jews.[3] The 'pragmatics of territoriality' as it is related to this semiotic – departure and the promise of return will be taken as a basis for an examination of territoriality in SCHINDLER'S LIST. The Jewish semiotic is one of the systems of signification which Deleuze and Guattari juxtapose to the so-called 'despotic regime', or the signifying semiotic which in their view is characterized by universal deception. As I will explain, the movement of deterritorialization which can occur within the despotic regime is based on the principle of the scapegoat. Due to the system's capacity to control signification, a specific sign can be charged (in the double sense of the word) with everything that was 'bad' in a given period. On the basis of the analysis of SCHINDLER'S LIST, I will suggest that the movement of deterritorialization imposed by the Nazis can be taken as a manifestation of the despotic regime.

The analysis of the structure of the film demonstrates that the progressive effacement of the territory on which the Jews are allowed to exist is commensurable with the progressive decimation of the Jewish population. The given historical conditions, then, which brought about the Holocaust and the systematic annihilation of the Jews exemplify the ultimate horror of a despotic regime. According to Deleuze and Guattari, the postsignifying system or the Jewish semiotic can be counterposed to the signifying semiotic of the despotic regime because within this system, the sign displays the capacity to voluntarily disattach from the center and set off down its own line of flight. The ability to disattach from the system opens up the connection with the countersignifying semiotic of the nomads, which I will discuss below. Nevertheless, Deleuze and Guattari also point to the negative aspect of the Jewish semiotic and its simultaneous connection with the despotic regime, due to the intrinsic striving of the Jews to return to the long-lost territory. Hence, in their view, the initially positive line of flight or deterritorialization becomes ultimately intertwined with the negative line of flight.

In this chapter I will suggest that the aspiration toward reterritorialization needs to be observed in terms of the historical period in which the de/re-territorialization occurs. While the notion of return principally implies a re-aquisition of the long-lost territory, in SCHINDLER'S LIST reterritorialization is elaborated as a possibility of overcoming deportation and ghettoization. As the analysis of the film shows, the movement of reterritorialization of the Jews can be juxtaposed to the movement of deterritorialization imposed by the Nazis. The arrival at the long-lost territory which marks the end of deportation will eventually put pressure on the myth of 'one people', and in that sense, SCHINDLER'S LIST will confront us with yet another face of history. In the film's closing, as I will explain, reterritorialization as the theological symbol of Judaism appropriated to depict the salvation of eleven hundred Jews (from absolute deterritorialization) is merging with specific signs that refer to another period in the history of the Jews: the Six-Day War and hence, the tenuous conditions in the present day Israel. By staging a tripartite overlap of returns in the film's closing, Spielberg, just as Deleuze and Guattari, problematizes the Jewish semiotic in terms of the positive and negative line of its movement. The ultimate question that emerges with the return to Israel is, what effect does the movement of reterritorialization have on the Jewish subject, to name but one agency? While the universalism inherent in mythical discourse is a way of affirming the identity in question, the overlapping of returns, lands and faces of history at the end of the film questions the notion of the Promised Land as a safe territory for all its inhabitants.[4]

The Jewish semiotic and the territoriality of signs

According to Deleuze and Guattari, semiotic systems depend on what they call assemblages: all assemblages are basically territorial, and hence, the first rule is to discover which territoriality they envelop. The assemblages determine that a given people, period or language can assure the predominance of one semiotic or another. Thus, Deleuze and Guattari make maps of the regimes of signs, depending on the case they are dealing with, that is, a social dimension, a pathological delusion or a historical event. The philosophers call any specific formalization of expression a regime of signs. A regime of signs constitute a semiotic system. There are, therefore, (at least) four semiotics which display very diverse characteristics: the signifying semiotic, the presignifying semiotic, the counter-signifying semiotic and the post-signifying semiotic. Within the realm of the signifying system, we can trace the movement of deterritorialization, but in each of the four signifying systems, this movement is blocked by the system itself; in other words, it is appropriated or absorbed by the system. The operation of the line of flight is the movement by which one leaves the territory, and this can be understood as deterritorialization. There are different cases of deterritorialization, but principally, the only possibility of a positive absolute deterritorialization is on the plane of the Body without Organs, which means outside of semiotic regimes. Deleuze and Guattari have introduced the notion of the 'abstract machine' which marks the plane of consistency, implying that it goes beyond language.[5] The abstract machine is deterritorialized and in itself is not physical or corporeal, any more than it is semiotic. It has no substance or form, and it operates by matter and function.

> The plane consists abstractly, but really, in relations to speed and slowness between uniformed elements, and in compositions of corresponding intensive affects (...). Consistency concretely ties together heterogeneous, disparate elements and assures the consolidation of fuzzy aggregates (...). In effect, consistency, proceeding by consolidation, acts necessarily in the middle, by the middle and stands opposed to all principles of finality.[6]

Here, in the middle, inscribed on this plane are events and incorporeal transformations such as becomings. According to Deleuze and Guattari, 'a becoming is the in-between, it constitutes a zone of proximity and indiscernability, a no-man's-land'.[7] The notion of the no-man's-land evokes the word utopia coined by Thomas Moore in 1516; the word means what is nowhere, and as Moore describes it, it is the island which is nowhere, the place which exists in no real place, a ghost city, a river with no water, a prince with no people. A becoming implies entering this extraterritoriality; or to put it in Deleuze and Guattari's terms, the entrance takes place into a zone of positive and absolute deterritorialization.

Juxtaposed to the zone of a positive absolute deterritorialization are the four regimes of signs which display very different characteristics. The first and most common regime is the signifying semiotic, and as I have mentioned above, its basic characteristic is universal deception. The regime is deceptive because it is regulative. It regulates the signifying circles, it controls interpretations, it facializes the center, and it governs the line of flight or the movement of deterritorialization. Within this line of thought, 'giving a face' to the signifier presupposes 'fixing' a meaning, but it also alludes to the intrinsic capacity of the signifier to generate lies, that is, to deceive. Within the realm of the signifying system we can trace the movement of deterritorialization, but as mentioned above, this movement is blocked by the system, or rather appropriated or absorbed by that system. This particularly concerns the principle of the scapegoat; because of the system's capacity to control signification, there is a continuous danger that a new becoming will be sent off into circulation, representing what Deleuze and Guattari call 'a new form of increasing entropy in the system of signs'.[8] The one who is tortured and who fundamentally loses his or her face, the one who is entering into becoming-animal, a becoming-molecular, becomes a scapegoat and comes to be charged with everything that was 'bad' in a given period, that is, 'everything that resisted signifying signs...'[9] Losing one's face as a way of entering into becoming-animal is in this case the first step before exclusion. Exclusion for the faceless, tortured person, or the scapegoat, appears inevitable for it incarnates that line of flight or deterritorialization the signifying regime cannot tolerate.[10] In the analysis of SCHINDLER'S LIST, I will take the movement of deterritorialization imposed on the Jews by the Nazis as the example of the negative line of flight produced via the system of universal deception.

To the regime of universal deception, or the signifying semiotic, Deleuze and Guattari counterpose three other semiotic systems: the presignifying semiotic, the counter-signifying semiotic and the post-signifying semiotic. The so-called primitive, pre-signifying semiotic is much closer to 'natural' codings operating without signs. Here, the overcoding which marks the privileged status of language operates diffusely: enunciation is collective, and the system encourages polyvocality of forms of expression particular to content. Forms of corporeality, gesturality, rhythm and dance, co-exist heterogeniously with the vocal form. Another regime of signs which they juxtapose to the signifying semiotic is the so-called counter-signifying semiotic. The representatives of the countersignifying semiotic are warlike and animal-raising nomads. Here the form of expression is the Number. In this counter-signifying regime, the imperial despotic line of flight (of the signifying regime) is replaced by a line of abolition; this specifies the ambition to destroy the empire.

Deleuze and Guattari place special emphasis on the post-signifying semiotic which is defined by a unique procedure, that of 'subjectification'.[11] While the signifying sign refers only to other signs, and the set of all signs to the signifier itself, the sign of this 'subjective regime' breaks its relation of significance with other signs. The split between the 'I' and a 'you', the constitution of the self at the expense of the other, can also be understood as a momentary death which Deleuze and Guattari describe as 'an absolute deterritorialization expressed in the black hole of consciousness and passion'.[12] On the one hand, the procedure of subjectification is decentering the sign, that is, the center of significance, is replaced due to the split of the subject into 'two faces turned away from each other'.[13] The subject of enunciation results from this point of subjectification and of the turning away. On the other hand, as Deleuze and Guattari argue, the subject of enunciation that sets out on the movement of deterritorialization recoils into the subject of the statement. Considering that in their view the subject of enunciation is the Althusserian State subject, the succession of proceedings is accompanied by what they call a 'a new form of priest and bureaucracy'.[14] The movement of deterritorialization is thereby marked by a continuous turning back/recoiling/reterritorialization, which makes the line of flight 'freed but segmented, remaining negative and blocked'.[15] In that sense, Deleuze and Guattari take the movement of reterritorialization and the striving of the Jews to return to the long-lost territory as an allegory of the production of subjectivity in language. The Jews thereby come to personify the recoiling subjects of enunciation.

In that respect they assert, 'in the case of Jewish people, a group of signs detaches from the Egyptian imperial network of which it was a part and sets off down a line of flight into the desert'.[16] According to Deleuze and Guattari, the Jews have taken upon themselves the task of following the most deterritorialized line, the line of the scapegoat. They have a strong determination to change its signs, to turn it into the positive line of their subjectivity, their Passion, their proceeding or grievance. This also includes making the line of separation their own, forging their path along it and dissociating the elements of the signifier. It is necessary to keep in mind the distinction they make between the existence in the middle, in the state of perpetual deferral, in no man's land, as is the case with the Jews, and the 'in-between' which constitutes the zone of becoming, or the Body without Organs. Furthermore, they point out that in the case of the post-signifying semiotic which affirms the Jewish identity there is a mix of semiotic regimes; on the one hand, as mentioned earlier, it is intimately related to the counter-signifying regime of the nomads, and on the other hand, especially because it is predicated on subjectification, it has an essential relation to the signifying semiotic itself. This is very much related to Deleuze and Guattari's contention that the regimes of signs cannot be strictly separated because the semiotic systems are constantly intermingling.

The connection between the Jewish semiotic and the counter-signifying semiotic, yields a positive line of flight, and accordingly, faciality undergoes a profound transformation. As they remind us, God turns away his face, not allowing anyone to see it. The subject, struck by the fear of the God, averts his or her face in turn. It is this double turning away that draws the positive line of flight, or deterritorialization. This is very different, Deleuze and Guattari emphasize, from the system of deception animating the face of the signifier, the interpretation of the seer and the displacement of the subject.

Hence, within the postsignifying regime, it seems that the line receives posi-tive signs, as though it were effectively occupied and followed by a people who find in it their reason for being or destiny. Nevertheless, even though the post-signifying regime is characterized by the seemingly positive line of flight, it is inevitably mixed with, as I have already mentioned, what they call the imperial despotic regime, in the sense that it strives toward reterritorialization. It is this signifying regime for which the Hebrews and their God would always be nostalgic: they want to 're-establish an imperial society and integrate with it, enthrone a king like everybody else, rebuild a temple that would finally be solid, erect the spiral Tower of Babel and find the face of God again: not just bring the wondering to a halt, but overcome the diaspora'.[17] In other words, for Deleuze and Guattari, the Jewish semiotic has negative implications due to its intrinsic striving to return to the long-lost territory. Within their line of thought becoming, Jewishness takes more than a state, more than re-acquiring a territory, and hence, the pertinent question is not how to affirm an identity, but rather how to lose it.

Distribution of territories in SCHINDLER'S LIST: despotic regime vs. the postsignifying regime

The intermingling of the signifying and the countersignifying semiotic that Deleuze and Guattari bring to the fore as constitutive of the postsignifying/ Jewish semiotic is pertinent for the discussion of SCHINDLER'S LIST because it announces a complex set of issues which emerge once the mythical land overlaps with present-day Israel.

The potentially negative line of flight bound up with reterritorialization will be addressed in the last part of the analysis, and it can be regarded as a consequence of the imposed deterritorialization which culminated with the Nazi regime. Therefore, the movement of deterritorialization as annihila-tion imposed by the despotic system forges the conditions for the voluntary act of deterritorialization. The bone of contention here is the 'nostalgia for the homeland' and the extent to which it simultaneously reveals a nostalgia for the imperial society. I would suggest that the negative view Deleuze and Guattari ascribe to the ambition of the Jews to overcome the diaspora be complemented with the specific historical conditions as these are spelled out in Spielberg's film, where the return to the promised land additionally refers to the overcoming of deportation, ghettoization and – most important of all – extermination.

As SCHINDLER'S LIST shows, reterritorialization becomes bound up with arriving at the territory where life would be possible. Spielberg is too cautious to leave it at that, however, and as we can gather from the analysis, with reterritorialization comes the impending danger of the negative line of flight. Before I engage in the discussion on the consequences of the return, I will first trace the manifestation of specific territorialities in SCHINDLER'S LIST. There are three lines of action in the film: the line of Oscar Schindler, the line of the Jews, and the line of the Nazis. Each of the lines pertaining to a specific character or group of characters is dependent and defined by concrete territories. This implies that the characters are dependent on the territories they inhabit and conversely, that the territories in question are dependent on the characters.

I. The Nazis: territorialism in progress or deterritorialization as a negative line of flight

The year is 1939, and the registering of the Jews arriving in Cracow has begun. They were ordered to leave their homes in the countryside and relocate to major cities, and for the moment, their new location is unknown. Their locus will be determined according to the list, hence, at the very outset, the Jews are related to the process of transfer and uprootedness. It is the time of the war. The text superimposed on the images informs us that the Polish army was defeated in two weeks, which implies that Poland as a territory has fallen under Hitler's control. From the scenes that follow, we realize that the new conditions have affected all levels of society.

2. Schindler's territorial expansion

One character who is quick to adapt to the new conditions is Schindler. The first convincing example is the night-club scene where Oskar Schindler is introduced; even though at the beginning of the sequence the Nazi officers of the highest rank are undoubtedly the most prominent guests and Schindler is only an outsider, he manages to insert himself into this territory and into the company of those who control it. This will prove quite useful for Schindler, for it will enable him to gain access to his own territory.

3. The Jews: territory suspended

While Schindler is depicted as the one who is on the rise, and hence, progressively acquiring the control of new spaces, the Jews are simultaneously being dispossessed of everything they own. At the point when they are waiting in lines to deliver their complaints to the Jewish Council, when laws are being issued that forbid them to practise their religion, to conduct their businesses or take part in any cultural institutions, Schindler is making preparations for his big enterprise: He wants to have a factory. He asks the

Jewish investors to put up all the money, and he is offering Itzhak Stern, a Jewish accountant, the job of plant manager and the opportunity to run the company for him.

Maintaining a favorable position amongst the Nazi officers takes more than good social skills, or acceptable political conviction; in other words, it costs money. These men need to be constantly appeased with exquisite presents, the kind one can get only on the black market. Schindler will find his best black market contact amongst the Jews; but curiously enough, the initial deal with Leopold Pfefferberg will be closed in the space of a Catholic church. There are two interesting things we accidentally learn about this holy territory: firstly, it only figures as a 'house of god', for there are secret and prohibited transactions going on; and secondly, while Jews are obliged to wear the Yellow Star in all public places, the church is one territory they can enter only if they remove the star.

The doom of the Jews, marked by the state of suspension and transition, is underscored in the extremely wide shot where a huge crowd of people laden with luggage is crossing a bridge. We immediately learn that it is March 20, 1941, the deadline for entering the Ghetto. At this stage, when the status of the Jews is on the verge of a total decline, Schindler is unmistakably emerging as a direct profiteer of the new state of things. This contrast is even elaborated through parallel editing: while a well-to-do Jewish family, the Nussbaums, is evicted from their apartment and forced into the over-crowded territory of the Ghetto, Schindler is expanding his territory and moving into a spacious apartment. Confronted with the demise of their living conditions, the Nussbaums ask themselves whether things could possibly get worse, while Schindler, stretching out on a king size bed, concludes that things could not be better. The meeting organized by Stern with the potential investors that is to take place in Schindler's car is another assertion of Schindler's territorial expansion at the expense of the Jews. The 'negotiation' is a one-way process, for Schindler's alleged partners do not have a say in the matter. They can only accept or refuse his proposal. Their concerned faces framed in the rear view mirror as they are struggling to comprehend the potential benefit of Schindler's highly exploitative scheme most clearly reveal their disadvantageous position. They are not only cornered and without any manoeuvring space, their position within Schindler's enterprise, just as in the mirror, is literally a fictive one.

If there was hope amongst the Jewish people that in spite of hunger and poverty the Ghetto could be a safe territory, with hindsight we could conclude that this hope was in fact a cherished illusion. At this point, the Nazis are issuing new lists whose purpose is the decimation of the Ghetto population. With the new laws declaring forced labor for the Jews, which means they are practically turned into slaves, survival is becoming contingent on one's professional skills. The new lists separate the essential workers from those who are considered superfluous. Needless to say the Nazi war machine had no use for people who were too old to work, or too ill, but they even had less use for Jewish intellectuals. Rabbis, professors, writers, painters, musicians could at any moment be ordered into a truck and be taken away to a concentration camp.

One possibility to frustrate the deportations from the Ghetto at this particular stage is to have a blue card or, rather, a profession that can facilitate the Reich economy. The other options to obtaining a blue card are much more complicated, involving either the acquisition of forged work certificates or the direct intervention of the employer. In any case, whoever can prove to the Nazis that s/he is an essential worker may have some kind of temporary guarantee that s/he is on safe grounds. Considering that Schindler's deal with the Jewish investors did go through, with Itzhak Stern as the financial manager, Schindler's enamel factory DEF is in immediate need of a work force. Schindler's decision to hire Jewish instead of Polish workers is based on very simple calculations. The Jews themselves do not get paid, and hiring them, therefore, is a matter of profit. Stern is the one who is supplying Schindler's newly acquired territory with a workforce, and he is especially engaged in furnishing the dispensable inhabitants of the Ghetto with documents which certify that they are essential occupants of Schindler's territory – metal press operators, metal polishers, metal workers of all profiles. As a German and a member of the Nazi party, Schindler is the person who is enjoying the financial profit, and his major task is to provide a 'face' for the factory that is appealing to the Nazis. This is literally the case in the film, for it is in fact Stern who is making sure that this territory will remain operative and that Schindler's social contacts with the Nazis will have a productive effect on the business.

According to the depiction of the current state of things in the film, there seems to be only two paths outside the territory of the Ghetto – one leads to Schindler's factory, the other to the concentration camps. We soon realize how incommensurable these two options are; while momentarily there is a group of 350 workers on their way to Schindler's factory, there are already long chains of cattle wagons taking people away toward death. The scene in which Schindler manages to prevent the deportation of Stern underscores this disproportion: the fact that he can save Stern attests to Schindler's power, but his intervention demonstrates at the same time how extremely limited his capacity to act as a savior actually is.

4. The liquidation of the ghetto: territory erased

As a juxtaposition to Schindler's enamel factory, another territory is introduced in 1943 – the Plaszow labor camp, run by Amon Goeth. In the labor camp, any of the workers can be executed at random; killing is part of Goeth's daily routine carried out from the balcony of his villa, on the hill, overlooking the camp. It is important to note that the camp territory by Goeth's villa had been a Jewish cemetery until two years earlier; shattered gravestones were used to pave the path at the camp's entrance, the mortuary building was used as the commandant's stables. With the arrival of Goeth, the Ghetto will for a brief moment emerge as a space in between the two opposing territories, the Plaszow camp on one side and Schindler's factory on the other. This situation which underscores the absence of a solid ground seems to be at the same time the condition of Jewish existence. Goeth's plan to liquidate the ghetto and force its inhabitants into his labor camp implies doing away with the last territory on which the Jewish population was allowed to exist. The Ghetto havoc is marked with the Nazi troopers storming through the streets fully prepared to carry out a series of horrific deeds – executions, deportations, tormenting and humiliating the Ghetto inhabitants. There is screaming in panic, failed attempts to run away, desperate search for places to hide. Not even the people who have a working permit are safe from murder and destruction; there is a calculated madness in this operation, and human lives seem to be spared only by chance.[18]

5. Schindler's 'haven': deterritorialization as a positive line of flight

Having witnessed the Ghetto massacre, Schindler is determined to preserve control of his own territory. The scene following the liquidation of the Ghetto depicts Schindler alone in his office, looking through the glass wall onto the empty platform; the occupants of his territory have disappeared. Although Schindler cannot save all the people, his struggle to save a specific group, the population of his territory, that is, 'his Jews', is what evokes comparison with Moses. Maintaining territorial control is a preparation for the ultimate act Schindler will perform – buying his workers from Goeth and taking them away to Brinnlitz.

From this point on a new ground is forged: with the arrival at Brinnlitz the three lines of action, as they are dependent on the characters and the territories, the line of Schindler, of the Jews and of the Nazis, converge into one. Arrival at this territory can be understood as a version of the arrival at a utopistic place, and this is already staged in the scene where Schindler is leading the women released from Auschwitz to the premises of his Brinnlitz factory. There, on the in-between territory, the Jews are encouraged to practise their religion, and the Nazis living under the same roof can hear the Hebrew prayers, but the entire atmosphere of Schindler's territory as outside of the 'real world' prevents them from taking regular measures. They sit quietly in their quarters and listen. Lastly, the inhabitants of this territory manage to keep up the pretence that the factory is producing ammunition, while in actuality its function is to preserve human lives.

6. The movement of reterritorialization

The 'utopian' features of the Brinnlitz factory are additionally confirmed in the scene that follows: The war is over, Schindler's Jews are ready to leave the Brinnlitz factory, and on the basis of the elaboration of the scene it is possible to conclude that the 'Promised Land' can be seen from the factory premises. When the survivors ask the Russian soldier where they should go, he tells them not to go East or West. In response to their question where they could get food, he points to the right, but in the reverse shot which immediately follows, it appears that he is also pointing to the left. According to the soldier, in the off-screen space, somewhere between right and left, there is a city. In the next shot we see a large group of people on the horizon walking toward the camera, with the land vast and undefined dominating in the foreground. At this point, we acquire information about Goeth and Schindler: the former is the ultimate representative of evil, and as the one who has committed crimes against humanity he is hanged. Schindler, on the other hand, is pronounced a righteous person. The survivors remain in the middle of these two extreme poles, walking through the promised territory.

The Return to the 'Jerusalem of Gold' and the impending negative line of flight

I would suggest that the movement of reterritorialization in the case of SCHINDLER'S LIST entails the arrival 'home' in a triple sense: home can be understood as an actual place, but it also signifies a symbolic space. The condition for the return to the actual home is dependent on the symbolic function of the term, but the negotiation between the two is dependent on the notion of home as the mind, where the memory of all the departures and returns is stored. Reterritorialization, or arrival at the Promised Land, is thereby suspended between the inside and the outside, between myth and reality. In quite a bold move Spielberg historicizes the mythical territory and complicates this tension even further. Firstly, the act of deterritorialization imposed by the Nazis clearly differs from the voluntary flight that took place in ancient Egypt, and secondly, the recourse to the people's anthem of Israel alludes to the tenuous conditions awaiting at 'home'.

More precisely, with the arrival of the survivors to the Land, in the film's closing, Neomi Shemer's song 'Jerusalem of Gold' is sung off-screen. Since the song is not listed in the film's credits, it is useful to add that it won the Israeli National Song Festival in 1967, just weeks before the Six-Day War started.[19] It was immediately embraced by the people for its nostalgic tone, drawing on the images of Jerusalem as a deserted city, which stands alone divided by the wall. By the end of the war, Israel had conquered enough territory to triple the size of the area it controls and this enabled Israel to unify Jerusalem. Shemer's song became the hymn of the paratroopers, and a suggestion was made that the words of the song be changed in accordance with the new state of things in Jerusalem. Finally, the words were not changed, but two new verses were added which invested the song with a more optimistic tone, speaking of the end of desolation and the return to the Dead Sea and the Jericho Road. In the closing of SCHINDLER'S LIST, the original version of the song is heard.[20] What needs to be taken into consideration here is the imaginary status of the Land as it is complemented with the song that had such a formative function for the people of Israel. Such an emphatic dissociation of the sound and image echoes a series of contrary and almost irreconcilable poles.[21]

Deleuze and Guattari's theorizing of the Jewish semiotic can be understood in terms of the procedure of subjectification inspired by the Zionist myths of an 'exiled territorial nation' longing to return not only to its soil but also to the Absolute Subject from which it was deterritorialized. Relating the de/re-territorialization of the Jews to a single biblical event cancels out a series of important historical factors which testify amongst other to the connection between deterritorialization and annihilation.[22] At the same time, however, what needs to be taken into consideration is that the state of Israel as a potentially Jewish territory does not immediately solve the question of Jewish identity, but on the contrary urges new questions.[23] The analysis of the structure in SCHINDLER'S LIST in regard to the territories the characters inhabit demonstrates that the territory of arrival can be traced within the line of narrative which marks the 'middle ground', a space which is neither 'right' nor 'left', and according to the effect of continuity editing, it emerges as an imaginary space. Secondly, on the basis of the clash between the Land as a theological symbol and Land as a concrete place, it is possible to conclude that the process of reterritorialization is an ongoing process, and that in many ways it is still not complete. Therefore, in the case of SCHINDLER'S LIST, the recourse to myth can ultimately help us articulate the Jewish subject as both inside and outside the territory as a signifier of identity. The process is continuously in the making, because it involves subjects whose identity is dependent both on their cultural present as well as their cultural memory.

Spielberg's film points to the multiple levels that a Jewish semiotic entails, that is, in new historical conditions we are dealing with a different set of assemblages. This accordingly implies that the movement of re-/de-territorialization needs to be considered in relation to the specific historical conditions. By structuring the events and the dynamics between the characters in terms of the territory they inhabit, SCHINDLER'S LIST demonstrates that the act of deterritorialization imposed by the Nazis urgently requires a counter-movement or rather the voluntary line of flight away from the despotic regime. With the threat of the Holocaust, however, existing without a territory wasn't an option, deterritorialization was synonymous with death. From this perspective, reterritorialization acquires different implications from those proposed by Deleuze and Guattari, because the return to the Promised Land infers safety and hence, life.

In other words, the erasure of territory can ultimately be associated with the annihilation of the Jewish race. The negative connotations Deleuze and Guattari trace in the Jewish semiotic have to do with the theological symbols of Judaism such as exile and the nostalgia for the lost homeland, and this is what they describe as a movement forward which is continuously blocked by the desire to return 'home.' Once the arrival at the Promised Land is attained, however, the concept of deterritorialization needs to be reconsidered, more precisely, the positive and the negative line of flight need to be renegotiated. The no-man's-land, or the middle ground becomes the point where new limits of what is thinkable and possible have to be re-invented. Within those conditions, deterritorialization from the subject of the 'system' which tends to prescribe the 'imaginable' is more than urgent.[24] The structuring of the territories in SCHINDLER'S LIST through the opposition between good and evil, left and right, utopia and death infers that via this opposition a middle ground is procured – the third term is an empty place, an u-topos, an impression of a face, or rather a screen on which the face of history is mapped out. Territorial and hence, in Deleuzian terms negatively charged, this face of history nevertheless reminds us that to view and negotiate our cultural present, we need to eventually step out of the past and the future, possibly even into a zone of positive absolute deterritorialization.

12 'Forty Acres and a Mule Filmworks'

– DO THE RIGHT THING – 'A Spike Lee Joint': Blocking and Unblocking the Block

Laleen Jayamanne

> The block where the bulk of the film takes place should be a character in its own right. I need to remember my early years for this.[1]

> Neither origin nor destination, 'home' is an effort to organise a 'limited space' that is never sealed in, and so it is not an enclosure but a way of going outside.[2]

> Colours do not move a people. Flags can do nothing without trumpets.[3]

The block

An Australian student once told me that she thought DO THE RIGHT THING (1989) looked a bit like *Sesame Street*, and when I first saw the film I felt too as if it had been shot on a set, maybe because I have never seen it on the big screen, or maybe because its opening credit sequence shot on a sound stage colours the rest of the film.[4] Anyway, both these images conjure up for me the memory of the endless summers on 6th Street between Avenues A and B of New York's East Village where I lived, when Francis Ford Coppola shot GODFATHER II in 1973, on our block, with Italian-looking extras drawn from our very mixed neighbourhood. Our block, not all bright and cheerful, made more sombre by the period set is, post GODFATHER II, densely tree-lined, the deal for the use of the block.

As they are not for Coppola, the actual coordinates of his chosen block are clearly vital for Lee's work. At the time the rumor was that Coppola could not film in Little Italy because of the mafia, so our block agreed to stand in for it in exchange for the trees, a rarity in the East Village. Spike Lee's journal of DO THE RIGHT THING records that the film was shot on Stuyvesant Avenue, between Lexington and Quincy in Brooklyn, and that despite the economically helpful suggestions from Universal Studios to shoot it on their back lot or in DC or Baltimore, with a non-union crew, Lee was insistent on the real location in Bedford-Stuyvesant, a Brooklyn ghetto.[5] This seemingly traditional neorealist imperative is especially intriguing because Lee then converts the real location to make it look like a set. It is legend that he hired Minister Farrakhan's security men, the Fruit of Islam, to clean the block of the two crack houses, that he painted the facades in vibrant Afro-Caribbean colour, and that the sidewalks and stoops were rubbish and drug-freed. So why does he take an actual location and make it look so clean and artificial that some critics thought he was being evasive, not dealing with real stuff, like drugs and crime? This chapter will try to approach this question obliquely by attempting to understand what Spike Lee's cinematic project is, by looking at the aesthetics of DO THE RIGHT THING.

Nearly ten years after its controversial US reception as a violent film inciting violence, or a polemical film that stages the debates on violence, one of the things that strikes me as a teacher of cross-cultural perspectives on cinema is the way in which it unfailingly engages Australian students, though largely by no means exclusively Anglo-Celtic.[6] It is usual for polemical films, say like Jean-Luc Godard's 60s Dziga Vertov films, to become poignantly dated when viewed after their moment has passed. This is not so with DO THE RIGHT THING. It does stand up beyond its moment of reception, and I shall argue that this is because of the way in which Lee marks and reinvests the block with aesthetic value.

Marking the block

Toni Morrison in a recent Australian Broadcasting Corporation interview said that she was not really interested in polemics, that what she was trying to do in her writing was something else.[7] Instead of pursuing this something else, Jana Wendt, the interviewer, diligently pursued the tack of race relations and asked a naïve question as to when Morrison might include white characters in her books; the equivalent question that plagued Lee at least until he made CLOCKERS was, 'When are you going to deal with drugs?' Morrison's reply, delivered softly, slowly and very gently and politely, was 'You can't imagine what a racist question that is.' Wendt was visibly shaken by this response which in its semantics was an accusation but in its delivery was more an exhilarating cross-cultural encounter. Morrison's reply to a naïvely ethnocentric and (unwittingly) violent question was not in a tit-for-tat mode. It was not, 'You are racist!' but rather 'You can't imagine how racist....' delivered at a speed and in a tone, pitch and timbre which unwound the rhythm of the urbane question and answer mode of the interview itself. What I saw was a transformation of the violence of white innocence into something else. I feel I learnt more about interracial exchange and of the relativisation of whiteness from its normative status through this change of rhythm and the ensuing brief pause, than through all of the information generated through the relaxed punctual rhythm of the questions and answers.

Spike Lee's films engage with polemics. He is himself a savvy polemicist/publicist and a good actor of a very particular deadpan kind. How else can one walk up to the podium (with John Singleton), address the glittering Oscar audience, read out the names of the nominees for a prize and announce the winner without smiling, even once; completely deadpan, vocally and facially; and then just leave without really acknowledging the Hollywood audience? 'I wanna be him.' DO THE RIGHT THING does of course have strong polemical moments. According to some opinion it was not nominated for the Oscar for best picture because of its putative violence, and the fact that Bruce Beresford's film DRIVING MISS DAISY, about the heart-warming friendship between a Southern Jewish woman and her African-American chauffeur, won the award instead certainly confirms the limits of Hollywood liberalism. But I do not think that DO THE RIGHT THING nor Lee's cinematic project can be entirely subsumed within an adversarial mode. He too, like Morrison, is after something else, less ephemeral than polemics, in his own fashion. As Lee himself says, 'I'm looking for a place, a home, where I can make the films I want to make without outside or inside interference'.[8]

What is evident in DO THE RIGHT THING is a preoccupation with aesthetics that tends to be overlooked in the critical writing (though not I think in its enthusiastic public reception), in the quick move to deal with the violence in the film. When I first saw the film, after every one else had seen it, after having read about its volatile public reception in the US, I remember waiting for the infamous violence, which was a long time in coming. What I experienced for long periods of the film was a leisurely pace, more like a stroll with the camera up and down a block which every now and then was punctured by sharper fragmented aural or visual rhythms. The camera is at times in tune with Mookie, one of its main characters (played by Lee), who works to the rhythm of a stroll, a to-ing and fro-ing, a dillying and a dallying. Critics tend to move to the violent moments fast (that is to say, narrativise the film) and forget to register the non-eventful leisurely moments that are plentiful and rich in neorealist detail. Examples of this are Jade simply combing Mother-Sister's hair, her Mother-Sister just hanging out the window casting her acerbic gaze at life passing by while Da Mayor serenades her, the children playing in the water of the fire hydrant, drawing pictures on the bitumen, buying ice blocks from the vendor, the chorus of three men drinking, laughing, peeing, yarning away their time, the posse of youth hanging around, Radio Raheem walking down the block being greeted by them and by Señor Mr Love Daddy at the local store-front radio station, Love Daddy's roll-call of African-American artists, and Mookie and Teena playing with an ice cube instead of doing 'the nasty'. All these elements introduce a variety of tones, moods and rhythms to the film. I am drawn to the film via its intricate and banal (summertime) rhythms rather than by its narrative, perhaps because once upon a time, I too, like Mother-Sister, simply watched life pass by on 6th Street between avenues A and B for what felt like an eternity.

These moments cited above and many more create a kind of drifting and do not have cumulative narrative drive. Attempting to narrativise them always makes one move too fast, much too fast, to the burning of the pizzeria as the main narrative event. Because of the-day-in-the-life-of-a-block structure of the film, much of what happens does not line up in a cause-effect sequence obeying the rules of sensory-motor action. In being drawn into the film by its rhythmic work, I feel there is an affinity between Toni Morrison's vocal modulations, as though she was singing while speaking (I have never experienced how talking could be like singing until I heard Morrison speak on Australian television), and the rhythmic modulations of Lee's film, which tempts me to think of it as a sort of opera of the everyday, where everyday speech, movements, gestures and color are made rhythmic and expressive.

Here are a few unnoted examples: in the climactic scene of the burning of the pizzeria, the hilarious Max Sennett Keystone Cops slapstick rhythm injected into the firemen's movements, making them tumble and fall as the pressure of the fire hose swells with rushing water. It is not only I who saw this bit of slapstick in an unlikely place, in the middle of a terrible event. Mister Señor Love Daddy also yells as the out-of-control fire hose sprays his storefront glass window, giving him reason enough to change shirts. This surprising slapstick moment is one among other a-metrical rhythms, transforming this climactic event from a sensory-motor action to something closer to an optical drama.[9] The gesture that stands out in this regard for its enigmatic quality (performed by Mookie just before he takes the garbage can, empties its contents and throws it through the pizzeria window, thus casting the first stone instigating the riot) is the palms of his two hands held together, slowly sliding down his face, making his closed eyes open. The gesture itself is a familiar one – I do it when I am tired – but it is enigmatic in that heated context, marking the moment when Mookie moves from being an observer to becoming a catalyst. But the gesture itself breaks any sense of sensory-motor rhythm that might coordinate the scene and actions, because it is too slow, too quiet, too difficult to name. This rhythmic variation is not a familiar technique of building tempo and suspense by varying speed (slow then fast), but rather injects durations that cannot be homogenised in a sweeping movement. That odd gesture converts Mookie into a mediator between a perception and a possible action; he embodies an affect which is difficult to name but can be felt in the movement of his hands and the opening of his eyes. One final example: the delicious rhythmic verbal and gestural give and take between Sal of Sal's Famous pizzeria and his racist son Pino (at the very beginning of the film), at the end of which, exasperated by his son's racist attitude, he exclaims, 'I'm going to kill someone today'. What does impel Sal to 'kill' Radio Raheem's boom box at the end of the film is the rhythm and volume of Public Enemy's 'Fight the Power', blaring out once too often. We would lose something if we thought that as in a good, well-made play the presence of a gun or baseball bat in the first act must lead to it paying off somewhere in act three. Between the impulse to want to kill someone, incited by his own son's bigotry and intransigence, and the 'killing' of the radio and of Radio Raheem, there is no causal link or inevitability. The terrible act occurs fortuitously, just as the infamous stray bullets in neorealist cinema. For despite protestations from Mookie at the end of a long hot day's work, Sal decides to let the last customers come in, be this for reasons of goodwill or wanting to make a few more dollars after they have closed shop.

Lee's obsession with the block is not a 'realist' one like Coppola's, whose East 6th Street set for GODFATHER II was created as a meticulous image of Little Italy as it was once upon a time, with every little bottle in every store front authentically labelled for historical verisimilitude, for just maybe five minutes of screen time for the street scenes, where such detail was invisible. If anything, Lee is a neorealist in the Deleuzean sense of loosening the sensory-motor rhythm of the movements that constitute the film.

Under the pressure of intense heat, color, close-up shots, rhythmic gesture and speech acts, Spike Lee's block floats in the situation, just as the action (such as it is) floats in the situation; in other words, the set and action are not organised according to a sensory-motor logic. For a long stretch of its two-hour duration nothing much happens, except that people just hang around, go up and down the block, look, talk, look for trouble, just listening to music, drinking, combing hair, just passing the time. To say that the set floats in the situation implies that it has an autonomous existence; to say that the action floats in the situation means that the action and situation do not mesh so tightly that you see only the foreground of action and not the background on which it is performed. But more importantly, when the fit between the situation and the action is not tight or sensory-motor driven, the action itself has a certain freedom, which I would want to call a rhythmic freedom from the necessity of the situation.

It is this rhythmic, aesthetic freedom that I want to trace by focusing on the role of 'Fight the Power' by considering it the refrain of DO THE RIGHT THING. My aim is to understand how and with what Lee rolls his joint, demarcates his territory and constructs a dwelling of his own. To do this I now need to call up a cluster of concepts from Deleuze and Guattari's chapter '1837: Of the Refrain' in *A Thousand Plateaus: Capitalism and Schizophrenia:*

> The role of the refrain has often been emphasised: it is territorial... Bird songs: the bird sings to mark a territory. The Greek modes and Hindu rhythms are themselves territorial, provincial and regional. The refrain may assume other functions, amorous, professional or social, liturgical or cosmic: it always carries earth with it; it has a land (sometimes a spiritual land) as its concomitant; it has an essential relation to the Natal, a Native. A musical 'nome' is a little tune, a melodic formula that seeks recognition and remains the bedrock or ground of polyphony (cantus firmus).[10]

The concepts of refrain, milieu, territory, territorialization and deterritorialization and the interval or the in-between are essential to understanding the complex process of making a dwelling by expressive markings. Ronald Bogue in his 'Rhizomusicosmology,' offers a lucid exposition of the chapter I use here: 'Using studies of birdsong as their guiding inspiration, Deleuze and Guattari treat the refrain as any kind of rhythmic pattern that stakes out a territory.'[11] A territory thus marked is characterised by three aspects: a point of stability, which could be a *pacing* or rhythm, like a child singing in the dark to calm himself; a *circle of property*, like a cat spraying the corners of a space around it to claim possession; an *opening* to the outside like a bird's song at dawn which opens its territory to other milieus and the cosmos at large. In 'Crazy talk is not enough,' Meaghan Morris offers an unusual entry point into understanding this process of 'home making' as a temporal act, by focussing repeatedly, but at varying speeds, on the Deleuzo-Guattarian image of the child in the dark, gripped with fear, singing to calm herself. The three moments of territorialization, a point of stability, a circle of property and an opening to the outside, she points out, are not sequential but simultaneous spatio-temporal operations of every territory that a refrain demarcates.[12] The distinction between milieu and territory is important in understanding the process of territorialization and deterritorialization.

The elements from which territories are formed are milieus and rhythms which themselves are created out of chaos. A milieu is a coded block of space-time, a code being defined by 'periodic repetition'[13]. The repetitive vibrations of a milieu are measured, but they are not rhythmic, for rhythm takes place between two milieus or between milieu and chaos. Measure may be regular, but rhythm 'is the Unequal or Incommensurable...' operating 'not in a homogeneous space-time, but with heterogeneous blocks.'[14] The importance of an interval or the in-between for rhythm to arise is made clear by this, and it may be more apparent by now that I have chosen the vocabulary of block, blocking and unblocking (because they are terms immanent to the film itself), instead of Deleuze and Guattari's terms, territorializing and deterritorializing.

So if one takes the enabling milieu of DO THE RIGHT THING as hip-hop, then one could say that 'Fight the Power''s own vibrations are interfered with and used by Lee as a milieu component with which to stake out a filmic territory.[15] Its sonic markings create the filmic territory; the territory does not exist prior to the marking. What characterises this territorializing marking is the increasing expressivity of rhythm, and the emergence of expressive qualities; colour, odor, sound silhouette. 'A territory borrows from all the milieus; it bites into them, seizes them bodily (although it remains vulnerable to intrusions). It is built from aspects or portions of milieus.'[16] A component torn off a milieu acquires a power to mark or express only when it becomes autonomous from prior functions, and 'acquires a temporal constancy and a spatial range that make it a territorial, or rather territorializing, mark: a signature'.[17] Bogue says that 'autonomy is evident as well in the shifting relations that link various qualities within the territory'.[18] It is sound as an expressive quality that I will pursue here because it has an unparalleled power in this film as a transformative force, both creative and destructive. Deleuze and Guattari speak eloquently of the ambiguity of this process:

> Sound invades us, impels us, drags us, transpierces us. It takes leave of the earth, as much in order to drop us into a black hole as to open us up to a cosmos. It makes us want to die. Since its force of deterritorialisation is the strongest, it also effects the most massive of reterritorializations, the most numbing, the most redundant. Ecstasy and hypnosis. Colours do not move a people. Flags can do nothing without trumpets... The potential fascism of music.[19]

Some Sonic Blocks

The DJ, Mister Señor Love Daddy, is also the observer-narrator-voice-over within the film, intervening in its actions through his control of the sonic waves of the radio station, I Love Radio. The block's temporal coherence is marked and varied by Love Daddy's intermittent interruptions into the-day-in-the-life-of-the-block. His rapping begins the film after the credit sequence, in a tight close-up of an alarm clock, microphone and lips yelling out 'Waaaake up! Wake up! Wake up! Wake up! up ya wake! up ya wake! Up ya wake!... I have today's forecast, HOT.' He also ends the 24 hours of the film with a farewell song to the dead Radio Raheem and signs off the film with 'We love you brother'. He cuts in and out of the day in hip-hop style, sound-editing his mode of speech, inverting phrases and repeating them which creates the reversible relations of nonsense and a non-uniform time, 'a time of flux, of multiple speeds and reversible relations'.[20] His long roll-call of African-American artists stretches time and layers it with the sounds that the proper names invoke and evoke. It is in these ways that DJ Love Daddy plays with rhythm and time, and it is his structural centrality that in part helps create the fluidity, layering and cutting up (of time) in the film. According to Tricia Rose, fluidity, layering and cutting are the three main formal techniques she finds common to all three forms of hip-hop expression, graffiti, break-dance and rap.[21]

When Radio Raheem walks into Sal's Famous Pizzeria for the first time on the hottest day of that summer, with his ghetto blaster blaring out Public Enemy's 'Fight the Power', Sal intones rhythmically, 'No music, no Rap, no music, no music, no music'. It's not that he doesn't like music, he just does not like Rap, for he says, 'what happened to nice music with words you could understand?' And it is also not that he doesn't have rhythm because his banning of Radio Raheem's music in his pizzeria is done with gestural and rhythmic flair, 'No music, no music, no music'. So it is not a black-white thing, everyone on the block is given over to a speaking which is marked by a rhythmic contagion.

Even the Korean shop owners, a husband and wife team, enter the spirit under duress, learning to say 'mother-fucker' as a rhythmic thing, thus eliciting a smile of bemused appreciation from Radio Raheem himself when he berates them for not knowing the date on the batteries he purchases from them and for not speaking English properly. It is at such moments that a character such as Radio Raheem gets individuated beyond a familiar type, a delicious moment of cross-race learning-the-lingo on the job, which makes Radio Raheem go from 'don't you speak English mother-fucker?' to 'you all right, mother-fucker'. By then the Korean man has begun to chant 'mother-fucker' as a little refrain. And perhaps it is this informal learning of street lingo that helps the Korean shop keeper to come up with another little crucial refrain, as the black mob turns to his shop after having set fire to Sal's 'Famous'. The Korean with a broom in hand attempts to shoo away the black mob with, 'I no white, I no white, I black, I black, you me same'. Which makes the black mob leader, the crusty ML, go, 'Same! me black, open your eyes mother-fucker!', at which point Sweet Dick Willy and Coconut Sid intervene, and one of them says, 'Leave the Korean alone, he's all right', as they crack up laughing and even ML sees the black humour in this instant construction of racialised identity under duress and decides that 'he's all right'. In a previous scene, when ML was grumbling about the Koreans' enterprise in setting up a business as soon as they got off the boat, it is Sweet Dick Willy who adds the biting line that the blacks also got off a boat many years ago, thus trying to dampen the impulse to find racialised scapegoats for the apathy of one's own ethnic group.

Towards the end of the film this Korean shopkeeper is prominent among the black youth who run after the police car carrying away Radio Raheem's dead body, banging on it in anger at his murder by a cop. This scene is so brief that it was only after watching the film maybe ten times or more, that I noticed for the first time that the baton pushing the Korean man away from the speeding police car is held by a black cop; and on further viewing it became clear that it is a African-American female cop, along with her white mate, who are clearing the way for the getaway police car. There is a brief instant when the white male cop on frame left and the black female cop on frame right, in fact frame with their outstretched batons an African-American youth and the Korean as the police car speeds away into the night. 'What can I say, say what I can, like Mister Señor Love Daddy, I say; I saw it, it I saw, and my mouth was opened.' And I might add that I saw it at the correct speed, not by looking at it frame by frame, though I must confess that I did slow the film down to police the gender of the black cop. I wonder why no one else wrote about this micro-moment, given the range of discussion which focused on the violence of this film. Surely this moment is evidence enough to show that the film is no simple tract inciting black people to riot, as some white critics chose to interpret it. This hidden moment is also perfectly consistent with the complicated and unpredictable ways in which intraracial and interracial relations are blocked out in the film. So it is not a unique moment tucked away for the perceptive critic to feel good about being able to decipher it. It is perhaps a more harrowing example of the not easily visible complexities of African-American experience which, it is the aim of Lee's 'Forty Acres and a Mule Filmworks' enterprise to make audible, visible and legible. The past of American racist history and Hollywood's complicity with it is, of course, firmly memorialised in the branding of Lee's production company as 'Forty Acres and a Mule', the sum of wealth promised, though not always given, to the emancipated slaves.

While Lee's project is thus under the sign of history, it seeks a certain relief from the burden of history and the weight of memory, via his logo, 'A Spike Lee Joint', which signals the weightless and memoryless floating realm of commodity and sign production of late twentieth-century America. Familiar Civil Rights-inspired 1960s phrases of an emergent 'Black' identity – 'My people, my people,' 'Brother, brother brother,' 'Brothers and sisters,' 'Power to the people,' 'Black power' – are now deployed through hip-hop, in such a way that their semantic inadequacy is assumed, even as their phatic performative value, for those who so choose to recycle clichés with style, is abundantly clear. Lee populates his sonic block with a collection of African-American types (the elderly Mother-Sister, with echoes of a Southern familial past; the old Da Mayor, a gentleman alcoholic; Mookie, the irresponsible young black father who sponges on his sister Jade, the responsible sister and voice of reason; Radio Raheem with his inseparable boom box; Bugginout, always looking for some trouble; the posse of youth; the eloquent chorus of black men just hanging out at the corner; the black mother beating the shit out of her son who just escaped being run over by an ice-cream van and furiously defending her right to bring up her son as she thinks fit) so as to explore their lack of commonality and their erratic communality. In setting intraracial differences within a wider series of interracial differences, Lee highlights humorously how racism is not the prerogative of any one ethnic group, as in the hilarious racial slur sequence constructed as a rap session, where a member of each ethnic community characterises another through stereotypes of habit, food and taste. And as it is directly addressed to the viewer, the spectator too is implicated in this robust rhythmic display of racist venom.[22]

A sonic brick: 'Fight the Power' as refrain and signature tune

Unlike any other piece of music in the film, Public Enemy's 'Fight the Power' works as repetitively as the poor mule would have had to if it ploughed the forty acres. Both the title of the film and the title of this song (DO THE RIGHT THING, 'Fight the Power') are imperatives with a habitual familiar quality to the point of being clichés. This is why when Da Mayor stops Mookie on one of his delivery rounds to say, 'Doctor, always try to do the right thing!', Mookie asks 'That's it?' to which Da Mayor replies 'That's it' and Mookie goes 'I got it, I'm gone'. This is Lee's way of telling us (and it's true some needed to be told) don't waste your time looking for the 'right thing', it is the red herring in the picture, the film's not that simplistic; 'c'mon, c'mon, lets get this mule movin, mmmmm, damn!'

The film begins and ends with 'Fight the Power.' It is heard twelve times in all, within the course of the film; at the beginning and the end as non-diegetic sound while being repeated ten times in the body of the film, always as the only sound blasting out from Radio Raheem's boom-box. Each person or group hearing this refrain has a reaction to it, which in each instance is different from Radio Raheem's absolute identification with the song and the radio. Both of these together form a mobile sonic block, his abode, territory and signature tune. So this song as recurrent refrain constructs two poles in the film, one consisting of its intrinsic non-diegetic quality as it works with or against the image and the other consisting of the response or force of the diegetic listener. This variability of functions and the multiple repetitions of the song as refrain effect qualitative transformations in the film. It is the temporal (aesthetic) power of this refrain that I wish to explore now by first sketching out its repeated appearance on the block.

1. After the long opening credit sequence in a MTV-style rendition of 'Fight the Power' with Rosie Perez' b-boy dance, it is first heard intradiegetically when the hip-hop posse greets Radio Raheem. After the usual phatic rap greetings, Ella and two of the boys do an unusual routine, turning themselves into 'onlookers' commenting on Radio Raheem's appearance and laughing like cartoon characters while he looks on in an enigmatic close-up. A strangely difficult scene to read because of this instant transformation of participants into observers and commentators, a shift one becomes more accustomed to as the film proceeds. This instant switching of functions, evident in other scenes as well, slackens, I think, further the already loose sensory-motor mechanisms of the film.

2. From this scene Radio Raheem moves further down the block and is greeted by the other agent of hip-hop, Mister Señor Love Daddy, so hip-hop's MTV image is acknowledged, used and returned (in a complicated move) to the block, its place of origin.

3. When we next hear Radio Raheem, the fire hydrant is flowing in full force, and members of the posse stop the flow of the water so that he and his radio can pass by undrenched. We now enter a rhythm marked by an impeding of flows, in this instance of water, later of the song.

4. When the refrain next emerges in the ghetto-blaster sound skirmish between 'Fight the Power' and the Puerto Rican boy's Latin Salsa rhythms, the two musics vie with each other without any clear victory; a result of the sensory-motor slackening of tension through the mixing of different musical rhythms, it seems.

5. In Radio Raheem's fifth appearance on the block, he greets Mookie, reduces the volume of his refrain, puts the radio down and tells a story about the two hands; 'LOVE' and 'HATE' engraved on his knuckledusters.

6. From then on the refrain's flow is impeded on each of the five times it is heard because people hate its sound, or the sheer volume, or its endless repetition. Radio Raheem goes to Sal's with it on full blast and gets the 'no music' rap from Sal, which makes him turn off the volume reluctantly.

7. The refrain gets distorted when the batteries run down, leading Radio Raheem into the 'Don't you speak English, motherfucker', routine with the Korean shopkeepers.

8. When the refrain is recharged by twenty batteries, the chorus of men close their ears and curse the music in unison as Radio Raheem goes past them at full blast.

9. Radio Raheem and Bugginout discuss boycotting Sal's pizzeria, late into the night with the song blaring out, which elicits an abusive 'Cut out that rap music, I've been trying to get some mother-fucking....' from a neighbouring apartment. Even Bugginout asks Radio Raheem why he plays only one song, and he replies 'I like nothing else' and agrees to boycott Sal. He adds movingly, 'Tellin me, Radio Raheem, to turn down my box and he didn't even say please'. (That 'please', kills me.)

10. Radio Raheem and Bugginout go into Sal's with the refrain at full blast on the hottest night of that summer, demanding that Sal put up some brothers on the wall of fame, and Sal yells out to shut the 'jungle music', the 'nigger radio', then smashes the radio with a baseball bat adding, 'I just killed your fucking radio', thus setting off a riot which ends in the murder of Radio Raheem by the cops, and the burning of the pizzeria by its clients. The refrain is heard one last time, as non-diegetic sound, when the camera scans the debris of the pizzeria which includes Radio Raheem's smashed boombox. This second non-diegetic appearance, so different in affect from its empowered opening MTV rendition, offers a powerful and lucid montage critique, if one cares to take note of it. It leaves me with a question, what power has been fought in this act of destruction?

Ten times

The repeated sonic markings of the block by Radio Raheem's ten appearances with 'Fight the Power' transforms him into a 'territorial motif' in Deleuze and Guattari's terms, or a 'rhythmic character' in Olivier Messiaen's terms, where it is not the character who has rhythm but rather the rhythm itself which becomes a character. To understand this notion of 'rhythmic character', one must know that for Messiaen as well as Deleuze and Guattari, there is a fundamental difference between metre and rhythm: 'metre presupposes an even division of a uniform time, rhythm presupposes a time of flux, of multiple speeds and reversible relations'.[23] According to Bogue, from whom I take this citation, one of Messiaen's chief techniques for generating ametrical rhythms is what he calls 'added values' ('short values added to any rhythm whatever, whether by a note, or by a rest, or by the dot'.[24] And his notion of 'rhythmic characters' is an extension of this idea.

By progressively modifying a figure through the addition or subtraction of rhythmic values, the composer can develop rhythmic characters whose dynamic relationships are like those of characters on the stage.[25] Let us imagine a scene in a play between three characters: the first acts in a brutal manner by hitting the second; the second character suffers this act, since his actions are dominated by those of the first; lastly, the third character is present at the conflict but remains inactive. If we transpose this parable into the field of rhythm, we have three rhythmic groups; the first, whose note-values are always increasing, is the character who attacks; the second, whose note-values decrease, is the character who is attacked; and the third, whose note-values never change, is the character who remains immobile.[26]

In music, with its very solid mathematical base, one can unambiguously speak of increased or diminished value, but in this film the register is not mathematics but emotions, so the concept of *varied* value' is more appropriate.[27] I suggest that we read 'Fight the Power' as the beat and the different reactions to it as the 'varied values' which make it a rhythmic rather than metrical character. It is now necessary to ask, what can a 'rhythmic character' of this kind do? This necessity is provoked by the power that a rhythmic character or motif has to connect the territory with forces both within and without. These forces, according to Deleuze and Guattari, are those of inner impulses or drives as well as external circumstance. As every territory has a centre of intensity (which is both within and without the territory, embodied for instance in the idea of an imagined or lost homeland, or the natal, always at hand yet difficult to reach, to which, for example, lobsters and salmon swim against great odds to spawn), where its forces come together; in this film we reach this burning hearth on the sound waves transmitted by Radio Raheem, as rhythmic character.[28]

A hesitant, faint refrain

'One ventures from home on the thread of a tune that is always in danger of breaking.'[29]

There are three impossibilities that I think Spike Lee negotiates or straddles
in developing his cinema and the terms of his independence.
1. Spike Lee can't not make films,
2. Spike Lee can't make Hollywood films,
3. Spike Lee can't not make films with Hollywood.
Stone- wAAAAAAAAAAAAAAAAAAAAAAAAAAAAAAAAAAAAAll![30]

As the pizzeria burns, the Fire Brigade arrives, and a cop calls out on a loud-
speaker for the mob to 'please go home', to which Mookie, standing on the
shattered block, replies, 'This is our home'. This barely audible retort brings
home to me pointedly and poignantly what Deleuze and Guatarri call the
ambiguity of the natal, the lost or unknown homeland. The two elders on
the block, Da Mayor and Mother-Sister, seem to know this only too well
when they say to each other on the morning after, 'Hope the block's still
standing.' 'We're still standin.' This is the ambiguity of the natal as it appears to an African-American; the lost homeland, the promised land, and its
embodied memory in a song or a name, Mother-Sister.

Raymond Bellour once said, at the 1982 Australian Screen Studies Association conference in Melbourne, that Hollywood cinema is a machine for
the manufacture of the couple. So Lee too gives us his odd romantic couple
(Ossie Davis and Ruby Dee, two African-American actors of an older generation who have in fact been husband and wife for 40 years), two figures who
seem anachronistic in a hip-hop space. Mother-Sister always 'watchin an
waitin', while Da Mayor sweeps the sidewalk for a dollar from Sal, buys
beer with it and sweet-talks Mother-Sister who spurns him. When the riot
begins, Mother-Sister is the first to shout 'burn it down, burn it down', and
when it burns, it is she who screams 'no, no, no, no,' with the same hysteria,
while it is Da Mayor's embrace that calms and comforts her. When they both
wake up the morning after in Mother-Sister's apartment, finally reconciled,
Lee certainly is reworking in his own way the Hollywood (American)
dream of the couple and at the same time paying tribute to two fine African-
American actors of an older generation who could never have been a cinematic romantic couple within the terms of that cinema.[31] So two of the key
means of symbolically marking and creating community, death and 'mar-
riage', have come to pass, though in an untimely way, with elders remarry-
ing and a youth dying. The territory held together by such events holds

together fragilely, they cannot be foundational events as in classical cinema, especially when the strongest image of community manifests itself in a riot which destroys something as basic as a business that feeds the block. 'Fight the Power' as refrain has marked a block, created territorial motifs and counterpoints to it; gathered a rhythmic force of hatred and absolute devotion, LOVE and HATE, shattering the block, plunging it into a black hole called 'Race Riot' by the white media and politics.

Lee's film does not conclude with the 'riot' but rather on the morning after. Lee revisits the site of the riot, a pervasive media-saturated image of contemporary Afro-American and Anglo-American relations hitting a stone wall. How then does Lee revisit the burnt-down pizzeria? On the lines of a hesitant, unpredictable, rhythmic movement, both vocal and gestural, Sal scrunches up five hundred dollars (Mookie's salary and more), into little pellets, throwing them at Mookie, one at a time, with excessive force. Mookie throws back two hundred at Sal because, as he says, his salary is only two hundred and fifty. Then they improvise a little rhyme to accompany the gestural refrain of throwing paper pellets, not unlike children playing on SESAME STREET:

Sal: Keep it.
Mookie: You keep it.
Sal: You keep it.
Mookie: You keep it.
Sal: You keep it.
Mookie: You keep it.

You will hear a metrical beat if you only hear the repetition of the same phrase, a mimicry, not much else. But if what you hear are differences, i.e., minutely 'varied values' of gesture, inflection, pitch, timbre, emphases, trying to establish some equilibrium, call it a pacing, in the midst of terrible chaos, then you may at the same time see a shifting line of property and an emerging thin fragile line leading to an outside, opening a channel. If we can see these, we may be able to hear a halting, hesitant, not-quite-yet refrain, but nevertheless a refrain which tries to invent a small gesture of sociability in a black hole. For this kind of cross-cultural move a little mimetic play seems useful.[32]

This is a version of a chapter in my forthcoming book, *Towards Cinema and Its Double: Crosscultural Readings – 1980-1999*, published by Indiana University Press 2001. With kind permission of Indiana University Press.

Notes

Notes to: Introduction

1 Pipilotti Rist, from her installation PAMALA. Text (with difference and repetition) in the catalogue and on CD of the exposition REMAKE OF LE WEEKEND. Cologne: Oktagon, 1998.

2 Hannah Arendt, 'Philosophy and Politics', part III of 'Philosophy and Politics: The Problem of Action and Thought after the French Revolution'. In *Social Research*, vol. 57/1, 1990, pp. 73-103.

3 'The Politics of Gilles Deleuze', symposium organised for ASCA (Amsterdam School of Cultural Analysis), University of Amsterdam, Spring 1999.

4 Gilles Deleuze, *Negotiations*. Trans. Martin Joughin. New York: Columbia University Press, 1990 (motto).

5 Richard Rorty, *Achieving our Country. Leftist Thought in Twentieth-Century America.* Cambridge, Mass. and London: Harvard University Press, 1998, p. 9.

6 *Achieving our Country*, p. 7.

7 *Achieving our Country*, p. 29. Discussing the ideas of Dewey and Whitman extensively is beyond the scope of this book.

8 *Achieving our Country*, pp. 100/101.

9 *Achieving our Country*, p. 78.

10 *Achieving our Country*, p. 79.

11 Many others have criticised Rorty as well on these points. Cf. Peter Berkowitz in *Commentary* and George Will in *Newsweek*. Will states that Rorty's book itself radiates with contempt for the country because he seems to despise most Americans for 'sadism' and 'cruelty' (see for Berkowitz and Will <http://www.infiltec.com>). In 'Utopia Limited: An Anthropological Response to Richard Rorty' Stacey Meeker argues that *Snow Crash*, for instance, is not only a novel of self-hatred, but also a way of working through cultural phobias. In this case the exploration of our fear of the market, providing a necessary contrast between those who have mastered the market (the former Americans) and the Raft people. Ultimately, Meeker argues, this is healthier than the utopian denial of Rorty (*Anthropoetics*, IV/2 (fall 1998/winter 1999). In 'Richard Rorty and the Future of the Left' David Horowitz attacks Rorty from a Jewish 'Right conservative' position. He objects that Rorty fails to see that some of the gains in political correctness of the cultural left has simply redirected many prejudices, for instance towards Jews. Rorty also does not know the work of many 'Right conservatists' who have thought 'long and hard about the problems of poverty' (*Salon Magazine*, 5/4/98; <http://www.frontpagemag.com/dh/1998/future.htm>).

12 In his book *Professional Correctness: Literary Studies and Political Change* Stanley Fish discusses in another way the relationship between theory and political practice. Like Rorty he critisises the 'political' turn to cultural studies (of literary studies). But contrary to Rorty he does not propose to re-establish (piecemeal) political action of the left, but to stick to the basic task of the academic discipline: literary studies should first and foremost ask: 'What does this poem (or play or novel) mean?' Although Fish

does not deny that there is a relationship between theory and the political, it is not the task of the academician to deal with it. 'Let the cobbler stick to his last,' Fish seems to argue. This is a clear and traditional (Aristotelian) position, but it does not give any insights into the indirect relationship between theory and politics that I would like to explore. Stanley Fish, *Professional Correctness: Literary Studies and Political Change.* New York: Clarendon, 1995. See for this quote:<I> http://www.gseweb.har-vard.edu/~heph/fa99.htm>, p. 6.

13 Luuk van Middelaar, *Politicide: De moord op de politiek in de Franse filosofie (Politicide: The Murder of Politics in French Philosophy).* Amsterdam: Van Gennep, 1999.

14 *Politicide,* p. 104. My translation from the Dutch.

15 As indicated before, Rorty looks at the work of Dewey and Whitman, in which a uto-pian dream of commonality is an organising principle. According to Van Middelaar, the only contemporary French thinker that offers a good solution out of the political impasses of theory and philosophy is Claude Lefort. Lefort goes back to Machiavelli to think about social conflict and the role of the state in controling these conflicts. As with Whitmen and Dewey in the case of Rorty, this is not the place to analyse Lefort's proposals. See also Paola Maratti's 'Against the Doxa', note 12 (this volume).

16 See, for instance, Gilles Deleuze and Félix Guattari, *A Thousand Plateaus: Capitalism and Schizophrenia.* Trans. Brian Massumi. London: the Athlone Press, 1988, pp. 505-506; and Gilles Deleuze and Claire Parnet, 'Politics' in *Dialogues.* Trans. Hugh Tomlinson and Barbara Habberjam. New York: Columbia University Press, 1987.

17 Paul Patton, *Deleuze and the Political.* London and New York: Routledge, 2000, pp. 104-105.

18 *Deleuze and the Political,* p. 105.

19 Patton explains: 'Critical freedom thus concerns those moments in a life after which one is no longer the same person. It is the freedom to transgress the limits of what one is presently capable of being or doing, rather than just the freedom to be or do those things. In the course of a life, individuals make choices which may significantly affect the range, nature or course of their future actions: the decision to become a parent, to embark upon one particular career or course of study, or to leave one's country of birth and live in another culture, are all cases of significant actions upon one's future actions. (...) Deleuze and Guattari do not offer a concept of a person but a concept of assemblage which can be applied equally to social or to personal identity.' (*Deleuze and the Political,* p. 85).

20 *Deleuze and the Political,* p. 87.

21 Gilles Deleuze and Michel Foucault, 'Intellectuals and Power'. Trans. Donald Bouchard and Sherry Simin. Donald Bouchard (ed.), *Michel Foucault: Language, Coun-ter Memory, Practice: Selected Essays and Interviews.* Ithaca: Cornell University Press, 1977. Reprinted in Russel Ferguson et al. (eds.), *Discourses: Conversations in Postmodern Art and Culture.* New York and Cambridge: The New Museum of Contemporary Art and MIT Press, 1990, pp. 9-10.

22 'Intellectuals and Power', p. 9.

23 Gilles Deleuze and Félix Guattari, *What is Philosophy?* Trans. Graham Burchell and Hugh Tomlinson. London: Verso, 1994, p. 218.

24 *What is Philosophy?,* p. 218.

25 *What is Philosophy?,* p. 99.

26 *What is Philosophy?,* p. 97.

27 *A Thousand Plateaus*, p. 216/217. Quoted by Busk.
28 In the chapter 'Nomads, Capture and Colonisation' Paul Patton looks at the nomadic war machine, which he prefers to call 'machines of metamorphosis' (because they have nothing to do with actual war, but everything with change). He takes the example of Australia where Aboriginal people, both as 'real' and 'conceptual' nomads, have a different relation to territory than the sedentary people who colonised their land. It is through this different relation to territory, Patton argues, that 'throughout the history of European colonisation, a recurrent form of justification for the expropriation of inhabited land has been the claim that the indiginous inhabitants were not sufficiently settled or had not tilled the land in a manner that made them rightful owners.' (*Deleuze and the Political*, p. 119). And 'the war machine that in the last few decades is at work is the 'native title jurisprudence as it continues to develop in Australia and Canada' which is 'a machine of constitutional metamorphosis'. (p. 131).
29 *Negotiations*, motto.
30 Manuel Castells, *The Rise of the Network Society*. Massachusetts and Oxford: Blackwell, 1996.
31 Gilles Deleuze, *Cinema 1: The Movement-Image*. Trans. Hugh Tomlinson and Barbara Habberjam. London: The Athlone Press, 1986 and *Cinema 2: The Time-Image*. Trans. Hugh Tomlinson and Robert Galeta. London: The Athlone Press, 1989.
32 In his book *Gilles Deleuze's Time Machine* (Durham and London: Duke University Press, 1997) David Rodowick gives a very profound analysis of Deleuze's film books. For an excellent example of a more formal analysis of 'applied Deleuzism', Ian Buchanan's analysis of BLADE RUNNER in his book *Deleuzism: A Metacommentary*. Edinburgh: Edinburgh University Press, 2000, pp. 127-140. In my book *The Matrix of Visual Culture: Working with Deleuze in Film Theory*, I work with both the formal concepts of Deleuze's cinema books and other Deleuzian concepts to see what one can do with Deleuze in respect to contemporary (Hollywood) cinema (Stanford: Stanford University Press, 2001 – forthcoming).
33 As indicated before, in *Achieving our Country* Rorty does not consider the many failures of the Left's direct engagements with politics, even though he proposes a more modest and pragmatic 'piecemeal' form of direct engagement ('I think the Left should get back into the business of piecemeal reform within the framework of a market economy, p. 105).
34 Interestingly, at the end of his article, Barbrook quotes Alexandre Kojève to counter Deleuzoguattarianism. Kojève, according to Van Middelaar, is precisely the cause of all philosophical trouble in practice.
35 In 'Intellectuals and Power' Deleuze and Foucault both talk about this changed role of the intellectual who is no longer representing anyone and knows that everybody is capable of expressing themselves. Foucault still uses the term 'the masses', which might imply some vanguardism nevertheless. See on this point Renato Janine Ribeiro, 'Les Intellectuels au Pouvoir' in Eric Alliez (ed.), *Gilles Deleuze: une vie philosophique*. Le Plessis-Robinson: Institut Synthélabo, 1998, pp. 391-402. In his preference for modernist masterpieces of cinema, Deleuze can be accused of some purism and elitism as well with respect to his cinema books.
36 *The Time-Image*, pp. 126-155 and pp. 215-224.

37 This term is used by Mark Dery to indicate the technophile, transcendental desire to leave the body (and earth) by technological revolution. See Mark Dery, *Escape Velocity: Cyberculture at the End of the Century*. London: Hodder and Stoughton, 1996.

38 *Deleuze and the Political*, pp. 83-87.

39 *The Time-Image*, pp. 215-224.

40 In *The Time-Image* Deleuze refers several times to this socio-linguistic term from Austin to indicate in which way cinema can have performative and actual power. African cinema, for instance, or the Brazilian cinema of Glauber Rocha are 'acts of story-telling' that go beyond a return to myth of a past people: 'Story-telling is not an impersonal myth, but neither is it a personal fiction: it is a word in act, a speech-act through which the character continually crosses the boundary which would separate his private business from politics, and which *itself produces collective utterances* (...) capable of raising misery to a strange positivity, the invention of a people' (p. 222). When Deleuze discusses the changing and increasingly complex relationship between image and sound (his example is the cinema of Marguerite Duras), he elaborates further on the speech-act and the different types of speech-acts which can be distinguished (p. 252). Finally, Deleuze also mentions the speech-act in relation to modern 'characters' in cinema ('psychological automaton') that he defines in relation to speech-acts and no longer, as before, by motor-action (here Deleuze refers to Bresson's 'puppets', p. 266). In 'The Fifth Element and the Fifth Dimension of the Affection-Image' I refer to the possible speech-acts in Luc Besson's film THE FIFTH ELEMENT (in Anu Koivunen and Astrid Söderbergh (eds.), *Cinema Studies into Visual Theory?* Turku: University of Turku, 1998, pp. 93-107). In her article 'Sharing Technologies' (this volume) Maaike Bleeker refers to the specific way in which the conceptual persona in philosophy can produce 'speech acts' in producing movement in thought.

41 'The paradox of this pure becoming, with its capacity to elude the present, is the paradox of infinite identity (the infinite identity of both directions or senses at the same time – of future and past (...)'. Gilles Deleuze, *The Logic of Sense*. Trans. Mark Lester with Charles Stivale. New York: Columbia University Press, 1990, p. 2.

42 The concept of the rhizome is developed by Deleuze and Guattari to indicate the non-hierarchical, unpredictable, 'grass roots' way of thinking that they propose (as opposed to 'tree-like' thinking that believes in roots and hierarchical patterns of thought). It is a very political concept that questions established thought and power structures and promotes unexpected encounters between a multitude of fields, disciplines and people. See the first plateau of *A Thousand Plateaus*.

Notes to 1: Redescriptive Philosophy

1 Richard Rorty, 'Derrida and the Philosophical Tradition' in *Truth and Progress: Philosophical Papers*, Volume 3. Cambridge: Cambridge University Press, 1998, pp. 327-50.

2 Richard Rorty, 'Unsoundness in Perspective', *Times Literary Supplement*, June 17, 1983, p. 620.

3 'Unsoundness in Perspective', p. 619.

4   For example, in 'Habermas and Lyotard on Postmodernity' in *Essays on Heidegger and Others: Philosophical Papers* Volume 2. Cambridge: Cambridge University Press, 1991, pp.172-3. Elsewhere, Rorty points to the possibility of convergence with pragmatism in suggesting that 'James and Dewey were not only waiting at the end of the dialectical road which analytic philosophy traveled, but are waiting at the end of the road which, for example, Foucault and Deleuze are currently travelling' (*Consequences of Pragmatism*. Minneapolis: University of Minnesota Press, 1982, p.vxiii)

5   Umberto Eco, with Richard Rorty, Jonathan Culler and Christine Brooke-Rose, 'The Pragmatist's Progress' in Stefan Collini (ed.), *Interpretation and Overinterpretation*. Cambridge: Cambridge University Press, 1992, p. 105.

6   Gilles Deleuze & Félix Guattari, *A Thousand Plateaus: Capitalism and Schizophrenia*. Trans. B. Massumi, Minneapolis: University of Minnesota Press, 1980, p. 4.

7   Gilles Deleuze & Félix Guattari, 'Rhizome'. Trans. P. Foss and P. Patton, *I&C*, 8, Spring 1981, p. 67.

8   Richard Rorty, 'Derrida and the Philosophical Tradition', *Philosophical Papers*, Volume 3, p. 329.

9   Richard Rorty, *Contingency, Irony, and Solidarity*. Cambridge: Cambridge University Press, 1989, p. 75

10 Gilles Deleuze: 'The theory of thought is like painting: it needs that revolution which took art from representation to abstraction. This is the aim of a theory of thought without image', in *Difference and Repetition*. Trans. P. Patton, London: Athlone, 1994, p. 276. Editor's note: see also Paola Marrati's 'Against the Doxa' in this volume.

11 Gilles Deleuze, *Nietzsche and Philosophy*. Trans. Hugh Tomlinson, London: Athlone, 1983, p. 95.

12 *Nietzsche and Philosophy*, p. 104.

13 Ibid.

14 *Nietsche and Philosophy*, p. 103.

15 *Difference and Repetition*, p.162.

16 *Difference and Repetition*, p.164

17 *Contingency, Irony, and Solidarity*, p. 77.

18 Gilles Deleuze & Félix Guattari, *What is Philosophy?* Trans. Hugh Tomlinson and Graham Burchell, New York: Columbia University Press, 1994, p. 5.

19 *What is Philosophy?*, p. 34.

20 'The following definition of philosophy can be taken as being decisive: knowledge through pure concepts', in *What is Philosophy?*, p. 7. Editor's note: Catherine M. Lord in 'The Lady Sits Between Two Long Windows, Writing' and Maaike Bleeker in 'Sharing Technologies' (both this volume) elaborate on the relationships between philosophy, art and science.

21 *What is Philosophy?*, p. 22.

22 *What is Philosophy?*, p. 79.

23 *What is Philosophy?*, p.18.

24 *Difference and Repetition*, p. 188. The equivalence of transcendental problems and pure events is reaffirmed in Deleuze's account of the logical genesis of propositions in his book *The Logic of Sense*. Trans. Mark Lester with Charles Stivale, Constantin Boundas (ed.), New York: Columbia University Press, 1990, p. 123.

25 *The Logic of Sense*, p. 19.

26 *What is Philosophy?*, p. 127.

27 Another example which Deleuze frequently uses to illustrate this difference is Blanchot's distinction between death as a realisable event towards which 'I' may have a personal relation and death as an impersonal and inaccessible event towards which 'I' can have no relation. See *The Logic of Sense*, pp. 151-2 and *Difference and Repetition*, p. 112.

28 *What is Philosophy?*, p. 110.

29 *What is Philosophy?*, p.156.

30 *What is Philosohy?*, pp.32-3.

31 Elizabeth Anscombe, *Intention*. Oxford: Blackwell, 1959.

32 Ian Hacking, *Rewriting the Soul, Multiple Personality and the Sciences of Memory*. Princeton, N.J.: Princeton University Press, 1995, p. 239.

33 *Rewriting the Soul*, p. 243.

34 *A Thousand Plateaus*, p. 81.

35 *Contingency, Irony, and Solidarity*, p. 74.

36 Critical engagement with current self-evidence regarding the nature of events may take a variety of forms. Baudrillard's ironic theory-fiction provides a purely negative manner of problematizing the common sense representation of historical events. In his third and final essay on the Gulf War, he argues that what took place was not a war since the military operations undertaken on either side demonstrated such enormous disparities in technology and strategy that direct encounters between opposing forces rarely took place and the overall effect was more in the nature of a police operation than a war. Baudrillard is not simply making a rhetorical point which relies upon an essentialist concept of war. Rather, he points to the fundamental indeterminacy in the pure event of armed conflict. New forms of military technology have made possible a type of engagement at a distance which no longer fits existing descriptions of war. The real is in advance of its representations, Baudrillard might say. Deleuze and Guattari might say that a new concept is required in order to give expression to the new type of event which took place in the Gulf. See Jean Baudrillard, *The Gulf War Did Not Take Place*. Trans. Paul Patton. Sydney: Power Institute Publications/ Bloomington: Indiana University Press, 1995.

37 Michel Foucault, 'Polemics, Politics and Problematizations: An Interview', in Paul Rabinow (ed.) *The Foucault Reader*. New York: Pantheon Books, 1984, p. 384.

38 Michel Foucault, 'Questions of Method'. *I & C* no.8, Spring 1981, p. 6.

39 H. J. Saatkamp, Jr (ed.), *Rorty and Pragmatism: The Philosopher Responds to His Critics*. Nashville and London: Vanderbilt University Press, 1995, p. 198.

40 *What is Philosophy?*, p. 112. This definition of the untimely is a direct quotation from Nietzsche's, 'On the Uses and Disadvantages of History for Life', *Untimely Meditations*. Trans. J.P. Hollingdale, Cambridge: Cambridge University Press, 1983, p. 60.

41 *What is Philosophy?*, p. 99.

42 *Contingency, Irony, and Solidarity*, p. 3.

43 *What is Philosophy?*, p. 108.

44 *Contingency, Irony, and Solidarity*, p. 78.

45 'Le "je me souviens" de Gilles Deleuze' – Interview with Didier Eribon, *Le Nouvel Observateur*, 16-22 November, 1995, pp. 114-5.

46 For a more detailed discussion of some of these vocabularies and an exploration of the ways in which they might enable effective redescription, see Paul Patton, *Deleuze and the Political*. London and New York: Routledge, 2000.

47 *Contingency, Irony, and Solidarity*, p. 9.
48 *What is Philosophy?*, p. 111.
49 *What is Philosophy?*, cf. p. 82.
50 *Contingency, Irony, and Solidarity*, pp. 88-91.
51 Richard Rorty, *Achieving Our Country: Leftist Thought in Twentieth Century America*, Cambridge, Mass.: Harvard University Press, 1998, p. 91.
52 *Contingency, Irony, and Solidarity*, p. 63.
53 *Contingency, Irony, and Solidarity*, pp. 64, 65.
54 Michel Foucault, 'What is Enlightenment?' in Paul Rabinow (ed.) *The Foucault Reader*. New York: Pantheon, 1984, p. 46.
55 Gilles Deleuze, *Negotiations 1972 –1990*. Trans. M. Joughin, New York: Columbia University Press, 1995, p. 171.

Notes to 2: The Lady Sits Between Two Long Windows, Writing

1 Virginia Woolf, *The Waves*. London: Penguin, 1971, p. 14.
2 Gilles Deleuze and Félix Guattari, *What is Philosophy*? Trans. Graham Burchell and Hugh Tomlinson. London: Verso, 1994, p. 66.
3 *What is Philosophy?*, pp. 35-61; pp. 163-201. The plane of immanence is dealt with in part 1, the plane of composition is the topic of part 2, 'Philosophy, Science, Logic, and Art', pp. 117-218.
4 *What is Philosophy?*, pp. 192-193.
5 *What is Philosophy?*, pp. 36-37.
6 *What is Philosophy?*, pp. 192-196.
7 *What is Philosophy?*, p. 66.
8 Ibid.
9 *What is Philosophy?*, p. 198.
10 Mieke Bal (ed.), 'Introduction,' in *The Practice of Cultural Analysis*. Stanford: Stanford University Press, 1999, p. 2. Following reference on p. 12. See also Jonathan Culler, *Literary Theory*. Oxford: Oxford University Press, 1997.
11 As Jonathan Culler insists, theory is *per se* interdisciplinary. It involves a 'discourse with effects outside an original discipline,' *Literary Theory*, p. 15. By close proximity, cultural analysis comes to function as that 'site' for the self-reflexivity of all disciplines (Culler in *The Practice of Cultural Analysis*, p. 346).
12 For an accessible and comprehensive essay on 'cultural analysis' see the 'Introduction' to *The Practice of Cultural Analysis*. See also Mieke Bal, *Double Exposures*. London: Routledge, 1996 (chapter one) and *ASCA Brief 1*. Amsterdam: ASCA, 1994, pp. 1-2.
13 These terms are fully scrutinised in Mieke Bal, *Narratology*. Toronto: University of Toronto Press, 1997.
14 See J.W. Graham (ed.), *The Waves: Two Holograph Drafts*. London: Routledge, 1976. In the first holograph version pp. 1-299, the 'ur' form of Bernard is a nameless, female and omniscient narrator.
15 *The Waves*, pp. 12-14.

16 *The Waves*, p. 245. My emphasis.
17 Deleuze and Guattari, *A Thousand Plateaus: Capitalism and Schizophrenia*, Trans. Brian Massumi. London: The Athlone Press, 1988, p. 245.
18 *What is Philosophy?*, p. 64.
19 *What is Philosophy?*, pp. 61-68.
20 I use the word 'force' advisedly, pinpointing it as a function of 'meaning'. According to the *OED*, meaning designates not just a set of correspondences between signifier and signified. Intention, and by close association force, are part of the term's matrix.
21 Mieke Bal, 'Self-Reflection as a Mode of Reading,' in *Reading 'Rembrandt': Beyond the Word/Image Opposition*. Cambridge: Cambridge University Press, 1991, pp. 247-285.
22 *Reading 'Rembrandt'*, pp. 247-248.
23 *Reading 'Rembrandt'*, pp. 283-285.
24 *A Thousand Plateaus*, p. 261.
25 *The Waves*, p. 247.
26 The plane of immanence is therefore sometimes called 'plane of consistency'.
27 'What is a Concept' in *What is Philosophy?* (pp. 15-34) gives a comprehensive exploration of what comprises concepts, namely, that they are the bedrock of philosophy, not science or the arts, and that they do not build bridges to other concepts; rather, they are self-referential to their own construction. Concepts have consistencies, that of 'endoconsistency' and 'exoconsistency' (p. 22).
28 The topic of specular identification is succinctly explored in Jacques Lacan, 'The Mirror Phase', *Ecrits: A Selection*. Trans. Alan Sheridan. London: Routledge, 1977, pp. 1-3.
29 *The Waves*, p. 187.
30 Mieke Bal, *Reading 'Rembrandt'*, p. 255.
31 *The Waves*, p. 254.
32 *The Waves*, p. 168.
33 Readers of Derrida will recognise in my use of 'cutting edge' a resonance with Derrida's deployment of the word 'cut' in 'The Sans of the Pure Cut'. See *The Truth in Painting*. Trans. Geoff Bennington and Ian McLeod. Chicago: Chicago University Press, 1987, pp. 83-90. What is cut is the field of a discourse. One example is the separation of text from context. But the incision is so fine, it is almost imperceptible. The lady's windows might provide such a cut between the conceptual and affective functions of writing, one so fine it is hard to discover and isolate. Such a cut, however, also has a provisional if not illusory function. In reading *The Waves*, my argument is that however razor-sharp and indiscernible a line may be, it is constantly moving, just as the de-territorializing borderlines of the plane of consistency are. The position of the cut will not be final.
34 *The Waves*, p. 204.
35 Two relevant examples would be works by Shoshana Felman, *The Literary Speech Act: Don Juan with J.L. Austin, or Seduction in Two Languages*. New York: New York University Press, 1984 and *Jacques Lacan and the Adventure of Insight*. London and Cambridge, Mass.: Harvard University Press, 1987.
36 Gilles Deleuze and Félix Guattari, *Anti-Oedipus: Capitalism and Schizophrenia*. London: The Athlone Press, 1984. In place of psychoanalysis, Deleuze and Guattari call for 'schizoanalysis' and the recognition that the concept of desiring machines, rather than individuals, can challenge the Freudian 'desire' which locates and imprisons subjectivity as a construct of the nuclear family.

37 Sigmund Freud, 'A Child Is Being Beaten,' *The Standard Edition of the Complete Works*, Volume 7. London: Penguin, 1973, p. 23-48. *A Thousand Plateaus*, p.264.

38 *A Thousand Plateaus*, pp. 239-241.

39 *A Thousand Plateaus*, p. 260.

40 Gilles Deleuze & Félix Guattari, *Anti-Oedipus: Capitalism and Schizophrenia*. Trans. Robert Hurley et al. London: The Athlone Press 1984, p. 296. Emphasis by Deleuze and Guattari.

41 *Anti-Oedipus*, p. 251.

42 *A Thousand Plateaus*, p. 274.

43 *A Thousand Plateaus*, p. 252.

44 Virginia Woolf quoted in Ann Oliver Bell (ed.), *The Diary of Virginia Woolf*, Volume 3. London: Penguin, 1980, pp. 209-210.

45 *The Diary of Virginia Woolf*, p. 274.

46 *The Waves*, p. 220

47 *The Waves*, p. 231.

48 *What is Philosophy?*, p. 35.

49 *What is Philosophy?*, p. 36.

50 *What is Philosophy?*, p. 23.

51 *What is Philosophy?*, pp. 16-19.

52 'Introduction,' *The Practice of Cultural Analysis*, pp. 1-14.

53 *The Practice of Cultural Analysis*, p. 7.

54 *The Practice of Cultural Analysis*, pp. 7-9.

55 *The Practice of Cultural Analysis*, p. 9.

56 *The Practice of Cultural Analysis*, p. 34.

57 *The Practice of Cultural Analysis*, p. 177.

58 Ibid.

59 *The Practice of Cultural Analysis*, p. 199.

60 *The Practice of Cultural Analysis*, p. 219.

61 Ibid.

62 In my book *The Intimacy of Influence* (Amsterdam: ASCA Press, 1999), I argue that a new type of artist and cultural analyst will emerge. I suggest that the next century belongs to those who practice in more than one domain, be it academics who make films and write novels, or actresses and film-makers who produce performances and stories which also function as cultural analysis. For the practice of art as cultural analysis or cultural analysis as art, I have coined the following: the practice of 'Renaissance Modernism'.

Notes to 3: Sharing Technologies

1 Gilles Deleuze and Félix Guattari, *What is Philosophy?* Trans. by Graham Burchell and Hugh Tomlinson. London/New York: Verso, 1994, p. 216. Emphasis by Deleuze and Guattari.

2 *What is Philosophy?*, p. 218.

3 WHEN YOU SEE GOD TELL HIM; premiere September 15th 1995, Stadsschouwburg Heerlen, the Netherlands. Choreography: Itzik Galili; Music: Scott Johnson; Soliloquy from *How it Happens*, written by I.F. Stone; Performed by Jennifer Hanna and Itzik Galili.

4 George Lakoff and Mark Johnson, *Metaphors We Live By*. Chicago: University of Chicago Press, 1980; *Philosophy in the Flesh. The Embodied Mind and its Challenge to Western Thought*. New York: Basic Books, 1999.

5 *What is Philosophy?*, p. 210.

6 Ibid.

7 *What is Philosophy?*, p. 65.

8 Editor's note: see on the conceptual persona also 'The Lady Sits Between Two Long Windows, Writing' by Catherine M. Lord (this volume).

9 *What is Philosophy?*, p. 69. My emphasis.

10 Gilles Deleuze with Claire Parnet, L'ABÉCÉDAIRE DE GILLES DELEUZE. Paris: Vidéo Editions Montparnasse, 1996.

11 *What is Philosophy?*, p. 4.

12 *What is Philosophy?* p. viii of the translator's introduction.

13 Ibid.

14 *Metaphors We Live By*, p. 5.

15 Ibid.

16 *What is Philosophy?*, p. 212.

17 *What is Philosophy?*, p. 66.

18 'You know, I have so little to say here this evening, but there's so many things that have been said over and over again that need to be said again and again. And, it's too small a planet – it grows smaller and smaller all the time in terms of travel time. We are becoming one family. We share each other's technology and culture and poetry and philosophy. And we have to begin to think of ourselves as a family. We have to begin to enjoy the differences in the human family like we enjoy the differences in a garden of flowers. And there's a race on – and the real race and the real ideological conflict is between those universalists who want to think in terms of mankind and those reversions to barbarity and tribalism, who are still hung up in ancient, anachronistic hatreds like we see in Ulster, like we see in Israel, Palestine. That we can see in so many parts of the world. Without a system of world law we're lost. And we can't have a system of law without a sense of community. And we can't have a sense of community without the underpinning of recognition of ourselves as part of one family. And there is very little time to muster this broader vision against the ancient, conditioned reflexes and psychoses of mankind and his homicidal tendencies. But either we learn to live together, or we die together. Is it necessary – is it necessary...' From a lecture given by I.F. Stone at the Ford Hall Forum. Broadcast on National Public Radio on April 12, 1983.

19 L'ABÉCÉDAIRE

20 *What is Philosophy?*, p. 203. Emphasis by Deleuze and Guattari.

21 *What is Philosophy?*, p. 204.

22 *What is Philosophy?*, p. 209.

23 *What is Philosophy?*. p. 210.

24 With special thanks to Catherine Lord for pointing out to me the creative potential of the conceptual personae.

Notes to 4: The Metaphor Made Flesh

1 David Cronenberg in Chris Rodley (ed.), *Cronenberg on Cronenberg*. Toronto: Alfred A. Knopf, 1992, p. 168.
2 *Cronenberg on Cronenberg*, p. 59.
3 *Cronenberg on Cronenberg*, p. 58.
4 Cronenberg in André S. Labarthe, CINÉMA DE NOTRE TEMPS – DAVID CRONENBERG: I HAVE TO MAKE THE WORD BE FLESH (TV portrait), Paris: AMIP/La Sept Arte/INA, 1999.
5 CINÉMA DE NOTRE TEMPS – DAVID CRONENBERG.
6 CINÉMA DE NOTRE TEMPS – DAVID CRONENBERG.
7 William Burroughs, *Naked Lunch*. New York: Grove Press Inc., 1966, p. 9.
8 David Cronenberg in *Cronenberg on Cronenberg*, p. 82.
9 Gilles Deleuze & Félix Guattari, *A Thousand Plateaus: Capitalism and Schizophrenia*. Trans. by Brian Massumi. Minneapolis: University of Minnesota Press, 1987, p. 151.
10 Gilles Deleuze, *Cinema 2: The Time-Image*. Trans. by Hugh Tomlinson & Robert Galeta. London: The Athlone Press, 1989, p. 189.
11 Ibid.
12 *The Time-Image*, p. 173.
13 *A Thousand Plateaus*, pp. 149-150.
14 *A Thousand Plateaus*, p.154. Editor's note: In 'Is Bess a Bike?' (this volume) Frans-Willem Korsten discussed the BwO in respect to Lars von Trier's main characters in BREAKING THE WAVES.
15 *A Thousand Plateaus*, p. 158.
16 *A Thousand Plateaus*, p. 164.
17 *A Thousand Plateaus*, p. 153.
18 *A Thousand Plateaus*, p. 159.
19 *A Thousand Plateaus*, p. 161.
20 *A Thousand Plateaus*, p. 160.
21 *A Thousand Plateaus*, p. 163.
22 *A Thousand Plateaus*, p. 165.
23 Cronenberg in *Cronenberg on Cronenberg*, p. 80.
24 In, for example, Robin Wood, 'An Introduction to the American Horror Film' (1979), reprinted in Bill Nichols (ed.), *Movies and Methods*. Berkeley, Los Angeles and London: University of California Press, 1985, pp. 195-220.
25 Cronenberg on The David Cronenberg homepage (interview in *The London Evening Standard*): <www.netlink.co.uk/users/zappa/cronen.html>
26 The David Cronenberg homepage (from *Mondo 2000*)
27 Cronenberg in *Cronenberg on Cronenberg*, p. 145.
28 *Cronenberg on Cronenberg*, p. 29.
29 Ibid.
30 *Cronenberg on Cronenberg*, p. 82.
31 The character Allegra Geller in EXISTENZ.
32 *Cronenberg on Cronenberg*, pp. 128-129.
33 Cronenberg in Chris Rodley, 'Game Boy'. London: *Sight and Sound*, April 1999.

34 The David Cronenberg homepage (interview by Jim Emerson).
35 The official EXISTENZ homepage: <www.existenz.com>.
36 *Cronenberg on Cronenberg*, p. 144.
37 *Cronenberg on Cronenberg*, pp. 111-113.
38 Cronenberg in CINEMA DE NOTRE TEMPS – DAVID CRONENBERG.
39 The EXISTENZ homepage.
40 Cronenberg in *Cronenberg on Cronenberg*, p. 9.
41 Cronenberg in CINEMA DE NOTRE TEMPS – DAVID CRONENBERG.
42   Cronenberg in *Cronenberg on Cronenberg*, p. 90.
43 *A Thousand Plateaus*, p. 161.
44 Steven Shaviro, *The Cinematic Body*. Minneapolis and London: University of Minne-
    sota Press, 1993, pp. 143-144.
45 The David Cronenberg homepage (interview by Lukas Barr).
46 Ibid.

Notes to 5: Micropolitics

1   My translation of 'Il est vrai que la philosophie ne se sépare pas d'une colère contre
    l'époque, mais aussi d'une sérénité qu'elle nous assure.' (Gilles Deleuze, *Pourparlers*.
    Paris: Les Editions de Minuit, 1990, p. 7.) Official translation: 'Philosophy's always
    caught between an anger with the way things are and the serenity it brings.' (Gilles
    Deleuze, *Negotiations 1972-1990*. Trans. Martin Joughin. New York: Columbia Univer-
    sity Press, 1995, unnumbered page after 'contents'.)
2   My translation of 'C'est que nous ne croyons pas à une philosophie politique qui ne
    serait pas centrée sur l'analyse du capitalisme et ses développements' (*Pourparlers*, p.
    323). Official translation: 'You see, we think any political philosophy must turn to the
    analysis of capital and the ways it has developed.' (*Negotiations*, p. 171.)
3   For the following passage see *Negotiations*, pp. 169-182.
4   *Negotiations*, p. 180.
5   My translation of 'Dans un régime de contrôle, on n'en a jamais fini avec rien.' (*Pour-
    parlers*, p. 237). Offical translation: 'In a control-based system nothing's left alone for
    long' (*Negotiations*, p. 175).
6   My translation of 'Il n'y a pas lieu de demander quel est le régime le plus dur, ou le
    plus tolérable, car c'est en chacun d'eux que s'affrontent les libérations et les
    asservissements. (...) Il n'y a pas lieu de craindre ou d'espérer, mais de chercher de
    nouvelles armes.' (*Pourparlers*, pp. 241-242). Official translation: 'It's not a question of
    asking whether the old or new system is harsher or more bearable, because there is
    conflict in each between the ways in which they free and enslave us. (...) It's not a
    question of worrying or hoping for the best, but of finding new weapons.' (*Negotia-
    tions*, p. 178).
7   Hans-Jørgen Schanz: *Karl Marx i tilbageblik efter murens fald* (*Marx in Retrospect after the
    Fall of the Wall*). Århus: Modtryk, 1994.
8   *Negotiations*, p. 171 (translation slightly modified: 'échelle agrandie' (*Pourparlers*, p.
    232) is in offical translation 'broader form' instead of 'larger scale').

9   This implies also a critique of a slightly caricatural idea among leftist-retorics about 'the Capitalists' some years ago: 'If an image of the master or an idea of the State is projected outward to the limits of the universe, as if something had domination over flows as well as segments, and in the same manner, the result is a fictious and rediculous representation.(...) Capitalists may be the masters of surplus value and its distribution, but they do not dominate the flows from which surplus value derives.' Gilles Deleuze and Félix Guattari, *A Thousand Plateaus: Capitalism and Schizophrenia.* Trans. Brian Massumi. London: The Athlone Press, 1988, p. 226.

10 *Marx-Engels-Werke*, bd. 24, p. 109 (quoted in *Marx in Retrospect*, p. 127). My translation from the Danish.

11 *Marx-Engels-Werke*, bd. 23, p. 604 (quoted in *Marx in Retrospect*, p. 129). My translation from the Danish.

12 Gilles Deleuze and Félix Guattari, *What is Philosophy?* Trans. Graham Burchell and Hugh Tomlinson. London/New York: Verso, 1994.

13 *What is Philosophy?*, p. 98. Emphasis by Deleuze and Guattari.

14 Following Marx the important thing about capital is not to have it, territorialize it, but to give it away again by investing it in a process of producing more value, meaning that capital is a deterritorializing movement.

15 *What is Philosophy?*, p. 99. Emphasis by Deleuze and Guattari.

16 I want to emphasize that Deleuze does not see the role of the intellectual as that of a 'vanguardist'. In his discussion with Foucault about the changed role of intellectuals, it is stated: 'In the most recent upheaval, the intellectual discovered that the masses no longer need him to gain knowledge'. ('Intellectuals and Power' in Russel Ferguson et al. (eds.), *Discourses: Conversations in Postmodern Art and Culture*. New York/ Massachusetts/London: The New Museum of Contemporary Art/MIT, 1990, p. 10. Reprinted from Michel Foucault, *Language, Counter-Memory, Practice*. Trans. Donald Bouchard and Sherry Simon, Ithaca: Cornell University Press, 1977). A similar anti-vanguardist point has also been made by Max Horkheimer and Theodor Adorno when they state in *Dialektik der Aufklärung* (Frankfurt: Fischer Taschenbuch Verlag, 1988; first published 1947) that they don't address the mass nor the individual person, but leave their thoughts behind to an 'imagined witness'. The untimely function (in a Nietschean sense) of a 'new people' as well an 'imagined witness' is crucial, precisely because these philosophers do not believe in any objective historical vanguard of progress for philosophy to turn to. Editor's note: in 'The Holy Fools' (this volume), Richard Barbrook has a different view on the idea of 'vanguardism'.

17 Editor's note: See also 'Against the Doxa' by Paola Marrati (this volume).

18 Marx quoted in *Marx in Retrospect*, p. 111. My translation from the Danish.

19 For example, the number of viewers can be measured and the rate of success be analyzed, but this does not offer an understanding of the media of television, which is not just repeating its own relative premises.

20 *What is Philosophy?*, p. 99. Emphasis by Deleuze and Guattari.

21 *Marx in Retrospect*, p. 11. My translation from the Danish.

22 *What is Philosophy?*, p. 100.

23 The concept of the event (*l'événement*) has a complex and central signification in Deleuze's works, to such a degree that the French philosopher F. Zourabichvili has called his book on Deleuze *Deleuze, une philosophie de l'événement* (Paris: PUF, 1994).

24 *Negotiations*, p. 171.

25 *Negotiations*, p. 175.
26 See Gilles Deleuze, *Expressionism in Philosophy: Spinoza*. Trans. Martin Joughin. New York: Zone Books, 1992. First published Paris: 1968 and Gilles Deleuze, *Spinoza: philosophie pratique*. Paris: Minuit, 1981. Revised edition, first publised 1970.
27 On the connections between Spinoza and Marx see Christopher Norris, *Spinoza and the Origins of Modern Critical Theory*. Oxford: Basil Blackwell, 1991. According to Norris, the French philosopher Louis Althusser used Spinoza to inform a special reading of Marx, whereby the Hegelian, idealistic traits of the early Marx could be separated from the Spinozistic inspirations of the later Marx. For Althusser, Spinoza was the one philosopher before Marx to think a 'metaphysical materialism' and, anticipating structuralism, to think strictly structuralistic. The interest in bringing together Marx and Spinoza is common in both Althusser and Deleuze. A third philosopher who has combined a critique of capitalism and negative thought inspired by Spinoza is Antonio Negri. See his profound study *The Savage Anomaly: The Power of Spinoza's Metaphysics and Politics*. Minneapolis: University of Minnesota Press, 1991. In 1990 he had an interview with Deleuze on societies of control, reprinted in *Negotiations*.
28 Michael Hardt, *An Apprenticeship in Philosophy: Gilles Deleuze*. London: UCL Press, 1993, p. 109. The book is a clear interpretation of Deleuze's inspiration from Bergson, Nietzsche and Spinoza.
29 Ibid.
30 Ibid. Tamsin Lorraine investigates in her book *Irigaray and Deleuze: Experiments in Visceral Philosophy* (Ithaca and London: Cornell University Press, 1999) a thought that proceeds from 'the inflection of mind and body' rather than their dualism. She argues from a feminist, ethical perspective, but she does not use Deleuze's readings of Spinoza. Nevertheless the synthesis she seeks between Irigaray and Deleuze is motivated by the need to formulate a 'dissolving' of strata, identities, systems, etc. (Deleuze), that does not lead to a dead end of personal fragmentation, but rather that is supported by a new 'open-ended' personal identity (Irigaray). This 'individual level' of Irigaray seems very similar to Deleuze's use of Spinoza on a collective level and his attempts to think a democracy that enable positive encounters, rather than a limiting order or a sad fragmentation. Lorraine's approach for for a reading of Deleuze and Irigaray on embodied subjectivity seems very relevant, and in a way, I would argue, the 'figure of thought' she is reaching for is already present in Deleuze's work. Editor's note: See 'How to Endure Intensity' (this volume) for another way of relating Deleuze and Irigaray.
31 *An Apprenticeship in Philosophy*, p. 111.
32 *A Thousand Plateaus*, p. 216.
33 *A Thousand Plateaus*, p. 219. Deleuze and Guattari are tributing here sociologist Gabriel Tarde (1843-1904) who was particularly interested in microsociology and for whom the concept of 'flows' consist of desires and beliefs.
34 See for an elaborate analysis of the role of desire and the 'politics of desire' of Deleuze and Guattari Paul Patton, *Deleuze and the Political*. London/New York: Routledge, 2000, pp. 68-77.
35 'And we extend our concept of number as in spinning a thread we twist fibre on fibre. And the strength of the thread does not reside in the fact that some one fibre runs through its whole lenght, but in the overlapping of many fibres.' Ludwig Wittgen-

stein, *Philosophical Investigations*. Oxford: Basil Blackwell, 1953, p. 32, paragraph no. 67.

36 *A Thousand Plateaus*, p. 216/217.

37 This difference is also described as the difference between a 'molar' and a 'molecular' level using terms from an older schism, expressing the operational incompatibility between the unity 'molecule' of physics and the unity 'mol' of chemistry, designing larger groups of molecules.

38 Editor's note: See also 'Against the Doxa' (this volume).

39 *A Thousand Plateaus*, p. 215.

40 *A Thousand Plateaus*, p. 215.

41 In a way Marx anticipates the mobile society of communication and control: 'By its nature capital strives beyond any spatial confinement. The creation of the physical conditions of the exchange – means of communication and transport – will become a necessity for it (the capital) to a much higher degree; the annihilation of space through time.' Karl Marx, *Grundrids. Volume 2*. Århus: Modtryk, 1978, p. 393. My translation from the Danish translation of Marx's *Grundrisse: Foundations of the Critique of Political Economy*.

42 Note the striking similarity with Marx' words in his Grundrisse: 'What is wealth... but the absolute development of its (the human being, MB) creative potential... (where the human being) does not seek to stay something that has already become, but is in the absolute movement of becoming.' My translation from the Danish (*Grundrids*, p. 362).

43 Philip Goodchild in his book *Deleuze and Guattari: An Introduction to the Politics of Desire*. (London: Sage Publications, 1996, pp. 211-213) makes a similar point. He concludes that the philosophy of Deleuze and Guattari has no privileged position (which I have called pragmatics); it presents itself as an ethical act and is opening itself up to infinite unconscious movements as an absolute (thus philosophically 'radical'). See on 'transcendental empiricism' Gilles Deleuze, *Difference and Repetition*. Trans. Paul Patton. London: The Athlone Press, 1994, p. xx and pp. 139-143. Editor's note: For a discussion of Deleuze's relation to Rorty's pragmatism, see 'Redescriptive Philosophy' by Paul Patton (this volume). On Deleuze and Guattari's critique of Rorty and communication see *What is Philosophy?*, p. 144.

44 Editor's note: Catherine Lord in 'The Lady Sits Between Two Long Windows, Writing' and Maaike Bleeker in 'Sharing Technology'(this volume) develop the 'Lady Writing' and 'The Dancer' as conceptual personae that function as go-betweens between the plane of immanence of philosophy and the plane of composition of art.

45 There is nothing romantic about this, only an indication of the intolerable in the world. For instance, the PLO has come into existence under Israeli oppression.

Notes to 6: Glamour and Glycerine

1 Gilles Deleuze and Félix Guattari, *Anti-Oedipus: Capitalism and Schizophrenia*. Trans. Robert Hurley, Mark Seem, and Helen Lane. London: The Athlone Press 1984, p. 274. First published Paris: Minuit, 1972.

2   Tyler Durden in FIGHT CLUB (David Fincher, USA: 1999).
3   Edward Norton's character is actually the nameless narrator. He takes on different names at different support groups (Rupert, Travis, Cornelius). In Tyler's house he finds magazines in which stories that could have been written by David Cronenberg (see 'The Metaphor Made Flesh' in this volume) are told from the point of view of organs: 'I am Jack's bowel'. After reading this, everytime the narrator goes to an intense experience he becomes his most intense affect: 'I am Jack's raging bile', 'I am Jack's cold sweat', 'I am Jack's lack of surprise', 'I am Jack's smurking revenge', 'I am Jack's inflaming sense of rejection'. On the official homepage Norton's character is referred to as Jack <http:www.foxmovies.com/fightclub>.
4   Gilles Deleuze and Félix Guattari, *A Thousand Plateaus: Capitalism and Schizophrenia*. Trans. Brian Massumi. London: The Athlone Press 1988 (first published by Les Editions de Minuit 1980).
5   See Richard Barbrook's 'The Holy Fools' (this volume).
6   Jonathan L. Beller, 'Capital/Cinema' in Eleanor Kaufman and Kevin Jon Heller (eds.), *Deleuze and Guattari: New Mappings in Politics, Philosophy, and Culture*. Minneapolis and London: University of Minnesota Press 1998, pp. 77-95. In 'Postmodernism, or the Cultural Logic of Late Capitalism' Fredric Jameson also emphasizes the importance of (audio-visual) culture in late capitalism (*New Left Review*, no. 146, 1984, pp. 53-94).
7   I want to emphasize that in this article I am not so much concerned with the formal analysis of the cinematographic image. In Deleuzian terms, for instance, FIGHT CLUB is actually a movement-image, an action-image, of the brain (see also notes 36 and 44). Elsewhere I develop the relations between 'form of contents' and 'form of expressions' of cinema (Patricia Pisters, *The Matrix of Visual Culture: Working with Deleuze in Film Studies*. Stanford: Stanford University Press, 2001 (forthcoming). Here I look at a broader level of micropolitics in relation to capital and cinema/audiovisual culture.
8   Manuel Castells, *The Information Age: Economy, Society and Culture*. Volume 1: *The Rise of the Network Society*; Volume 2: *The Power of Identity*; Volume 3: *End of Millenium*. Oxford and Massachusetts: Blackwell 1996. In 'Politics and Silicon Valley: Liberty.com', in *The Economist*, October 30th 1999, pp. 23-27, Castells's work is mentioned as the most significant study of cyber space and the economic, sociological and cultural aspects of contemporary society.
9   *The Network Society*, p. 172-193.
10 When reading about Castells's networks, it is difficult not to make a first connection to a Deleuzeguattarian concept, namely that of the rhizome. Since it is such an obvious link, I will not elaborate very much on this parallel between Castells and Deleuze and Guattari. The rhizome is a term that originates from biology, in which it means a system (network) of roots and leafy shoots that grow just above and just below the surface. Grass, for instance, is a rhizomatic plant. Deleuze and Guattari use this term to talk about the network structure of the mind ('we have grass in our heads') and the world in which we have come to live. They give examples of computer technology and microbiology (DNA) that make rhizomatic connections. The rhizome is also the central metaphor for their entire work and working method. From the beginning of their collaboration, Deleuze and Guattari have been thinking in terms of open (machinic) networks that depend on connections and consistencies. Society and thought seem to be organized in similar ways.

11 *The Network Society*, pp. 376-428. Informational flows are processed between 'mega-cities' and 'customized cottages' (Castells argues that Marshall McLuhan's global village has turned into many 'customized cottages'). Castells' view on space in late capitalism differs from the postmodernist view of Fredric Jameson. According to Jameson space in postmodernism has become flat, overdetermined and disorienting as in the film BLADE RUNNER. For a discussion of the Jameson in respect to BLADE RUNNER see Vivian Sobchack, *Screening Space: The American Science Fiction Film*. New Jersey and London: Rutgers University Press, 1987, pp. 223-305. However, both conceptions of new spatial configurations do not need to exclude each other. Overabundancy can lead to 'foldings' (to use another Deleuzian term) in space, e.g. from local to global.

12 *The Network Society*, pp. 429-468.

13 *The Network Society*, p. 471.

14 Gilles Deleuze, 'Control and becoming' and 'Postscript on Control Societies' in *Negotiations 1972-1990*. Trans. Martin Joughin. New York: Columbia University Press 1995, pp. 169-182. First published Paris: Minuit, 1990. See also Malene Busk's 'Micro-politics: Political Philosophy from Marx and Beyond' (this volume).

15 'Control and becoming', p. 172.

16 See Coco Fusco, 'At Your Service: Latinas in the Global Information Network' at <www.hkw.de/forum/forum1/doc/text/fusco-isea98.html>(dd. January 2000) and Michel Hardt, 'La société mondiale de contrôle' in Eric Alliez (ed.), *Gilles Deleuze: une vie philosophique*. Le Plessis-Robinsin: Institut Synthélabo 1998, pp. 359-375.

17 Desire (as micropolitics and schizophrenia elaborated further in relation to FIGHT CLUB) is to Deleuze what power is to Foucault. See for a comparison between Foucault's 'power' and Deleuze's 'desire' Paul Patton, *Deleuze and the Political*. London and New York: Routledge, 2000, pp. 49-67.

18 With 'representation' I mean here both the reflective capacity of cultural products (to mirror what happens in society) and the more participating and active aspect of representation (representations also construct actively society). This second aspect has been elaborated in cultural studies. See, for instance, Stuart Hall, 'New Ethnicities' in: *ICA-Document 7, Black Film British Cinema*. London: ICA, 1988, pp. 27-31.

19 *The Network Society*, p. 328.

20 *The Network Society*, p. 372.

21 *The Network Society*, p. 373.

22 Gilles Deleuze, 'Immanence, A Life...'. Trans. Nick Millet. *Theory, Culture & Society*, no. 14/2. London: Sage Publications 1997, pp. 3-7. First published Paris: Minuit, 1995; and Gilles Deleuze 'Le virtuel et l'actuel', a new text added to the last French Edition of Gilles Deleuze and Claire Parnet, *Dialogues*. Paris: Flammarion 1996 (first published 1977). The difference between the virtual and the actual is a difference of time: it is the present that passes that defines the actual; the virtual is defined by the past that conserves itself (note that we are dealing here with a non-linear Bergsonian conception of time as duration and the co-existing layers of time). See for more on the virtual and actual Patricia Pisters, 'The Fifth Element and the Fifth Dimension of the Affection-Image' in Anu Koivunen and Astrid Söderberg (eds.), *Cinema Studies into Visual Theory?* Turku: University of Turku 1998, pp. 93-107.

23 The more active conception of representation that was introduced by cultural studies is much closer to 'the culture of real virtuality'. However, cultural studies keeps the

distinction between real and virtual much more in place than the shifts that Castells and Deleuze are proposing.

24 *The Network Society*, p. 195-200.

25 *The Network Society*, p. 199.

26 Deleuze and Guattari, *What is Philosophy?* Translated by G. Burchell and Hugh Tomlinson. London/New York: Verso 1994 (first published by Les Editions de Minuit 1991). A third domain of thinking is science. Science thinks in functions.

27 Gilles Deleuze, *Cinema 1: The Movement-Image*. Trans. Hugh Tomlinson and Barbara Habberjam. London: The Athlone Press 1986 (first published by Les Editions de Minuit 1983) and *Cinema 2: The Time-Image*. Trans. Hugh Tomlinson and Robert Galeta. London: The Athlone Press 1989 (first published by Les Editions de Minuit 1985).

28 'Capital/Cinema', p. 82-83.

29 'Capital/Cinema', p. 91. In his book *Deleuzism: A Metacommentary* (Edinburgh: Edinburgh University Press, 2000) Ian Buchanan makes a similar point when he investigates in which ways Deleuze's work can actually account for the peculiar events and phenomenon of popular culture (cf. pp.175-189).

30 According to Deleuze the brain itself is the real 'connecting screen'. And if cinema wants to look for any 'models' it should look at the 'micro-biology of the brain.' Gilles Deleuze, *Negotiations*. Trans. Martin Joughin. New York: Columbia University Press, 1995, p. 60 and Gilles Deleuze, 'Le cerveau, c'est l'écran', *Cahiers du Cinéma*, March 1986. See also Gregory Flaxman (ed.), *The Brain is the Screen: Deleuze and the Philosophy of Cinema*. Minneapolis and London: University of Minnesota Press, 2000.

31 *The Network Society*, p. 68 and 75.

32 *Big Brother* was a true media event in the last three months of 1999 in The Netherlands and was soon sold to many other countries. Perhaps inspired by Peter Weir's film THE TRUMAN SHOW, commercial television production company John de Mol got the very smart idea to put nine people for 100 days in a house under 24 hours surveillance of 24 cameras (including cameras in the bathroom and infra-red cameras in the bedrooms) that could be followed on television and the internet. The popularity of this format has turned *Big Brother* into a global media phenomenon.

33 Jackie Stacey, *Star Gazing: Hollywood Cinema and Female Spectorship*. London and New York: Routledge 1994.

34 *Star Gazing*, p. 190.

35 On the website this is emphasized in banners showing well trained body parts, accompanied by slogans like: 'Uses stairmaster 60 minutes every day... has never had to run to save his life'; 'Benches 425 Lbs... has never written poetry'; 'Can do 500 crunches in 5 minutes... has never witnessed birth' See <http://www.foxmovies.com/fightclub>. It is as if Jack and Tyler speak to Victor Ward.

36 It is only at the end of the film that we realize that the fight, or 'duel' that is characteristic for the action-image (*The Movement-Image*, p. 142; 'The action in itself is a duel of forces, a series of duels: duel with the milieu, with the others, with itself') is not an external but an internal (virtual) fight. Even in an (at first sight unambiguous) action-image, the boundaries between actual and virtual seem to have disappeared. Another important indicator of 'the virtual but real' status of all the images, is Jack's insomnia. Jack has the impression 'everything becomes like a copy of a copy of a copy' and at many instances in the film he wonders if he's asleep or awake.

37 *Anti-Oedipus*, p. 227.

38 *Anti-Oedipus*, p. 245.

39 In postmodern theory Fredric Jameson has taken up Lacan's term of schizophrenia in order to indicate how in postmodernism there is a breakdown between signifiers, related to the inability of access to the Symbolic that has become too full and overdetermined. See 'Guliana Bruno: Ramble City: Postmodenism and BLADE RUNNER' in Annette Kuhn (ed.), *Alien Zone: Cultural Theory and Contemporary Science Fiction Cinema*. London: Verso, 1990, pp. 183-195. Schizophrenia is used here in a descriptive way (to describe the confusion of the postmodern condition). Although they recognize the 'vertigo' of signification, Deleuze and Guattari use the term in a much more political way (as a way of resistance to capitalism).

40 Eugene Holland, *Deleuze and Guattari's Anti-Oedipus: Introduction to Schizoanalysis*. London and New York: Routledge, 1999, p. x.

41 *Introduction to Schizoanalysis*, p. 3.

42 See, for instance, *A Thousand Plateaus*, pp. 505-506. Although the molecular takes place at the micro-level of the mind and the body, it is not restricted to the private and personal experience ('a delirium is world-historical, not familial' say Deleuze and Guattari in *Anti-Oedipus*).

43 *Anti-Oedipus*, p. 281. See for more elaborations on the Body without Organs the contributions of Eva Jørholt, Rosi Braidotti and Frans-Willem Korsten in this volume.

44 In LOST HIGHWAY Fred metamorphoses into Pete (but without a clear 'fight' between them). Here schizophrenia borders paranoia, and here too audiovisual technology like a cell phone and various videotapes play a significant role. In BEING JOHN MALKOVICH John Malkovich's brain is turned into a commodity and is literally populated by many people. In her essay 'The Duration of Oblivion: Deleuze and Forgetting in FIGHT CLUB and LOST HIGHWAY', Jennifer Heuson analyses how Fincher and Lynch present maps of the brain (the spatial movement-image of FIGHT CLUB) and the mind (the time-image of LOST HIGHWAY); she also demonstrates how the movement-image and time-image even become reversible in the splitting cerebral/spiritual paths both films present (MA-assignment; Department of Film and Television Studies, University of Amsterdam 2000).

45 In *Deleuze and the Political*, Paul Patton states: 'This kind of sudden shift towards a life which is lived at another degree of intensity is one possible outcome of what they call a line of flight. It is on this kind of line that critical freedom is manifest' (p. 87). Jack's schizophrenization can certainly be seen as such a 'sudden shift' towards another degree of intensity.

46 See Richard Barbrook, 'The Holy Fools' in this volume.

47 Gilles Deleuze, *Bergsonism*. Trans. Hugh Tomlinson and Barbara Habberjam. New York: Zone Books, 1988, p. 107. First published Paris: PUF, 1966.

48 *Anti-Oedipus*, p. xvi. See also Gilles Deleuze, *Spinoza: Practical Philosophy*. Trans. Robert Hurley. San Francisco: City Lights, 1988, p. 10. First published Paris: Minuit, 1981.

49 Aden Evens, Mani Haghighi, Stacey Johnson, Karen Ocaña, and Gordon Thompson, 'Another Always Thinks in Me,' in Elanor Kaufman and Kevin Jon Heller (eds.), *Deleuze and Guattari: New Mappings in Politics, Philosophy, and Culture*, pp. 270-280.

50 'Another Always Thinks in Me', p. 277. The quotations in this quotation are from Deleuze's *Difference and Repetition*.

51 At the end of the film Tyler tells Jack: 'You created me, you needed me'. And Jack an-swers: 'I don't need you any more'. He has learned to live 'at another degree of inten-sity'. It is also only at this point that Jack becomes fully aware of the importance of Marla (Helena Bonham Carter), the only woman in the film, who all the time has been his actual 'double', mirroring his own search for intensity (as opposed to the virtu-ality of Tyler).

52 After the revolution of schizophrenization, the next step would be to look at the ethics of such revolution. How to combine a Spinozian 'sustainability of life' and freedom of the other with the micro-political revolution of schizophrenization. This problem, however, requires a new essay. See, for instance, Rosi Braidotti's 'How to Endure In-tensity' (this volume).

53 André Parente, 'Le cinéma de la pensée ou le virtuel en tant que jamais vu' in Eric Alliez (ed.), *Gilles Deleuze, une vie philosophique*, pp. 555-564. See also John Rajchman, 'Y-a-t-il une intelligence du virtuel?' in the same volume, pp. 403-420.

54 'Capital/Cinema', p. 91.

55 I would like to thank Thomas Elsaesser, Michael Wedel and Wim Staat for their useful questions and remarks on an earlier version of this paper.

Notes to 7: Is Bess a Bike?

1   Gilles Deleuze and Félix Guattari, *A Thousand Plateaus*. Trans. Brian Massumi. Lon-don: The Athlone Press, 1988, p. 176.

2   *A Thousand Plateaus*, p. 181.

3   In the light of what I shall be arguing in relation to the film, the following is a relevant quotation: 'Each freed faciality trait forms a rhizome with a freed trait of landscapicity, picturality, or musicality.' (*A Thousand Plateaus,* p. 190). The idea to 'free' the male model of Christ through turning it into a female one is a modern con-cern and stands at the heart of a real struggle. See, for instance Fokkelien van Dijk-Hemmers and Athalya Brenner, *Reflections on Theology and Gender*. Kampen: Kok Pharos, 1994.

4   Jonneke Bekkenkamp, 'Breaking the Waves: Corporeality and Religion in a Modern Melodrama', Jonneke Bekkenkamp & Maaike de Hardt (eds.), *Begin with the Body*: *Corporeality, Religion and Gender*. Leuven: Peeters, 1998, pp. 134-157.

5   In The Netherlands, the discussion on BREAKING THE WAVES was largely initiated by feminist critics or feminist theologians. For instance, Jessica Prager-Stein presented a discussion between the writer Renate Dorresteijn and the theologian Irmgard Busch under the title '*Breaking the Waves*: Moving or Indigestible?' (*Fier*, no. 1/1, pp. 24-25). For the international controversy see, for instance, the reactionary review of Will Geeslin, and the resulting responses: <http://sac.uky.edu/~wwgeeso/sack/waves.html>.

6   Kaja Silverman, *The Threshold of the Visible World*. New York and London: Routledge 1996, p. 19. See also *Male Subjectivity at the Margins*. New York and London: Routledge, 1992, p. 130.

7   Gilles Deleuze & Félix Guattari, *Anti-Oedipus: Capitalism and Schizophrenia*. Trans. Helen Lane, Mark Seem & Robert Hurley. Minneapolis: University of Minnesota Press, 1984, p.34. Editor's note: see also chapter 6 'Glamour and Glycerine' in this volume.

8   An asymmetry in gender is certainly one characteristic of Deleuze and Guattari's work as was pointed out by Rosi Braidotti, e.g. in the article 'Meta(l)morphosis'. *Theory, Culture and Society*, no. 14/2, pp. 67-80. That asymmetry does not deny the possibility of acting out a schizoanalysis that takes gender seriously. See also Ian Buchanan & Claire Colebrook (eds.), *Deleuze and Feminist Theory*. Edinburgh: Edinburgh University Press, 2000. For a similar operation, see what Kaja Silverman did to the concept of 'screen', which was a creative amplification of Lacan's imagery. Screen is different from concrete looking and different from the look that produces us as subjects, the gaze. When stating that a film in its affects is at the heart of a rosette of screens, I mean to say that there are always many different screens operative.

9   'Le style documentaire et brutal que j'ai donné au film, et qui en fait l'annule et le contredit, implique que nous acceptons l'histoire en tant que telle'(Stig Björkman, 'Entretien avec Lars von Trier', *Cahiers du Cinéma*, no. 503, p. 24).

10 The image was produced by transferring the film to video, then working on the colors, then transferring the video back to film again. (Ibid.)

11 Ibid.

12 The chapter titles are: Prologue; 1: Bess Gets Married; 2: Life with Jan; 3: Life Alone; 4: Jan's Illness; 5: Doubt; 6: Faith; 7: Bess' Sacrifice; Epilogue.

13 The concept of 'intertextuality' is too often seen as a means for pinpointing textual genetics, or historical influence. This is certainly not how it is understood by Julia Kristeva, who develops the notion in thinking through Bakhtin's concept of dialogism. To enhance the content of the concept in Kristeva's sense, Ernst van Alphen proposes the notion of 'resonance' in his book *De toekomst der herinnering: essays over moderne Nederlandse literatuur* (*The Future of Memory: Essays about Modern Dutch Literature*). Amsterdam: Van Gennep, 1993.

14 The Dutch story on Brendan is called *De reis van Sinte Brandaan* (*The Journey of Saint Brendan*). For the study of *Brandaan*, see Wim Gerritsen, Doris Edel & Mieke de Kreek (eds.), *De Wereld van Sint Brandaan*. Utrecht: Hes, 1986, pp. 19-23.

15 *Anti-Oedipus*, p. 270.

16 Another Jesus who is flown in by helicopter is at the start of Fellini's la dolce vita; and in an earlier film by Von Trier, epidemic, a docter is flown in in a same way.

17 Eugene W. Holland, *Deleuze and Guattari's Anti-Oedipus: Introduction to Schizoanalysis*. London and New York: Routledge 1999, p. 28.

18 *Anti-Oedipus*, p. 8.

19 In terms of face there is a strong intertextual resonance with Fellini's LA STRADA and the face of Giulietta Masina; a film that could be analysed in comparable terms. In fact, when Von Trier was introducing Emily Watson (Bess) to the film, he showed her extracts of LA STRADA (See Marie-Anne Guérin, 'Emily Watson', *Cahiers du Cinéma*, no.506, 1996, p. 28).

20 Xandra Schutte, 'Filmlezen: Het Woord is vlees geworden' ('Film Reading: The Word has become Flesh). *De Groene Amsterdammer* (18-09-1996). My translation from the Dutch. Deleuze's analysis of Christ's conception of love is telling: 'he did not want to keep anything, not even the inviolable part of himself. There was something suicidal

about him.' (Gilles Deleuze, *Essays Critical and Clinical*, London and New York: Verso, 1998, p. 50).

21 *Introduction to Schizoanalysis*, p. 21.

22 See for example: Marie-Ann Guérin, 'Emily Watson'. *Cahiers du Cinéma* no. 506, 1996, p. 28; Frédéric Strauss, 'A la vie, á la mort'. *Cahiers du Cinéma* no. 506, 1996, pp. 27 and 29; Patricia Pisters, Liefde doet wonderen: Breaking the Waves'. *Skrien* no. 209, 1996, pp. 11-13; 'What's Love Got to Do with It?' in Mieke Bal et al. (eds.), *Visions and Voices of Otherness*. ASCA Brief. Amsterdam: ASCA Press 1996, pp. 61-72; Renate Dorrestein in Jessica Prager-Stein, 'Breaking the Waves: Ontroerend of onverteerbaar'. *Fier* no. 1:1, 1998, pp. 24-25.

23 See *Anti-Oedipus*. See also Paul Patton, *Deleuze and the Political*. London and New York: Routledge, 2000; especially chapter 5 'Social Machines and the State', pp. 88-108.

24 See *Introduction to Schizoanalysis*, p. 64.

25 On despotism and god, see *Anti-Oedipus*, p. 197.

26 See *Anti-Oedipus*, pp. 262-271 and pp. 356-361; see also *Introduction to Schizoanalysis*, p. 87.

27 *A Thousand Plateaus*, pp. 115-116.

28 *A Thousand Plateaus*, p. 153. Editor's note: See Eva Jørholt's 'The Metaphor Made Flesh' for BwO's in the work of filmmaker David Cronenberg.

29 *A Thousand Plateaus*, p. 151.

30 For the relation between face and landscape, see *A Thousand Plateaus*, p.173.

31 For Cynthia Fuchs, see <http://www.addict.com/issues/2.12/html/hifi/Reviews/In_the_Frame/Breaking_the_Waves>. In this context Bess neatly fits the image that has been depicted by Andrea Dworkin in *Intercourse* (New York and London: Free Press, 1997) in which Dworkin argues that fucking is not innocent, or the epitome of love. In the current historical circumstances, Dworkin states, 'murder [...] is the sex act or it is sexual climax' (p. 7). For criticism and theory on the gendered asymmetry in relation to film, see Mary Ann Doane, *The Desire to Desire: The Woman's Film of the 1940's*. Bloomington: Indiana University Press, 1987. Mary Ann Doane, *Femmes Fatales: Feminism, Film Theory, Psychoanalysis*. New York/London: Routledge, 1991; Teresa de Lauretis, *Alice Doesn't: Feminism, Semiotics, Cinema*. Bloomington: Indiana University Press, 1984.Teresa de Lauretis, *Technologies of Gender: Essays on Theory, Film, and Fiction*. Bloomington/Indianapolis: Indiana University Press, 1987. Kaja Silverman, *The Threshold of the Visible World*. New York/London: Routledge, 1996. Criticism that in my view repeats the problem is presented by Slavoj Zizek (1994) in his article 'Why is Woman Symptom of Man' (*The Metastasis of Enjoyment: Six Essays on Woman and Causality* (London and New York: Verso, 1994) where the difference between individual and type is completely obliterated, and psychoanalysis remains caught in a closed circle: produced by the historical circumstances that it tries to explain.

32 Mieke Bal, 'Body Politics' in *On Meaning-Making: Essays in Semiotics*. Sonoma, California: Polebridge Press, 1994, pp. 263-280.

33 For an overview of the discussion following strange days, see Patricia Pisters, *From Eye to Brain. Gilles Deleuze: Refiguring the Subject in Film Theory*. Amsterdam: PhD University of Amsterdam, 1998, pp. 106-107.

34 Joan Smith quoted in *From Eye to Brain*, p. 107.

35 For criticism on the function of art as redeeming, see especially Leo Bersani, *The Culture of Redemption*. Cambridge Mass. and London: Harvard University Press, 1990.

36 Gilles Deleuze, *Essays Critical and Clinical*. Trans. Daniel W. Smith and Michael A. Greco. London and New York: Verso, 1998.

37 This article profited immensely from the comments of Patricia Pister and Markha Valenta, for which I thank them. I also thank Ulrike Dietze for her responses.

Notes to 8: 'The Holy Fools'

1   Lewis Carroll, *Alice in Wonderland*. London: Pan, 1947, p. 69.

2   See Richard Barbrook and Andy Cameron, 'The Californian Ideology'. *Science as Culture* no. 26/6, 1996, pp. 44-72. See also <hrc.wmin.ac.uk>.

3   A TJ is a 'theory-jockey': Amsterdam slang for intellectuals who cut 'n' mix philosophies like DJs in a club.

4   DIY stands for 'do-it-yourself'. See Elaine Brass and Sophie Poklewski Koziell with Denise Searle (eds.), *Gathering Force: DIY culture – Radical Action for those Tired of Waiting*. London: Big Issue, 1997.

5   See the FAQ (Frequently Asked Questions) section on Rhizome (was www.rhizome.com, now www.rhizome.org).

6   'May '68 was a demonstration, an irruption, of a becoming in its pure state... Men's only hope lies in a revolutionary becoming: the only way of casting off their shame or responding to what is intolerable.' Gilles Deleuze, 'Control and Becoming', *Negotiations: 1972-1990*. Trans. Martin Joughin. New York: Columbia University Press 1995, p. 171.

7   Jacques Camatte, *The Wandering of Humanity*. Detroit: Black & Red, 1975, pp. 35-36.

8   See Félix Guattari, *Molecular Revolution: Psychiatry and Politics*. Trans. Rosemary Sheed. Harmondsworth, Middlesex: Penguin, 1984.

9   Gilles Deleuze and Félix Guattari, *A Thousand Plateaus: Capitalism and Schizophrenia*. Trans. Brian Massumi. London: The Athlone Press, 1988, pp. 149-166.

10 Alfred Douglas, *The Tarot*. London: Penguin, 1991, p. 43. This Gnostic vision of human freedom is remarkably close to the liberating role of insanity championed by the two philosophers.

11 See Félix Guattari, 'The Three Ecologies'. Trans. Chris Turner. *New Formations*, no. 8, 1987, pp. 131-147.

12 See Félix Guattari, 'Les Radios Libres Populaires' in *La Nouvelle Critique*, no. 115/296 (1978, pp.77-79) and his introduction to *Collectif A/Traverso*, 'Radio Alice, Radio Libre', translated in *Molecular Revolution: Psychiatry and Politics*.

13 Jean-Paul Simard, interviewed by Richard Barbrook. *Fréquence Libre*, April 1985; and Annick Cojean and Frank Eskenazi, *FM: la folle histoire des radios libres*. Paris: Grasset, 1986.

14 The vanguard was a military term used for the advance guard who opened up the path for the main army. Applied to politics, this phrase emphasised the leadership role of radical intellectuals within revolutionary organisations.

15 For a critique of New Left vanguardism, see Jo Freeman, 'The Tyranny of Structurelessness' in *CS. Untying the Knot: Feminism, Anarchism & Organisation.* London: Dark Star and Rebel Press, 1984.

16 See V.I. Lenin, *What Is To Be Done? Burning Questions of our Movement.* Beijing: Foreign Language Press, 1975; and Georg Lukács, *History and Class Consciousness.* London: Merlin, 1968.

17 See Louis Althusser, *Lenin and Philosophy and Other Essays.* London: New Left Books, 1971.

18 Above all, anarcho-communism was seen as the heir of those Left Communists who had fought for direct democracy organised through the Soviets against the dictatorship of the Leninist party. See Maurice Brinton, *The Bolsheviks & Workers' Control: 1917-1921.* London: Solidarity, 1970; and Ida Mett, *The Kronstadt Uprising 1921.* London: Solidarity, 1967.

19 See Jacques Camatte, *The Wandering of Humanity.* Of course, a much diluted variant of this attack on oppressive 'grand narratives' later formed the ideological basis for the self-styled post-modernists.

20 In classic New Left films like weekend and themroc, rebellion against a repressive and alienating urban society was symbolically represented through a return to primitive simplicity. Curiously, both films portrayed cannibalism as the ultimate expression of liberation from bourgeois morality!

21 See Gilles Deleuze and Félix Guattari, *A Thousand Plateaus,* pp. 149-166.

22 Apart from its emphasis on peasants rather than nomads, Khmer Rouge ideology was very similar to the anti-modernism espoused by Deleuze and Guattari. See Michael Vickery, *Cambodia: 1975-1982.* Hemel Hempstead: Allen and Unwin, 1984.

23 In contrast, most of their contemporaries gravitated towards either electoral politics or post-modern nihilism. See Jean-Pierre Garnier and Roland Lew, 'From The Wretched Of The Earth To The Defence Of The West: An Essay on Left Disenchantment in France' in *Socialist Register 1984: The Uses of Anti-Communism.* London: Merlin, 1984.

24 From 1930 to 1933, the Surrealists' journal was called *Le Surréalisme au service de la révolution.* See Helena Lewis, *Dada Turns Red: The Politics of Surrealism.* Edinburgh: Edinburgh University Press, 1990.

25 According to Nietzsche, the culturally impoverished masses were 'herd animals' compared to the 'eagles' of the artistic world.

26 Friedrich Nietzsche, *The Will to Power.* New York: Vintage, 1968. Deleuze commended Nietzsche for the 'positive task' of inventing the reactionary concept of the Superman. See Gilles Deleuze, *Nietzsche and Philosophy.* Trans. Hugh Tomlinson. London: The Athlone Press, 1983.

27 See Ken Knabb (ed.), *Situationist International Anthology.* California: Bureau of Public Secrets, 1981.

28 See Raoul Vaneigem, *The Revolution of Everyday Life.* London: Practical Paradise, 1972. The Situationists discovered the tribal gift economy in Marcel Mauss, *The Gift: The Form and Reason for Exchange in Archaic Societies.* London: Routledge, 1990.

29 See Warren O. Hagstrom, 'Gift Giving as an Organisational Principle in Science' in Barry Barnes and David Edge (eds.), *Science in Context: Readings in the Sociology of Science* Milton Keynes: The Open University, 1982.

30 See for a discussion of the Nepstar/MP3 debate my article 'The Regulation of Liberty: Free Speech, Free Trade and Free Gifts on the Net' <hrc.wmin.ac.uk>.

31 See Rishab Aiyer Ghosh, 'Cooking Pot Markets: An Economic Model for the Trade in Free Goods and Services on the Internet' <dxm.org/tcok/cookingpot/>.

32 See Keith W. Porterfield, 'Information Wants to be Valuable: A Report from the First O'Reilly Perl Conference' <netaction.org/articles/freesoft.html>.

33 See Eric C. Raymond, 'The Cathedral and the Bazaar' <tuxedo.org/~esr/writings/cathedral-bazaar/>.

34 See Netscape Communications Corporation, 'Netscape Announces Plans to Make Next-Generation Communicator Source Code Available Free on the Net' <netscape.com/newsref/pr/newsrelease558.html>.

35 Andrew Leonard, 'Let My Software Go!' <salonmagazine.com/21st/feature/1998/04/cov_14feature.html>.

36 Wired uses 'The New Economy' as a synonym for its neo-liberal fantasies about the digital future.

37 Alexandre Kojève, Introduction to the Reading of Hegel: Lectures on the 'Phenomenology of Spirit'. Ithaca NY: Cornell University Press, 1969, p. 243.

38 Henri Lefebvre, *Everyday Life in the Modern World*. New Brunswick NY: Transaction Publishers, 1984, p. 204.

Notes to 9: How to Endure Intensity

1 Moira Gatens and Genvieve Lloyd, *Collective Imaginings: Spinoza, Past and Present*. London and New York: Routledge, 1999.

2 This distinction between the visible and the sayable is crucial, among others, to Deleuze's reading of Foucault's work. See Gilles Deleuze, *Foucault*. Trans. Seán Hand. Minneapolis: University of Minnesota Press, 1988. First published Paris: 1986.

3 In L'ABÉCÉDAIRE DE GILLES DELEUZE. Paris: Vidéo Editions Montparnasse, 1996.

4 See Luce Irigaray, *Spéculum, de l'autre femme*. Paris: Minuit, 1974; Gilles Deleuze and Félix Guattari, *A Thousand Plateaus: Capitalism and Schizophrenia*. Trans. Brian Massumi. Minneapolis: University of Minnesota Press, 1987.

5 See for instance the chapter on 'Geophilosophy' in Philip Goodchild, *Deleuze and Guattari: An Introduction to the Politics of Desire*. London: Sage, 1996.

6 Genevieve Lloyd, *Part of Nature: Self-Knowledge in Spinoza's Ethics*. Ithaca: Cornell University Press, 1994.

7 Julia Kristeva, 'Women's Time' in N.O. Keohane et al.(eds.), *Feminist Theory: A Critique of Ideology*. Chigago: Chigago University Press, 1982.

8 See for instance, Gayatri Chakravorty Spivak, 'In a Word'. *Differences* 1/2, pp. 124-156.

9 Narco-philosophers such as Arthur and Marie-Louise Kroker, Nick Land and Jean Baudrillard.

10 Genevieve Lloyd, *Part of Nature*; and *Spinoza and the Ethics*. London and New York: Routledge, 1996; Lloyd and Gatens, *Collective Imaginings*.

11 *Part of Nature*, p. 106.

12 *A Thousand Plateaus*, chapter 10 (cf. on Cuvier and Geoffrey Saint Hilaire).

13 Brian Massumi, *A User's Guide to Capitalism and Schizophrenia*. Boston and Massachussets Institute of Technology Press, 1992.

14 Zygmunt Bauman, *Postmodern Ethics*. Oxford: Blackwell, 1993.

15 See Goodchild, *An Introduction to the Politics of Desire*.

16 Jeanette Winterson, *The Passion*. London: Bloomsbury, 1987.

17 Jackie Stacey, *Teratologies: A Cultural Study of Cancer*. London: Routledge, 1997.

18 Elisabeth Grosz, 'Darwin and Feminism: Preliminary Investigations for a Possible Alliance' in *Australian Feminist Studies*. Vol. 14/29, pp. 31-45.

19 Martin Amis, *Einstein's Monsters*. London: Penguin, 1987; Kathy Acker, 'The End of the World of White Men', in J. Halberstam and I. Livingston (eds.), *Posthuman Bodies*. Bloomington: Indiana University Press, 1995.

20 André Colombat, 'November 4, 1995: Deleuze's death as an event' in *Man and World*, Vol. 29/3, July 1996, pp. 235-249.

21 Goodchild, *An Introduction to the Politics of Desire*, p. 208.

22 See Grosz, 'Darwin and Feminism'.

23 Keith Ansell Pearson, *Viroid Life: Perspectives on Nietzsche and the Transhuman Condition*. London and New York: Routledge, 1997, p. 109.

24 Luce Irigaray, *Etique de la différence sexuelle*. Paris: Minuit, 1984.

25 See, for example, Dorothea Olkowski, 'Body, Knowledge and Becoming-Woman: Morpho-logic in Deleuze and Irigaray' in Ian Buchanan and Claire Colebrook (eds.), *Deleuze and Feminist Theory*. Edinburgh: Edinburgh University Press 2000, pp. 86-109; Tamsin Lorrain, *Irigaray and Deleuze: Experiments in Visceral Philosophy*. Ithaca and London: Cornell University Press, 1999.

26 *Viroid Life*, pp. 62-63.

27 *Viroid Life*, p. 68.

28 Dorothea Olkowski, *Gilles Deleuze and the Ruin of Representation*. Berkeley: University of California Press, 1999.

29 See for instance Martha Nusbaum, *Cultivating Humanity*. Cambridge: Harvard University Press, 1999; and Seyla Benhabid, *The Situated Self*. Cambridge: Polity Press, 1992.

Notes to 10: Against the Doxa

1 Gilles Deleuze and Félix Guattari, *What is Philosophy?* Trans. G. Burchell and H. Tomlinson. London: Verso, 1994, p. 206.

2 Gilles Deleuze and Félix Guattari, *Anti-Oedipus: Capitalism and Schizophrenia*. Trans. Robert Hurley, Mark Seem, Helen R. Lane. New York: Viking Press, 1977 and London: the Athlone Press, 1884; *Kafka. Towards a Minor Literature*. Trans. Dana Polan. Minneapolis: University of Minnesota Press, 1986; *A Thousand Plateaus: Capitalism and Schizophrenia*. Trans. B. Massumi. Minneapolis: University of Minnesota Press, 1987.

3 In particular from the existential Marxism of Sartre and the structuralist approach of Louis Althusser. See Mark Poster, *Existential Marxism in Postwar France. From Sartre to Althusser*. Princeton: Princeton University Press, 1975; and Antonio Negri, 'Gilles-

Félix', in *Gilles Deleuze. Immanence et vie*. Paris: Collège International de Philosophie, 1998.

4   Gilles Deleuze, *Nietzsche and Philosophy*. Trans. Hugh Tomlinson, New York, Columbia University Press, 1983; Gilles Deleuze, *Difference and Repetition*. Trans. Paul Patton. New York: Columbia University Press, 1994.

5   Gilles Deleuze and Michel Foucault, 'Les intellectuels et le pouvoir', in Michel Foucault, *Dits et Ecrits*, vol. II, Paris: Gallimard, 1994, p. 306-307. First published in *L'Arc* 49 (issue entitled: *Deleuze*), 1972. Trans. in M. Foucault, *Language, Counter-Memory, Practice*, Ithaca: Cornell University Press, 1977. Reprinted in Russel Ferguson et al. (eds.), *Discourses: Conversations in Postmodern Art and Culture*. New York/Massachusetts: The New Musuem of Contemporary Art/MIT, 1990, p. 9.

6   For an account of the politics implied in Deleuze's thought – in a different perspective from the one I will follow here – see François Zourabichvili, 'Deleuze et le possible (de l'involontarisme en politique)', in Eric Alliez (ed.), *Gilles Deleuze. Une vie philosophique*. Le Plessis-Robinson: Les Empêcheurs de penser en rond, 1998.

7   As Deleuze and Guattari put it: 'The two of us wrote *Anti-Oedipus* together. Since each of us was several, there was already quite a crowd.' *A Thousand Plateaus*, p. 3.

8   See E. Balibar, 'Les trois concepts de la politique: émancipation, transformation, civilité' in *La crainte des masses*. Paris: Galilée, 1997.

9   *A Thousand Plateaus*, p. 105.

10 Ibid.

11 These processes are indeed taking place, at least, in some countries, and their importance is perfectly acknowledged by Deleuze and Guattari, see *A Thousand Plateaus*, p. 291 sq.

12 *A Thousand Plateaus*, p. 115. See also Michael Hardt, 'The Withering of Civil Society' and Gary Genosko, 'Guattari's Schizoanalytic Semiotics: Mixing Hjemslev and Peirce', both in Eleanor Kaufman and Kevin J. Heller (eds.), *Deleuze and Guattari. New Mappings in Politics, Philosophy, and Culture*. Minneapolis: University of Minnesota Press, 1998; and Paola Marrati, 'Contro la doxa: filosofia e letteratura nell'opera di Gilles Deleuze' in S. Petrosino and M. Iofrida (eds.), *Filosofia e letteratura*. Roma: Bulzoni, 2000. Editor's note: The concept of faciality is elaborated in the context of an analysis of several regimes of signs which takes into account different forms of subjectivation and of social organization which is discussed more elaborately in the chapter on SCHINDLER'S LIST and the face of history in this volume.

13 *A Thousand Plateaus*, p. 209.

14 *A Thousand Plateaus*, pp. 177-178.

15 *A Thousand Plateaus*, p. 178.

16 On the contrary, Deleuze and Guattari emphazise the differences between a number of social, political and cultural '*agencements*'. The analysis of different forms of *agencements* is precisely one of the major issues of *A Thousand Plateaus*.

17 *A Thousand Plateaus*, p. 105.

18 The theme of an 'empty place' of the universal necessary to democracies has been elaborated by Claude Lefort. See Lefort, *Democracy and Political Theory*. Minneapolis: University of Minnesota Press, 1988. On the hegemonic logic constitutive of democracy see Ernesto Laclau, *Emancipation(s)*. London: Verso, 1996.

19 *A Thousand Plateaus*, p. 106.

20 See *Kafka. Toward a Minor Literature*.

21 *A Thousand Plateaus*, p. 291.

22 Gilles Deleuze, *Empiricism and Subjectivity: An Essay on Hume's Theory of Human Nature*. Trans. Constantin V. Boundas. New York: Columbia University Press, 1991.

23 See Gilles Deleuze and Claire Parnet, *Dialogues*. Trans. Hugh Tomlinson and Barbara Habberjam. New York: Columbia University Press, 1987.

24 'Man, as a dominating form, is majoritarian par exellence, whereas becomings are minoritarian.' *A Thousand Plateaus*, p. 291.

25 *A Thousand Plateaus*, pp. 291- 292.

26 Deleuze and Guattari state here their distrust of any easy provocation and their taste for sobriety: 'That is what Kierkegaard relates in his story about the "knight of the faith", the man of becoming: to look at him, one would notice nothing, a bourgeois, nothing but a bourgeois. That is how Fitzgerald lived: after a real rupture, one succeeds ...in being just like every body else. To go unnoticed is by no means easy. To be a stranger, even to one's doorman or neighbors.' *A Thousand Plateaus*, p. 279.

27 *A Thousand Plateaus*, pp. 279-280. We should notice here that the cosmic dimension of becoming is related to Deleuze's interpretation of Bergon. It is Bergson who cultivated the idea that philosophy could and should go beyond human experience. See Keith Ansell Pearson, *Germinal life. The Difference and Repetition of Deleuze*, chapter 1 'The Difference of Bergson: Duration and Creative Evolution'. London and New York: Routledge, 1999.

28 See *What is Philosophy?*, p. 110.

29 *A Thousand Plateaus*, p. 292. In *What is Philosophy?* Deleuze and Guattari reject the term 'utopia' precisely because it is dependent on History. Even when one opposes Utopia to History, the first is still subject to the second as an ideal.

30 An analysis of power – and especially in regard to Foucault – would be required.

31 *Difference and Repetition*, p. 129.

32 *Difference and Repetition*, p. 131.

33 On the political implications of an ontology of immanence, see P. Marrati, 'L'animal qui sait fuir. Gilles Deleuze: politique du devenir, ontologie de l'immanence', in M-L. Mallet (ed.), *L'animal autobiographique. Autour de Jacques Derrida*. Paris: Galilée, 1999.

34 Deleuze refers here to Descartes' *Recherche de la vérité par la lumière naturelle*. See *Difference and Repetition*, p. 170

35 *Difference and Repetition*, p. 131.

36 Ibid.

37 *Difference and Repetition*, p. 134.

38 *Difference and Repetition*, p.137. See also, *Nietzsche and Philosophy* where Deleuze interprets Nietzsche as having taken up the Kantian project of an immanent critique of reason without remaining prisoner, as did Kant, of the image of thought. See Daniel Smith, 'The Place of Ethics in Deleuze's Philosophy: Three Questions of Immanence' in *Deleuze and Guattari: New Mappings*.

39 *Difference and Repetition*, p. 139.

40 'Intellectuals and Power', p. 11.

41 On the participation of Deleuze to GIP, See Didier Eribon, *Michel Foucault*. Paris: Flammarion, 1991.

42 *What is Philosophy?*, p. 109. See also Gilles Deleuze, *Essays Critical and Clinical*. Trans. Daniel W Smith and Michael A. Greco, Minneapolis: University of Minnesota Press, 1997.

43 *What is Philosophy?*, p. 109.
44 *What is Philosophy?*, p. 110.

Notes to 11: SCHINDLER'S LIST and the Facing of History

1   In the edition that followed the film, the title of Keneally's novel was changed to *Schindler's List*.

2   'Deterritorialized existence' of the Jews as it can be traced via the theological symbols of Judaism is explored by a number of scholars, and an exemplary study is offered by Gershom Scholem in *The Messianic Idea in Judaism* (New York: Schocken Books, 1995). He asserts at the outset that 'in the history of Judaism its influence has been exercised almost exclusively under the conditions of the exile as a primary reality of Jewish life and Jewish history' (p. 2). He adds that within rabbinic Judaism as a social and religious phenomenon there are three forces which need to be taken into account: conservative, restorative and utopian. The conservative forces are directed toward preservation of that which was always in danger in the historical environment of Judaism, and hence toward construction and continuing preservation and development of religious law. The theme of exile as it is bound up with return is discussed in inspiring ways in James M. Scott (ed.), *Exile: Old Testament, Jewish and Christian Conceptions* (Leiden, New York and Cologne: Brill, 1997). Relevant here is a complementary collection of texts in J.H. Charlesworth et al. (eds.), *The Messiah: Developments in Earliest Judaism and Christianity* (Mineaplois: Fortress Press, 1995). In correspondence to Scholem's conception of Messianism as the 'Age to Come', the Messiah is bound up with memory of the past projected into the future. While Jewish Messianism can be theorized in terms of its restorative function, Scholem emphaizses that in its origins and by its nature it is a theory of catastrophe. According to Scholem, apocalypticism is complemented by the utopian view of realized redemption.

3   Gilles Deleuze and Félix Guattari, *A Thousand Plateaus: Capitalism & Schizophrenia*. Trans. Brian Massumi. London: The Athlone Press, 1996, pp. 111-149. As will be explained further in the next section of this chapter, Deleuze and Guattari distinguish (at least) four regimes of the sign: 1. The signifying regime of the sign in which each sign refers to another sign (each signifier refers to another signifier); 2. the primitive, presignifying semiotic, which is closer to 'natural' codings (cannibals; hunting nomads); 3. the countersignifying semiotic, which processes by arithmetic and numeration (warlike and animal raising nomads); 4. the postsignifying regime, which is defined by 'subjectification'. Deleuze and Guattari propose to make maps of regimes of signs. These regimes are always mixed and change over time and according to circumstances.

4   Emmanuel Levinas foregrounds this problem in *Beyond the Verse, Talmudic Readings and Lectures* and asserts that although the Jewish people were granted a state on account of their role as victims, peace on this territory is still far from attained (1994). In 'Moving Bodies, or The Cinematic Politics of Deportation', Samira Kawash discusses the position of the non-Israelis; she contends that the settling of Israel is achieved at

the expense of the Palestinian population, and in her view, the Palestinian identity is 'effaced, managed and contained'. In: Eleanor Kaufman and Kevin J. Heller (eds.), *Deleuze & Guattari: New Mappings in Politics, Philosophy and Culture* (Minneapolis and London: University of Minnesota Press, 1998, p. 131).

5   *A Thousand Plateaus*, p. 141.

6   *A Thousand Plateaus*, p. 507.

7   *A Thousand Plateaus*, p. 293.

8   *A Thousand Plateaus*, p. 116.

9   Ibid.

10 Spielberg's film amistad (1997) can be taken as an example of what could be understood as the principle of the scapegoat: in the opening of the film, before the mutiny takes place, the main character Sengbe (Djimon Hounsau) appears in mega close-ups, which creates the impression of his alien-like character and cancels the possibility of associating Sengbe with a human subject . In his cinema books Deleuze has related the close-up to both the face and facelessness ('effacement'). See Deleuze, *The Movement-Image*. Trans. Hugh Tomlinson and Barbara Habberjam. London: The Athlone Press, 1986, p. 100.

11 Deleuze and Guattari underscore the connection between subject and state subject as theorized by Althusser. 'Althusser clearly brings out this constitution of social individuals as subjects: he calls it interpellation (...) and calls the point of subjectification the Absolute Subject' (*A Thousand Plateaus*, p. 130). In their view, the production of subjectivity through language is not in fact a question of a linguistic operation, and they assert that a subject is never the condition of possibility of language or the cause of the statement. 'There is no subject,' they contend, 'only collective assemblages of enuciation' (*A Thousand Plateaus*, p. 130). In relation to the most essential distinction between the signifying regime and the subjective regime, Deleuze and Guattari point to their respective movement of deterritorialization they effectuate (*A Thousand Plateaus*, p. 133).

12 *A Thousand Plateaus*, p. 133.

13 *A Thousand Plateaus*, p. 137.

14 Ibid.

15 Ibid.

16 *A Thousand Plateaus*, p. 122.

17 *A Thousand Plateaus*, p. 123.

18 While watching the fierceness of the Ghetto massacre perversely joined, in specific scenes, with the Nazi passion for Bach (or Mozart), one recalls George Steiner's discussion in *The Extra-Territorial: Papers on Literature and the Language Revolution* on the 'puzzle of the dissociation between poetic humanism on the one hand and political sadism on the other, or rather, on their association in a single psyche' (London: Faber & Faber, 1972, p. 46).

19 The Six-Day War broke out on June 5, 1967, following three weeks of tension. After just six days of fighting, Israeli forces broke through the enemy lines and were in a position to march on Cairo, Damascus and Amman. With the victory, the territory of Israel had increased from 8,000 to 26,000 square miles. Apart from being able to unify Jerusalem, Israeli forces had also captured the Sinai, Golan Heights, Gaza Strip and the West Bank. Israel now ruled more than three-quarters of a million Palestinians. The extremely sensitive political issues that have necessarily come to the fore were

addressed by Israeli and Palestinian scholars. See for example, Evron Boas's chapter 'The Hebrew People versus the Palestinian People,' in *Jewish State or Israeli Nation?* (Bloomington: Indiana University Press, 1995) as well as Edward W. Said's 'Zionism from the Standpoint of its Victims,' in *The Questions of Palestine* (New York: Vintage Books, 1992).

20 I owe my gratitude to Aurel Pelleg for translating Nemer's song 'Jerusalem of Gold': Mountain air, clear as wine/ And the smell of pine/ Carried on the evening wind/ With the sound of bells. In the sleep of tree and stone/ Imprisoned in her dream/ The City that sits alone/ And in its heart, a wall. Chorus. Jerusalem of gold/ Of copper and of light/ To all your songs/ I am a violin. How the water wells dried/ The Market square empty/ And no one comes/ To the mountain of the house/ In the Old City. And in the caves that are in the rocks/ The winds howl/ And no one goes down to the Dead Sea/ On Jericho's road. Chorus. But today when I come to sing to you/ And to you to tie the crowns/ I am younger than your youngest sons/ Smaller than the last of the poets. Because your name burns the lips/ Like an angel's kiss/ If I'll forget you Jerusalem/ That is all of gold. Chorus. We are back at the water holes/ To the market square/ The horn is calling on the mountain of the house/ In the old city. And in the caves that are in the rocks/ A thousand shining suns/ And again we go down to the dead sea/ On Jericho's road.

21 In Deleuze and Guattari's view becoming-music is the most intense form of deterritorialization. They assert that 'music has a thirst for destruction, every kind of destruction, every kind of destruction, extinction, breakage, dislocation' (*A Thousand Plateaus*, p. 299). Whereas the refrain is essentially territorial, territorializing, or reterritorializing, music makes it a deterritorialized content for a deterritorialized form of expression' (*A Thousand Plateaus*, p. 300). When comparing music to painting they add that 'Music seems to have a much stronger deterritorializing force, at once more intense and much more collective, and the voice seems to have a much greater power of deterritorialization' (*A Thousand Plateaus*, p. 302). Interestingly enough, the song 'Jerusalem of Gold' emerges at the moment of 'reterritorialization' of the Promised Land; the clash between the mythical past and the historical present is thereby underscored, I would suggest, through the deterritorializing force of the song. For an elaboration of the complex relationship between film and becoming-music, see Patricia Pister's chapter 9, *From Eye to Brain, Gilles Deleuze: Refiguring the Subject of Film Theory* (Amsterdam: PhD University of Amsterdam, 1998).

22 In his study *Jewish State or Israeli Nation?* Evron Boas points out that this predicament 'arises only with the concatenation of several historical factors, and it may assume several forms: economic pressure and legal discrimination (as in most of Europe during the Middle Ages and in tsarist Russia in modern times); real persecution, including pogroms (as in Russia from 1881 to 1905); massacre and annihilation (as in Nazi Germany and the countries under its sway, and on a different level of brutality and totality, during the seventeenth-century Cossack revolt in Ukraine and the massacre of the Rhineland Jewish communities during the First Crusade in the eleventh century)'(p. 2).

23 This issue is addressed in Boyarin and Boyarin's discussion in 'Diaspora: Generation and the Ground of Jewish Identity,' where they assert that 'a Jewish subject-position founded on generational connection and its attendant anamnestic responsibilities and pleasures affords the possibility of a flexible and nonhermetic critical Jewish

identity' (*Critical Inquiry*, no.19, Summer 1993, p. 201). Similarly, Boas asserts that if Judaism is to continue to exist and if it is to remain sane, the myth of 'one people' needs to be abolished. In the first instance this myth of the one people refers to the necessity of acknowledging the fact that with secular Zionism the Jewish people is entitled to continue living in the Diaspora 'without feeling inferior to the Israeli nation, while the Israeli nation will stop viewing itself as the future of the Jewish people' ('Diaspora', p. 239). There are two elements Boas takes into consideration which involve the recent history: the first historical event which had a traumatic impact on the Diaspora and the Israeli people is the Holocaust. The other is the Arab siege of Israel. In schindler's list, as I have already suggested, both events are incorporated into the mythical return to the Promised Land: the arrival of the Holocaust survivors in the Promised Land is accompanied by the song 'Jerusalem of Gold' written just before the Six-Day War started. Both events, pertaining to our recent history, are bound up with the fulfilment of the mythical hope of the return to the 'homeland'. The myth facilitates the memory of the ancient land crucial for the formation of Jewish identity. By taking recourse to myth, or rather to the story of Jewish redemption, as it is bound up with territorialism and genealogy, the film engages in the process of facing history in a double sense: In the first place, the memory of the past projected into the future implies an overlapping of temporal continuums, but it also indicates an overlapping of 'lands'. Hence, in the film's closing there is a double arrival at stake. The promise of (the perpetually deferred) arrival at the Promised Land clashes with the arrival (prophetic promise fulfilled) in present-day Israel.

24 This concluding remark is additionally inspired by Paul Ricoeur's *Lectures on Ideology and Utopia* (ed. by George H. Taylor, New York: Columbia University Press, 1986); Ricoeur reminds us that since utopia is the view from 'nowhere', the literal meaning of the word ensures that we no longer take our present reality for granted. In that respect, utopia has a constitutive role in helping us rethink the nature of our social life: 'It is the "fantasy" of an alternative society and its exteriorization "nowhere" that works as one of the most formidable contestations of what is' (pp. 1-3). In Ricoeur's view, utopia acts not only to de-reify our present relations but to point to those possibilities that may yet be ours. He adds that the correlation of ideology and utopia offers the alternative to the failed model that opposes ideology to reality. What is important here is the productive character of imagination which encourages the exploration of what is possible. Because there is a positive as well as a negative side to both ideology and utopia, the polarity between the two sides of each term may be enlightened by exploring a similar polarity between the two terms. According to Ricoeur, this polarity between and within the two terms may be ascribed to some structural traits of what he calls cultural imagination. It is along these lines that Deleuze and Guattari's concept of de/re-territorialization can be further illuminated.

Notes to 12: 'Forty Acress and a Mule Filmworks'

1 Spike Lee with Lisa Jones, *Do the Right Thing: A Spike Lee Joint*. Fireside: New York, 1989, p. 29.

2 Meaghan Morris, 'Crazy Talk Is Not Enough'. Editorial essay, Special Issue on Deleuze and Dwelling. *Planning D: Society and Space* no. 14/4, 1996, p. 386.

3 Gilles Deleuze and Felix Guattari, *A Thousand Plateaus, Capitalism and Schizophrenia.* Trans. Brian Massumi. Minneapolis: University of Minnesota Press, 1987, p.348.

4 My thanks to Melissa McMahon for sharing her perception with me.

5 Lee and Jones, *Do the Right Thing*, pp. 55-56.

6 A favourable article on the film is W.J.T. Mitchell's 'The Violence of Public Art: DO THE RIGHT THING,' *Critical Inquiry* no. 16 (Summer 1990) and a hostile one is a response to it by Jerome Christensen, 'Spike Lee, Corporate Populist,' *Critical Inquiry* no. 17 (Fall 1991). Mitchell cites several of the main reviews that were hostile to the film and discusses the way the film moved from its regular commercial public sphere into culture-debating public art as a result of its controversial public reception. See especially pp. 891-897. See Mark A. Reid (ed.), *Spike Lee's Do The Right Thing*. Cambridge: Cambridge University Press, 1997.

7 ABC Television, UNCENSORED, 16 September 1998.

8 Lee and Jones, *Do the Right Thing*, p. 31. While the context of this quotation is Lee's hassles with the Hollywood studios, it can also be read as expressing his desire to construct a dwelling with aesthetic means.

9 It is rare to find critical writing that deals with Spike Lee's cinematic antecedents, which must surely include Sennett and Godard among others. Sharon Willis, in *High Contrast: Race and Gender in Contemporary Hollywood Film* (Durham and London: Duke University Press, 1998, p.167) says that a dominant white liberal tendency is to see Lee as a 'delegate speaking for a whole population'. What this tendency occludes is precisely aesthetic play, which does not obey the rules of discursive polemics.

10 Gilles Deleuze and Félix Guattari, *A Thousand Plateaus: Capitalism and Schizophrenia.* Trans. Brian Massumi. London: The Athlone Press, 1988, p. 312.

11 Ronald Bogue, 'Rhizomusicosmology,' *Substance* no. 66, 1991, pp. 85-101.

12 'Crazy Talk,' see note 2. I have found this article also indispensable in understanding how '1837: Of the Refrain' relates to other plateaus in the book and how it might contribute to feminist work on temporality and action.

13 *A Thousand Plateaus*, p. 384.

14 *A Thousand Plateaus*, p. 385.

15 Tricia Rose, *Black Noise: Rap Music and Black Culture in Contemporary America.* Hanover and London: Wesleyan University Press, 1994. I have found the cultural history of hip-hop in this book indispensable to understanding DO THE RIGHT THING, and the following quotation encapsulates this history. 'Rap music is a black cultural expression that prioritized black voices from the margins of urban America. Rap music is a form of rhymed storytelling accompanied by highly rhythmic, electronically based music. It began in the mid-1970s in the South Bronx, in New York City as part of hip-hop, an African-American and Afro-Caribbean youth culture composed of graffiti, break-dancing and rap music. Rappers speak with the voice of personal experience, taking on the identity of the observer or narrator', p. 4.

16 *A Thousand Plateaus*, p. 315.

17 Ibid.

18 'Rhizomusicosmology', p. 90.

19 *A Thousand Plateaus*, p. 348.

20 'Rhizomusicosmology', p. 93.

21 *Black Noise*, p. 4.
22 See Barbara Jean Field's, 'Slavery, Race and ideology in the United States,' in *New Left Review* no.181, 1990, pp. 95-119, for an account of the history and ideology of American racism. In such a sociological and historical context Lee's cross-cultural efforts are, I think, exemplary in their imaginative daring, generosity and biting/disarming humour.
23 'Rhizomusicosmology', p. 93.
24 Ibid.
25 'Rhizomusicosmology', p. 94.
26 Ibid.
27 I wish to thank Brian Rutnam for this formulation and for helping me understand two things about Messiaen's musical theory around three o'clock in the morning on Sunday 15th November 1998.
28 'Rhizomusicosmology', pp. 90-91.
29 'Crazy Talk,' p. 387. Morris comments perceptively on the importance of the moments of the impeding of flows and the fragility of the movement outwards by also discussing MURIEL'S WEDDING by P. J. Hogan.
30 These are the terms of Kafka's impossibility, though under different circumstances, as spelt out by Deleuze and Guattari in *Kafka, Towards a Minor Literature*. Trans. Dana Polan. Minneapolis: University of Minnesota Press, 1986, p. 16.
31 Hepburn and Tracy, as a prickly couple on screen and lovers off, come to mind as I think of African-American exclusion and Hollywood.
32 According to Lee, 'Universal's main concern... was the ending. Was it too open ended? How would audiences feel leaving the theatre? Will blacks want to go on a rampage? Will whites feel uncomfortable?' in *Do the Right Thing*, p. 281. See RUSH HOUR (1989) with Jackie Chan and Chris Tucker, for more elaborate, virtuoso, mimetic, cross-cultural moves, starring the Mandarin Kung-Fu tradition infused with American slapstick on the one hand, and contemporary African-American dance moves with hip-hop, street origins, on the other.

Bibliography

Eric Alliez, *Gilles Deleuze: une vie philosophique*. Le Plessis-Robinson: Institut Synthélabo, 1998.

Louis Althusser, *Lenin and Philosophy and Other Essays*. London: New Left Books, 1971.

Ernst van Alphen, *De toekomst der herinnering: essays over moderne Nederlandse literatuur*. Amsterdam: Van Gennep, 1993.

Martin Amis, *Einstein's Monsters*. London: Penguin, 1987.

Hannah Arendt, 'Philosophy and Politics: The Problem of Action and Thought after the French Revolution'. *Social Research*, vol. 57/1, 1990, pp. 73-103.

Elisabeth Ascombe, *Intention*. Oxford: Blackwell, 1959.

Mieke Bal, *Reading 'Rembrandt': Beyond the Word/Image Opposition*. Cambridge: Cambridge University Press, 1991.

Mieke Bal, 'Body Politic' in *On Meaning-Making: Essays in Semiotics*. Sonoma, Cal.: Polebridge Press, 1994, pp. 263-280.

Mieke Bal, *Double Exposures*. London: Routledge, 1996.

Mieke Bal, *The Practice of Cultural Analysis*. Stanford: Stanford University Press, 1999.

E. Balibar, *La crainte des masses*. Paris: Galilée, 1997.

Richard Barbrook and Andy Cameron, 'The Californian Ideology'. *Science as Culture*, no. 26/6, 1996, pp. 44-72.

Barry Barnes and David Edge (eds.), *Science in Context: Readings in the Sociology of Science*. Milton Keynes: The Open University, 1982.

Jean Baudrillard, *The Gulf War did not Take Place*. Trans. Paul Patton. Sydney: Power Institute Publications and Bloomington: Indiana University Press, 1995.

Zygmunt Bauman, *Postmodern Ethics*. Oxford: Blackwell, 1993.

Jonneke Bekkenkamp, 'Breaking the Waves: Corporeality and Religion in a Modern Melodrama'. Jonneke Bekkenkamp and Maaike de Haardt (eds.), *Begin with the Body. Corporeality, Religion and Gender*. Leuven: Peeters, 1998, pp. 134-157.

Ann Oliver Bell (ed.), *The Diary of Virginia Woolf*, Volume 3. London: Penguin, 1980.

Jonathan Beller, 'Capital/Cinema' in Eleanor Kaufman and Kevin Jon Heller (eds.), *Deleuze and Guattari: New Mappings in Politics, Philosophy, and Culture*. Minneapolis and London: University of Minnesota Press, 1998, pp. 77-95.

Seyla Benhabid, *The Situated Self*. Cambridge: Polity Press, 1992.

Leo Bersani, *The Culture of Redemption*. Cambridge Mass. and London: Harvard University Press, 1990.

Stig Björkman, 'Entretien avec Lars von Trier'. *Cahiers du Cinema* no. 503, 1996, pp. 23-25.

Evron Boas, *Jewish State or Israeli Nation?* Bloomington: Indiana University Press, 1995.

Ronald Bogues, 'Rhizomusicosmology'. *Substance* no. 66, 1991, pp. 85-101.

Donald Bouchard (ed.), *Michel Foucault: Language, Counter Memory, Practice. Selected Essays and Interviews*. Ithaca: Cornell University Press, 1977.

Daniel and Jonathan Boyarin Boyarin, 'Diaspora: Generation and the Ground of Jewish Identity.' *Critical Inquiry* no. 19, Summer 1993, pp. 693-723

Rosi Braidotti, 'Meta(l)morphoses' in *Theory, Culture and Society* vol. 14/2, 1997, pp. 67-80.

Elaine Brass et al. (eds.), *Gathering Force: DIY Culture – Radical Action for those Tired of Waiting*. London: Big Issue, 1997.

Maurice Brinton, *The Bolsheviks and Workers' Control: 1917-1921*. London: Solidarity, 1970.

Ian Buchanan and Claire Colebrook, *Deleuze and Feminist Theory*. Edinburgh: Edinburgh University Press, 2000.

Ian Buchanan, *Deleuzism: A Meta-Commentary*. Edinburgh: Edinburgh University Press, 2000.

William Burroughs, *Naked Lunch*. New York: Grove Press Inc., 1966.

Jacques Camatte, *The Wandering of Humanity*. Detroit: Black & Red, 1975.

Lewis Carroll, *Alice in Wonderland*. London: Pan, 1947.

Manuel Castells, *The Rise of the Network Society*. Massachusetts and Oxford: Blackwell, 1996.

James H. Charlesworth (et al., eds.), *The Messiah: Developments in Earliest Judaism and Christianity*. Fortress Press: Mineapolis, 1992.

Jerome Christensen, 'Spike Lee, Corporate Populist'. *Critical Inquiry* no. 17, Fall 1991.

Annick Cojean and Frank Eskenazi, *FM: la folle histoire des radios libres*. Paris: Grasset, 1986.

Jonathan Culler, *Literary Theory*. Oxford: Oxford University Press, 1997.

Gilles Deleuze, *Nietzsche and Philosophy*. Trans. Hugh Tomlinson. London: Athlone, 1983. First published Paris 1962.

Gilles Deleuze, *Bergsonism*. Trans. Hugh Tomlinson and Barbara Habberjam. New York: Zone Books, 1988. First published Paris: 1966.

Gilles Deleuze, *Expressionism in Philosophy: Spinoza*. Trans. Martin Joughin. New York: Zone Books, 1992. First published Paris: 1968.

Gilles Deleuze, *Difference and Repetition*. Trans. Paul Patton. London: Athlone, 1994. First published Paris: 1968.

Gilles Deleuze, *The Logic of Sense*. Trans. Mark Lester with Charles Stivale. Ed. Constantin Boundas. New York: Columbia University Press, 1990. First published Paris: 1969.

Gilles Deleuze, *Spinoza: Practical Philosophy*. Trans. Robert Hurley. San Francisco: City Lights, 1988. First published Paris: 1970.

Gilles Deleuze and Félix Guattari, *Anti-Oedipus: Capitalism and Schizophrenia*. Trans. Helen Lane, Mark Seem and Robert Hurley. Minneapolis: University of Minnesota Press, 1984. First published Paris: 1972.

Gilles Deleuze and Félix Guattari, *Kafka: Toward a Minority Literature*. Trans. Dana Polan. Minneapolis: University of Minnesota Press. First published Paris: 1975.

Gilles Deleuze and Claire Parnet, *Dialogues*. Trans. Hugh Tomlinson and Barbara Habberjam. New York: Columbia University Press, 1987. First published Paris: 1977.

Gilles Deleuze and Félix Guattari, *A Thousand Plateaus: Capitalism and Schizophrenia*. Trans. Brian Massumi. Minneapolis: University of Minnesota Press, 1987 and London: The Athlone Press, 1988. First published Paris: 1980.

Gilles Deleuze, *Cinema 1: The Movement-Image*. Trans. Hugh Tomlinson and Barbara Habberjam. London: The Athlone Press, 1986. First published Paris: 1983.

Gilles Deleuze, *Cinema 2: The Time-Image*. Trans. Hugh Tomlinson and Robert Galeta. London: The Athlone Press, 1989. First published Paris: 1985.

Gilles Deleuze, *Foucault*. Trans. Seán Hand. Minneapolis: University of Minnesota Press, 1988. First published Paris: 1986.

Gilles Deleuze, *Negotiations 1972 – 1990*. Trans. Martin Joughin. New York: Columbia University Press, 1995. First published Paris: 1990.

Gilles Deleuze and Félix Guattari, *What is Philosophy?* Trans. Graham Burchell and Hugh Tomlinson. London: Verso, 1994. First published Paris: 1991.

Gilles Deleuze, *Essays Critical and Clinical*. Trans. Daniel W. Smith & Michael A. Greco. London/New York: Verso 1998. First published Paris: 1993.

Gilles Deleuze, 'Immanence, A Life...'. Trans. Nick Millet. *Theory, Culture & Society*. No. 14/2, May 1997. First published Paris: 1995.

Jacques Derrida, *The Truth in Painting*. Trans. Geoff Bennington and Ian McLeod. Chicago: Chicago University Press, 1987. First published 1978.

Marc Dery, *Escape Velocity: Cyberculture at the End of the Century*. London: Hodder and Stoughton, 1996.

Fokkelien van Dijk-Hemmers and Athalya Brenner (eds.), *Reflections on Theology and Gender*. Kampen: Kok Pharos, 1994.

Mary Ann Doane, *The Desire to Desire: The Woman's Film of the 1940's*. Bloomington: Indiana University Press, 1987.

Mary Ann Doane, *Femmes Fatales: Feminism, Film Theory, Psychoanalysis*. New York and London: Routledge, 1991.

Andrea Dworkin, *Intercourse*. New York and London: Free Press, 1997 (1987).

Umberto Eco, with Richard Rorty et.al, 'The Pragmatist's Progress' in Stefan Collini (ed.), *Interpretation and Overinterpretation*. Cambridge: Cambridge University Press, 1992.

Didier Eribon, *Michel Foucault*. Paris: Flammarion, 1991.

Shoshana Felman, *The Literary Speech Act: Don Juan with J.L. Austin, or Seduction in Two Languages*. New York: New York University Press, 1984.

Shoshana Felman, *Jacques Lacan and the Adventure of Insight*. London and Cambridge, Mass.: Harvard University Press, 1987.

Russel Ferguson et al. (eds.), *Discourses: Conversations in Postmodern Art and Culture*. New York and Cambridge: The New Museum of Contemporary Art and MIT Press, 1990.

Barbara Jean Field, 'Slavery, Race and Ideology in the United States'. *New Left Review* 181, 1990, pp. 95-119.

Gregory Flaxman (ed.), *The Brain is the Screen: Deleuze and the Philosophy of Cinema*. Minneapolis and London: University of Minnesota Press, 2000.

Michel Foucault, 'Questions of Method'. *I & C* no. 8, Spring 1981, p. 6.

Jo Freeman, *CS. Untying the Knot: Feminism, Anarchsim & Organisation*. London: Dark Star and Rebel Press, 1984.

Sigmund Freud, *The Standard Edition of the Complete Works*, Volume 7. London: Penguin, 1973.

Jean-Pierre Garnier and Roland Lew, *Socialist Register 1984: The Use of Anti-Communism*. London: Merlin, 1984.

Moira Gatens and Genevieve Lloyd, *Collective Imaginings: Spinoza, Past and Present*. London and New York: Routledge, 1999.

W.P. Gerritsen, Doris Edel and Mieke de Kreek, *De wereld van Sint Brandaan*. Utrecht: Hes, 1986.

W.P. Gerritsen and S. Oppenhuis-de Jong (eds.), *De reis van Sint Brandaan*. Amsterdam: Prometheus/Bert Bakker 1994.

Philip Goodchild, *Deleuze and Guattari. An Introduction to the Politics of Desire*. London: Sage, 1996.

J.W. Graham (ed.), *The Waves: Two Holograph Drafts*. London: Routledge, 1976.

Elizabeth Grosz, 'Darwin and Feminism: Preliminary Investigations for a Possible Alliance'. *Australian Feminist Studies* no. 14 /29, 1999, pp. 31-45.

Félix Guattari, 'Les Radios Libres Populaires'. *La Nouvelle Critique*, no. 115/296, 1978, pp. 77-79.

Félix Guattari, *Molecular Revolution: Psychiatry and Politics*. Trans. Rosemayr Sheed. Harmondsworth, Middlesex: Penguin, 1984.

Félix Guattari, 'The Three Ecologies'. Trans. Chris Turner. *New Formations*, no. 8, 1987, pp. 131-147.

Marie-Anne Guérin, 'Emily Watson'. *Cahiers du Cinema* no. 506, 1996, pp. 28.

Ian Hacking, *Rewriting the Soul, Multiple Personality and the Science of Memory*. Princeton, NJ: Princeton University Press, 1995.

Judith Halberstam and Ira Livingston (eds.), *Posthuman Bodies*. Bloomington: Indiana University Press, 1995.

Stuart Hall, 'New Ethnicities'. *ICA-Document 7, Black Film British Cinema*. London: ICA, 1988, pp. 27-31.

Michael Hardt, *An Apprenticeship in Philosophy: Gilles Deleuze*. London: UCL Press, 1993.

Eugene Holland, *Deleuze and Guattari's Anti-Oedipus: Introduction to Schizoanalysis*. London and New York: Routledge 1999.

Max Horkheimer and Theodor Adorno, *Dialektik der Aufklärung*. Frankfurt: Fischer Taschenbuch Verlag, 1988. First published 1947.

Luce Irigaray, *Spéculum, de l'autre femme*. Paris: Minuit 1974.

Luce Irigaray, *Etique de la différence sexuelle*. Paris: Minuit, 1984.

Fredric Jameson, 'Postmodernism, or the Cultural Logic of Late Capitalism'. *New Left Review*, no. 1467, 1984, pp. 53-94.

Eleanor Kaufman and Kevin Jon Heller (eds.), *Deleuze and Guattari: New Mappings in Politics, Philosophy, and Culture*. Minneapolis and London: University of Minnesota Press, 1998.

Ken Knabb (ed.), *Situations International Anthology*. California: Bureau of Public Secrets, 1981.

Any Koinuven and Astrid Söderbergh (eds.), *Cinema Studies into Visual Theory?* Turku: University of Turku, 1998.

Alexandre Kojève, *Introduction to the Reading of Hegel: Lectures on the 'Phenomenology of Spirit*. Ithaca NY: Cornell University Press, 1969.

Julia Kristeva, 'Women's Time' in N.O. Keohane et al. (eds.), *Feminist Theory: A Critique of Ideology*. Chicago: Chicago University Press, 1982.

Annette Kuhn, *Alien Zone: Cultural Theory and Contemporary Science Fiction Cinema*. London: Verso, 1990.

Jacques Lacan, *Ecrits: A Selection*. Trans. Alan Sheridan. London: Routledge, 1977.

Ernesto Laclau, *Emancipation(s)*. London: Verso, 1996.

George Lakoff and Mark Johnson, *Metaphors We Live By*. Chicago: University of Chicago Press, 1980.

George Lakoff and Mark Johnson, *Philosophy in the Flesh. The Embodied Mind and its Challenge to Western Thought*. New York: Basic Books, 1999.

Teresa de Lauretis, *Alice Doesn't: Feminism, Semiotics, Cinema*. Blommington: Indiana University Press, 1984.

Teresa de Lauretis, *Technologies of Gender: Essays on Theory, Film, and Fiction*. Bloomington/Indianapolis: Indiana University Press, 1987.

Spike Lee with Lisa Jones, *Do the Right thing: A Spike Lee Joint*. New York: Fireside, 1989.

Henri Lefebre, *Everyday Life of the Modern World*. New Brunswick NY: Transaction Publishers, 1984.

Claude Lefort, *Democracy and Political Theory*. Minneapolis: University of Minnesota Press, 1988.

V.I. Lenin, *What is to Be Done? Burning Questions of our Movement*. Beijing: Foreign Language Press, 1975.

Helena Lewis, *Dada Turns Red: The Politics of Surrealism*. Edinburgh: Edinburgh University Press, 1990.

Genevieve Lloyd, *Part of Nature: Self-Knowledge in Spinoza's Ethics*. Ithaca: Cornell University Press, 1994.

Genevieve Lloyd, *Spinoza and the Ethics*. London and New York: Routledge, 1996.

Catherine Lord, *The Intimacy of Influence*. Amsterdam: ASCA Press, 1999.

Tamsin Lorraine, *Irigaray and Deleuze: Experiments in Visceral Philosophy*. Ithaca and London: Cornell University Press, 1999.

George Lukács, *History and Class Consciousness*. London: Merlin, 1968.

Paola Marrati, 'L'animal qui sait fuir. Gilles deleuze: politique du devenir, ontologie de l'immanence' in M-L. Mallet (ed.), *L'animal autobiographique. Autour de Jacques Derrida*. Paris: Galilée, 1999.

Paola Marrati, 'Contra la doxa: filosofia e letteratura nell'opera di Gilles Deleuze' in S. Iofrida (ed.), *Filosofia e letteratura*. Roma: Bulzoni, 2000.

Karl Marx, *Grundrids*. Århus: Modtryk, 1978.

Marcel Mauss, *The Gift: The Form and Reason of Exchange in Archaic Societies*. London: Routledge, 1990.

Luuk van Middelaar, *Politicide: De moord op de politiek in de Franse filosofie*. Amsterdam: Van Gennep, 1999.

W.J. T. Mitchell, 'The Violence of Public Art: DO THE RIGHT THING' in *Critical Inquiry* 16, Summer 1990.

Meaghan Morris, 'Crazy Talk is Not Enough'. *Planning D: Society and Space* no. 14/4, 1996.

Antonio Negri, *The Savage Anomaly: The Power of Spinoza's Metaphysics and Politics*. Minneapolis: University of Minnesota Press, 1991.

Antonio Negri, *Gilles Deleuze. Immanence et vie*. Paris: Collège International de Philosophie, 1998.

Christopher Norris, *Spinoza and the Origins of Modern Critical Theory*. Oxford: Basil Blackwell, 1991.

Martha Nusbaum, *Cultivating Humanity*. Cambridge: Harvard University Press, 1999.

Dorothea Olkowski, *Gilles Deleuze and the Ruin of Representation* Berkeley: University of California Press, 1999.

Paul Patton, *Deleuze and the Political*. London and New York: Routledge, 2000.

Keith Ansell Pearson, *Viroid life. Perspectives on Nietzsche and the Transhuman Condition*. London and New York: Routledge, 1993.

Patricia Pisters, 'Liefde doet wonderen: Breaking the Waves.' *Skrien* no. 209, 1996, pp.11-13.

Patricia Pisters, 'What's Love Got to Do with It?'. Mieke Bal et al. (eds.), *Visions and Voices of Otherness*. Amsterdam: ASCA Press, 1996, pp. 61-72.

Patricia Pisters, *From Eye to Brain: Gilles Deleuze: Refiguring the Subject in Film Theory*. Amsterdam: PhD University of Amsterdam, 1998.

Mark Poster, *Existential Marxism in Postwar France. From Sartre to Althusser*. Princeton: Princeton University Press, 1975.

Jessica Prager-Stein, 'Breaking the Waves: Ontroerend of onverteerbaar?' *Fier* no. 1:1, 1998, pp. 24-25.

Paul Rabinow (ed.), *The Foucault Reader*. New York: Pantheon Books, 1984.

Mark A. Reid (ed.), *Spike Lee's* DO THE RIGHT THING. Cambridge: Cambridge University Press, 1997.

Pipilotti Rist, *Remake of Le Weekend*. Cologne: Oktagon, 1998.

Chris Rodley (ed.), *Cronenberg on Cronenberg*. Toronto: Alfred A. Knopf, 1992.

David Rodowick, *Gilles Deleuze's Time Machine*. Durham and London: Duke University Press, 1997.

Richard Rorty, *Consequences of Pragmatism*. Minneapolis: University of minnesota Press, 1982.

Richard Rorty, 'Unsoundness in Perspective'. *Times Literary Supplement*, June 17, 1983, p. 620.

Richard Rorty, *Contingency, Irony, and Solidarity*. Cambridge: Cambridge University Press, 1989.

Richard Rorty, 'Habermas and Lyotard on Postmodernity' in *Essays on Heidegger and Others: Philosophical Papers*, Volume 2. Cambridge: Cambridge University Press, 1991.

Richard Rorty, 'Derrida and the Philosophical Tradition' in *Truth and Progress: Philosophical Papers*, Volume 3. Cambridge: Cambridge University Press, 1998, pp. 327-350.

Richard Rorty, *Achieving our Country. Leftist Thought in Twentieth-Century America.* Cambridge, Mass. and London: Harvard University Press, 1998.

Tricia Rose, *Black Noise: Rap Music and Black Culture in Contemporary America.* Hanover and London: Wesleyan University Press, 1994.

Edward Said, *Questions of Palestine.* New York: Vintage Books, 1980.

Hans-Jørgen Schanz: *Karl Marx I tilbageblik efter murens fald* (*Marx in Retrospect after the Fall of the Wall*). Århus: Modtryk, 1994.

Gerhom Scholem, *The Messianic Idea in Judaism.* Foreword by Arthur Hertzberg. New York: Schocken Books, 1995.

James M. Scott (ed.), *Exile: Old Testament, Jewish and Christian Conceptions.* Leiden, New York and Cologne: Brill, 1997.

Xandra Schutte, 'Filmlezen: Het woord is vlees geworden'. *De Groene Amsterdammer* 18- 9-1996.

Steven Shaviro, *The Cinematic Body.* Minneapolis and London: University of Minnesota Press, 1993.

Kaja Silverman, *Male Subjectivity at the Margins.* New York and London: Routledge, 1992.

Kaja Silverman, *The Threshold of the Visible World.* New York and London: Routledge, 1996.

Joan Smith, 'Speaking Up For Corpses'. Karl French (ed.), *Screen Violence.* London: Bloomsbury 1996, pp. 196-204.

Vivian Sobchack, *Screening Space: The American Science Fiction Film.* New Jersey and London: Rutgers University Press, 1987.

Gayatri Spivak, 'In a word', *Differences* 1/2, 1989, pp. 124-156.

H.J. Staatkamp, Jr (ed.), *Rorty and Pragmatism: The Philosopher Responds to his Critics.* Nashville and London: Vanderbilt University Press, 1995.

Jackie Stacey, *Star Gazing: Hollywood Cinema and Female Spectatorship.* London and New York: Routledge, 1990.

Jackie Stacey, *Teratologies: A Cultural Study of Cancer.* London: Routledge, 1997.

George Steiner, *The Extra-Territorial: Papers on Literature and the Language Revolution.* London: Faber & Faber, 1972.

Frédéric Strauss, 'A la vie, á la mort'. *Cahiers du Cinema* no. 506, 1996, pp. 27, 29.

George H. Taylor (ed.), *Lectures on Ideology and Utopia.* New York: Columbia University Press, 1986.

Raoul Vaneigem, *The Revolution of Everyday Life.* London: Practical Paradise, 1972.

Michael Vickery, *Cambodia: 1975-1982*. Hemel Hempstead: Allen and Unwin, 1984.

Sharon Willis, *High Contrast: Race and Gender in Contemporary Hollywood Film*. Durham and London: Duke University Press, 1998.

Jeanette Winterson, *The Passion*. London: Bloomsbury, 1987.

Ludwig Wittgenstein, *Philosophical Investigations*. Oxford: Basil Blackwell, 1953.

Robin Wood, 'An Introduction to the American Horror Film' (1979), reprinted in Bill Nichols (ed.), *Movies and Methods*. Berkeley, Los Angeles and London: University of California Press, 1985, pp. 195-220.

Virginia Woolf, *The Waves*. London: Penguin, 1971. First published 1931.

Contributors

Richard Barbrook is co-ordinator of the Hypermedia Research Centre of the University of Westminster, London, U.K. His book *Media Freedom: The Contradictions of Communication in the Age of Modernity* was published by Pluto Press (London 1995). He is the author of 'The Cyborg communist Manifesto' and co-author with Andy Cameron of *The Californian Ideology*. His writings about the Net and other related topics can be found on the Hypermedia Research Centre website: <www.hrc.wmin.ac.uk>

Maaike Bleeker is currently finishing her PhD, entitled *The Locus of Looking: Dissecting Visuality in the Theatre*, at the Amsterdam School of Cultural Analysis (ASCA) at the University of Amsterdam, the Netherlands. As co-founder of theatre group Het Oranjehotel, she also has a career as a dramaturge. Her academic work aims at rethinking theatre theory, paying special attention to the corporeal, the affective and the multi-sensuous dimensions of the theatrical experience. A case study from her work, entitled 'Death, Digitalization and Dys-Appearance: Staging the Body of Science' appeared in *Performance Research* 4, Summer 1999.

Rosi Braidotti is Professor of Womens's Studies at the University of Utrecht, The Netherlands, and visiting Professor at the Gender Institute, London School of Economics, UK. She has written on feminist theory, French philosophy and teratology, including the book *Nomadic Subject: Embodiment and Sexual Difference in Contemporary Feminist Theory* (1994) and the anthology *Between Monsters, Goddesses and Cyborgs* (1996), which she co-edited. Her next book is called *Metamorphoses: Towards a Materialist Theory of Becoming*, forthcoming with Polity Press.

Malene Busk is writing her PhD at the Department of History of Ideas at the University of Aarhus, Denmark, and is currently connected to ASCA, University of Amsterdam, The Netherlands. In her thesis with the working title *At Once Strict and Free. On Experiments with Microethical Thought in Deleuze and Adorno*, she is investigating Deleuze's ethics of affirmative thought in resonance with actualized aspects of Adorno's critical texts. She has published articles on Derrida's traces of death, Deleuze's concepts of thought, political philosophy and temporality and ethics of subjectivation.

Laleen Jayamanne teaches Cinema Studies in the Department of Art History and Theory, at the University of Sydney, Australia. She has made several short films including A SONG OF CEYLON (1985) and is the editor of *Kiss Me Deadly: Feminsim and Cinema for the Moment* (Power Publications, 1995). Her book *Cinema and Its Double: Crosscultural Readings – 1980-1999* will be published at Indiana University Press in 2001.

Eva Jørholt is associate professor at the Department of Film and Media Studies of the University of Copenhagen, Denmark. Her PhD thesis *Thinking Images: Film, Reality and Knowledge* (1996) was largely inspired by Gilles Deleuze's philosophical approach to film studies. She is currently working on a research project which investigates the relationship between African cinema and the oral story-telling tradition.

Frans-Willem Korsten is an assistant professor at the University of Leiden in the Department of Literary Studies. His PhD is entitled *The Wisdom Brokers: Narrative's Interaction with Arguments in Cultural Texts*. His current research and recent publications address interactions between the humanities and sciences, Dutch-Indonesian literature, relations between film and literature, and seventeenth-century drama.

Catherine M. Lord is a postdoctoral researcher in literature, theory and cultural analysis. She teaches in the English and Film Department of the University of Amsterdam. Her PhD thesis *The Intimacy of Influence* is published by ASCA University Press (1999). In addition to her scholarly work, she is a stage performer and writer.

Paola Marrati teaches philosophy and esthetics at several universities. Currently she is a research fellow at the Faculty of Philosophy of the University of Tilburg, The Netherlands. She studied in Pisa and Paris with Jacques Derrida and in Strassbourg with Lacoue-Labarthe. Her publications include articles on Levinas, Heidegger, Deleuze and the book *La genèse et la trace: derrida, lecteur de Husserl et Heidegger* (1998).

Paul Patton teaches Philosophy at the University of Sydney. He is the author of *Deleuze and the Political* (Routledge, 2000). He also edited *Deleuze: A Critical Reader* (Blackwell, 1996) and translated Deleuze's *Différence et Répétition* into English (Athlone, 1994).

Patricia Pisters teaches at the Department of Film and Television Studies of the University of Amsterdam. Her book *The Matrix of Visual Culture: Working with Deleuze in Film Theory* will be published at Stanford University Press in 2001. She co-authored with Hannah Bosma *Madonna: De Vele*

Gezichten van een Popster (Prometheus, Amsterdam 1999) and writes regularly in various media about film, television and media culture.

Sasha Vojkovic currently has a postdoctoral teaching fellowship at the Centre for Cultural Studies at the humanities faculty of the University of Science and Technology of Hong Kong. Her PhD dissertation is entitled *Fathers, Sons and Other Ghosts: Subjectivity in the New Hollywood Cinema*. She is affiliated to the Amsterdam School of Cultural Analysis and the Department of Film and Television Studies of the University of Amsterdam and has published in *ASCA-Brief*, *European Journal for Semiotics* and *Parallax*.

Index